Recent Results in Cancer Research 89

Pain in the Cancer Patient

Pathogenesis, Diagnosis and Therapy

Edited by
M. Zimmermann P. Drings G. Wagner

With 67 Figures and 57 Tables

Springer-Verlag
Berlin Heidelberg New York Tokyo 1984

Professor Dr. Manfred Zimmermann
II. Physiologisches Institut, Universität Heidelberg
Im Neuenheimer Feld 326, 6900 Heidelberg 1, FRG

Professor Dr. Peter Drings
Krankenhaus Rohrbach,
Klinik für Thoraxerkrankungen
der Landesversicherungsanstalt Baden
Amalienstrasse 5, 6900 Heidelberg 1, FRG

Professor Dr. Gustav Wagner
Deutsches Krebsforschungszentrum
Im Neuenheimer Feld 280, 6900 Heidelberg 1, FRG

Sponsored by the Swiss League against Cancer

ISBN-13:978-3-642-82030-4 e-ISBN-13:978-3-642-82028-1
DOI: 10.1007/978-3-642-82028-1

Library of Congress Cataloging in Publication Data. Main entry under title: Pain in the cancer patient. (Recent results in cancer research; 89) Bibliography: p. Includes index. 1. Cancer Complications and sequelae-Addresses, essays, lectures. 2. Pain-Treatment-Adresses, essays, lectures. I. Zimmermann, M. (Manfred), 1933– . II. Drings, P. (Peter). III. Wagner, Gustav, 1918– . IV. Series: Recent results in cancer research; v. 89, [DNLM: 1. Pain 2. Neoplasms. W1 RE106P v. 89 QZ 200 P144] RC261.R35 vol. 89 [RC262] 616.99'4s 83-16818 [616.99'40472]

Softcover reprint of the hardcover 1st edition 1984

2125/3140–543210

Preface

Pain is unfortunately not an early symptom in neoplastic diseases. When it occurs, however, as it so often does in the advanced stages of the disease, then it can be particularly severe. Many physicians are not able to treat such pain efficiently with the standard methods familiar to them. Even in the oncological clinic, it is common for cancer patients not to receive adequate treatment of their pain; the therapeutic efforts are directed principally at the cancer, the pain often being neglected. This book fills a gap in the literature and should enhance the awareness of pain of all those who deal with cancer patients.

For the patient, the symptoms of the disease are usually the direct cause of suffering, and pain is often the most severe symptom. The pain may be potentiated by knowledge of the threat posed by the cancer, or may itself considerably increase the patients existing anxiety. Thus there is a vicious circle of pain and psychological factors which will reduce the patient to a state of despair and distress. It is, therefore, obvious that efficient pain therapy is of utmost significance to the patient, who will judge the doctor's ability to provide medical assistance according to the degree of pain relief achieved. The patient's quality of life will also depend critically on the relief obtained.

Treatment of pain, therefore, has to form an essential part of the therapeutic approach to the cancer patient, but unfortunately this is not a generally accepted attitude, and most handbooks of oncology do not deal adequately with the problem of pain. The data presented in this volume show that virtually all patients can be given sufficient relief by appropriate application of known principles of pain treatment. It is, therefore, necessary to teach doctors which methods are best used. Of course, the selection of therapy has to be based on evaluation of the pathogenetic mechanisms involved in the pain. The success of the therapy depends on careful diagnosis of the factors causing the pain, and this book provides some attempts to clarify and classify the pathological and pathophysiological mechanisms concerned. More research is required into these mechanisms in order to improve our concepts of cancer pain and its therapy. This volume provides a critical overview of the presently available methods for treatment of chronic pain in cancer patients, and will hopefully stimulate workers in the fields of research and therapy of chronic pain to increase their efforts toward the further elucidation of the problems.

The editors owe their thanks to Miss Hannelore Ehlers for her competent editorial assistance and to Dr. Thomas Thiekötter and the staff of Springer-Verlag for their continuous encouragement and patience during the editorial process.

Heidelberg, October 1983

For the Editors
M. Zimmermann

Contents

M. Zimmermann and P. Drings:
Guidelines for Therapy of Pain in Cancer Patients 1

J. J. Bonica:
Management of Cancer Pain 13

H. Pompey:
The Telos and Ethos of Pain and Suffering 28

K. Hill:
Pathological Anatomy of Cancer Pain 33

W. Jänig:
Neurophysiological Mechanisms of Cancer Pain 45

F. Lembeck:
Pharmacology of the Primary Nociceptive Neuron 59

G. Wagner:
Frequency of Pain in Patients with Cancer 64

R. Hartenstein and W. Wilmanns:
Clinical Pain Syndromes in Cancer Patients and Their Causes 72

M. Berger and F. Gerstenbrand:
Analysis of Cancer Pain by the Neurologist 79

W. Schreml:
Pain in the Cancer Patient as a Consequence of Therapy (Surgery, Radiotherapy, Chemotherapy) 85

R. Wörz:
Control of Cancer Pain with Analgesics Acting in the Central Nervous System 100

M. Zenz:
Epidural Opiates for the Treatment of Cancer Pain 107

T. D. Walsh:
Opiates and Respiratory Function in Advanced Cancer 115

R. Kocher:
The Use of Psychotropic Drugs in the Treatment of Cancer Pain 118

P. Porges:
Local Anesthetics in the Treatment of Cancer Pain 127

U. Drechsel:
Treatment of Cancer Pain with Neurolytic Agents 137

J. Siegfried, A. Kühner, and V. Sturm:
Neurosurgical Treatment of Cancer Pain 148

A. Braun and K. Rohe:
Orthopedic Surgery for Management of Tumor Pain 157

W. Queißer:
Chemotherapy for the Treatment of Cancer Pain 171

R. Ziegler:
Calcitonin: Analgesic Effects 178

A. Szücs, B. Csillik, and E. Knyihár-Csillik:
Treatment of Terminal Pain in Cancer Patients by Means of Iontophoresis of Vinca Alkaloids 185

H. Kuttig:
Radiotherapy of Cancer Pain 190

R. H. Adler and W. Hemmeler:
Psychological Treatment Modalities for Pain in Cancer Patients 195

T. D. Walsh and C. M. Saunders:
Hospice Care: The Treatment of Pain in Advanced Cancer ... 201

Subject Index 212

*List of Contributors**

Adler, R. H. *195*[1]
Berger, M. *79*
Bonica, J. J. *13*
Braun, A. *157*
Csillik, B. *185*
Drechsel, U. *137*
Drings, P. 1
Gerstenbrand, F. *79*
Hartenstein, R. *72*
Hemmeler, W. *195*
Hill, K. *33*
Jänig, W. *45*
Knyihár-Csillik, E. *185*
Kocher, R. *118*
Kuhner, A. *148*
Kuttig, H. *190*
Lembeck, F. *59*
Pompey, H. *28*
Porges, P. *127*
Queißer, W. *171*
Rohe, K. *157*
Saunders, C. M. *201*
Schreml, W. *85*
Siegfried, J. *148*
Sturm, V. *148*
Szücs, A. *185*
Wagner, G. *64*
Walsh, T. D. *115, 201*
Wilmanns, W. *72*
Wörz, R. *100*
Zenz, M. *107*
Ziegler, R. *178*
Zimmermann, M. *1*

---

* Addresses given at beginning of each contribution
1 Page on which contribution begins

Guidelines for Therapy of Pain in Cancer Patients

M. Zimmermann[1] and P. Drings[2]

[1] II. Physiologisches Institut, Universität Heidelberg, Im Neuenheimer Feld 326, 6900 Heidelberg 1, FRG
[2] Krankenhaus Rohrbach, Klinik für Thoraxerkrankungen der Landesversicherungsanstalt Baden, Amalienstrasse 5, 6900 Heidelberg 1, FRG

It is obvious from several of the contributions to this monograph that pain is a most important symptom and problem for many cancer patients because of the great impact it has on their psychological state. Pain has a twofold signal function: It indicates to the patient that a threatening process is going on in the body and it reflects how efficiently the physician is treating the disease. Even a pain not related to the cancer may be attributed to malignancy by the patient and thus can enhance the emotional concern. A chronic pain not sufficiently treated might itself become an illness. Pain therapy is, therefore, of the utmost importance, even if it is merely palliative and does not contribute to the cure of the primary disease. We have learned from the contributions to this monograph that most, if not all, of the pain due to cancer can be efficiently treated – there is no need for a patient to suffer pain! The basic principles of efficient pain therapy are quite simple. However, it seems that the attitude of modern medicine – technological rather than humanitarian – hinders the insight into what the physical and psychic essentials are in alleviating pain and suffering.

Here we will outline some basic principles on how and by whom the pain in cancer patients might best be treated. These guidelines are directed toward providing the patient with the maximum life quality even if disease prognosis is poor. Much can be done to prevent and alleviate pain. It is least disturbing for the patient if pain therapy is performed at home.

Who Should Treat Pain in the Cancer Patient?

The treatment of pain can best be performed by the joint efforts of physicians, the family and friends, and the patient himself. One of the physicians responsible for the control of pain and other symptoms is the family doctor. He is in close contact with the patient for most of the time during the disease and thus holds a key position. The family doctor should, therefore, have sufficient knowledge on how to treat the pain effectively. Unfortunately, practitioners are often not familiar with modern concepts of pain diagnosis and therapy, and, thus, it is of the utmost importance that they acquire such knowledge.

The other physician who will be concerned with the cancer patient for a limited period of time is the oncologist treating the cancer. Apart from his interest in curative treatment, the oncologist should also be concerned with the concomitant treatment of pain. The criticism has often been raised that the oncologist overemphasizes the cancer treatment and neglects the pain, whereas for the patient the order of importance is often the reverse. This neglect of pain by the oncologist need not be. Recently, many oncologists have accepted that pain is a major problem and that they are in a crucial position to relieve the symptoms of the

Recent Results in Cancer Research. Vol. 89

disease, even if only by palliative measures (De Vita et al. 1982). Thus, it would be best if the oncologist could consider both the primary disease and the pain and find an appropriate balance in his therapeutic strategies.

An experienced specialist for pain diagnosis and therapy should be available in every oncological department. His field could be any discipline commonly involved in oncology. In the light of the present impetus with regard to pain, it is most likely that an anesthesiologist would be most interested in pain. This specialist on matters involved with pain should have the following tasks:

- Advising the oncologist on how to incorporate pain therapy and prophylaxis into the plan of cancer therapy
- Analyzing the etiology and probable pathogenesis of pain
- Providing the symptomatic or palliative therapy of pain that is least burdensome for the patient but maximally efficacious
- Applying special methods of pain therapy according to his field of expertise, e.g., by local anesthetic or neurolytic blocks, peridural opiates
- Coordinating specialist therapy of pain if required, e.g., radiotherapy, general surgery, neurosurgery, hormone therapy, chemotherapy
- Providing advice about pain treatment for the family doctor during home care of the patient.

The family and friends of the patient can have a significant impact on the patient's pain by giving emotional support and not allowing him to fall into a state of distress and social isolation. The security provided by a friendly, communicative, but not overreacting family environment helps to improve greatly the benefit a patient derives from any symptomatic therapy. Unfortunately, a family that adapts badly often gives rise to neurotic behavior greatly aggravating pain.

Thus, the joint efforts of the family doctor, the oncologist, the pain specialist, the patient and his family may provide the optimum background for the specific medical therapeutic approaches against pain. These allied efforts will be competent and efficient in preserving or restoring the quality of life for the patient, which so much depends on pain relief.

Diagnosis and Concepts for Pathogenesis of Cancer Pain

A considerable number of pathogenetic mechanisms for cancer pain have been proposed (see articles by Jänig and by Hartenstein and Wilmans, this volume). Although they provide reasonable explanations for the various types of cancer pain, they are still for the most part hypothetical where no appropriate research has actually confirmed them. However, the careful assessment and diagnosis of the pain could yield at least a working hypothesis about the pathogenetic mechanisms causing it, and this can help the doctor to develop a rational strategy for the therapy. Thus, the following questions should be clarified:

- Localization of pain – unilateral, midline, diffuse large area, bone?
- Does the pain depend on movement?
- Is an inflammatory process involved?
- Is a nerve, plexus, or spinal root irritated by a tumor or by the deformation of vertebrae due to metastases?
- Is there ischemia by arterial occlusion?
- Can a distinct nerve be determined conducting pain information, e.g., by diagnostic local anesthesia?

- Is pathophysiology of the sympathetic efferent system involved?
- Is hypertonus of skeletal muscle involved?
- Is smooth muscle spasm involved?
- Is a neuropathy involved, due to irradiation or chemotherapy?
- Is depression or anxiety a factor enhancing the pain?

The answers will give at least some hints toward a rational approach to pain therapy. For example, the pain of osseous metastases producing prostaglandins can be efficiently treated with antiinflammatory drugs. Diffuse bone pain, e.g., by widely distributed metastases in the spine, usually cannot be relieved by a chordotomy, however, a low dose of large-area X-irradiation might give long-lasting relief. Pain due to sympathetic disturbances will respond to a sympathetic block. Pain related to muscle hypertonus can be treated by local anesthesia of trigger points, or by physical therapy.
Thus, as is true for any other causes of pain, an intelligent diagnosis of causal factors and logical therapeutic considerations are to be preferred to a purely phenomenological and empirical approach, which could involve the risk of a series of inappropriate measures. However, both insufficient and exaggerated treatments should be avoided because both will be a burden to the patient and will evoke his doubts in the physician's skill and competence.

A Pain Diary for the Assessment of Pain

Apart from the diagnosis by the physician, self-evaluation of the pain should be performed by the patient. An appropriate assessment can be obtained using a pain questionnaire.

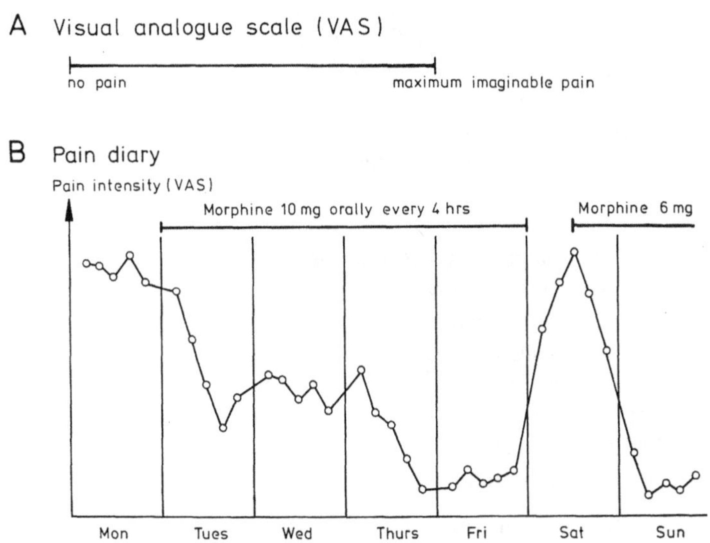

Fig. 1A, B. Assessment of pain intensity by the patient. **A** The patient is asked to indicate the intensity of his pain on the visual analogue scale (VAS). This is a line, the end points being referred to as *no pain* and *maximum imaginable pain*. The patient indicates the intensity of his perceived pain on this scale. **B** The value of a patient's pain intensity measured on a VAS at regular intervals is plotted against time, over a week. These VAS values from the pain diary show the pain-relieving effect of orally administered morphine, 10 mg and 6 mg, respectively, every 4 h

However, the questionnaire should be more straightforward and shorter than those used for scientific analysis of pain evaluation. It should be aimed at showing the time-course of pain development in a patient and the efficacy of therapy. Thus, the questionnaire should involve a simple method for subjective pain rating, such as the visual analogue scale (VAS) (Fig. 1A). Most patients can indicate their actual pain intensity on this VAS between the reference points "no pain" and "maximum imaginable pain". Pain ratings performed several times a day would yield a pain diary. These repeated pain ratings can be arranged to a graphic display of the time-course of pain intensity, reliably indicating the effects of a therapy (Fig. 1B). Such a display of pain ratings would unambiguously reveal the best of several attempts of therapy.

Apart from the diary of pain intensity rating, the questionnaire should contain a schema of the body onto which the patient can draw the area(s) of pain it should also include some; basic information concerning the quality of pain and some anamnestic data. Most patients will accept keeping a pain diary, since they realize that in this way their problems are being taken seriously by the physician and that communication with the physician is intensified with regard to their problems. Patients might, therefore, expect improvement in therapy from their efforts with the pain diary.

Because of its simplicity the pain questionnaire we are proposing will be of limited value in sophisticated psychological pain research. However, its benefit for the patient might be considerable because of the documented effects of therapy.

Order of Therapeutic Measures

In many cases of pain due to cancer, the following order of therapeutic measures would be recommended although a different sequence of events might be appropriate according to the individual diagnosis of the patient:

- Transcutaneous nerve stimulation
- Antiinflammatory drugs
- Local anesthetic blocks (e.g., trigger points)
- Sympathetic blocks with local anesthetics
- Psychotropic drugs
- Hormone therapy
- Narcotic analgesics (oral administration)
- Palliative radiotherapy
- Chordotomy (percutaneous)
- Neurolytic and cryogenic nerve blocks
- Palliative surgery and bone protection
- Hypophysectomy
- Epidural opiates
- Deep brain stimulation.

Of course, the noninvasive measures that can be administered by the home physician are the methods of first choice and only if these prove to be inefficient might specialist therapy be recommended. However, a careful screening of the patient should be performed in order to avoid empirical polypragmas with many inefficient and frustrating attempts at therapy. These will have considerable distressing effects on the patient, thereby increasing his sensitivity to the pain. On the other hand, the prospective life span of the patient should also be a crucial determinant when selecting the analgesic therapy. For example, epidural opiates or neurolytic nerve blocks are not appropriate for analgesic therapy aimed at providing pain relief for more than a few months.

Transcutaneous Nerve Stimulation

Repetitive electric stimulation of peripheral nerves triggers inhibitory systems in the central nervous system. Therefore, transcutaneous nerve stimulation (TNS) has been used effectively to treat pain of many origins, such as stump pain or musculoskeletal pain. It has been claimed that the severe pain due to nerve compression by a tumor might not be a case for efficient treatment with TNS. This seems reasonable, according to the critical reviews in this field. However, not all pain in cancer patients is of this severe type. Some forms of less severe pain might be secondary to a tumor, such as cutaneous hyperpathia in a zone of sympathetic dysfunction due to a tumor, musculotendinous pain due to reflex hypertonus of skeletal muscle, or neuralgia due to a polyneuropathia subsequent to chemotherapy. Several of these paraneoplastic pains might well respond to TNS, and even a postherpetic neuralgia occurring in a cancer patient may be effectively treated. Therefore, this method giving rise to no risk and side effects should be recommended, depending on the diagnosis of the causes of pain.

The use of a portable stimulator by the patient might have a considerable psychological benefit: the patient is able to switch on the stimulator and adjust the degree of stimulation himself. Thus, he will experience that he can control the pain himself. The assurance of self-control is an important psychological factor for many patients. This influence might be sufficient reason to recommend the use of a stimulator in addition to other analgesic therapy, e.g., an anti-inflammatory analgesic drug. Unfortunately, some patients might react adversely to the possibility of self-control depending on factors of personality.

Non-narcotic Analgesic Drugs

The term "mild analgesics" for this group of drugs is inappropriate since it suggests that these analgesics will be useful only for mild or weak pain. This is not the case, however; there is much evidence now that several forms of severe chronic pain can be efficiently treated using these drugs. Even the severe pain induced by bone metastases can be satisfactorily treated with a non-narcotic drug such as aspirin.

The drugs, for which acetylsalicylic acid is a prototype, have their dominant mechanism of action in the periphery, although some influence might also exist on the central nervous system. Others have their main impact on the central nervous system, e.g., Nefopam.

According to current knowledge, the main mechanism of action of the anti-inflammatory analgesics is to interfere with the endogenous pain-producing substances, such as are released during an inflammatory process. It is known that prostaglandins, bradykinin, serotonin, histamine, and many other substances are factors contributing to the pain caused by inflammation. Interference with the biosynthesis or action of these substances might, therefore, result in pain relief.

Currently, the emphasis of research and of concepts of function is on the well-established inhibition of prostaglandin synthesis by several of these anti-inflammatory drugs. However, the correlation between the potencies of these drugs to inhibit prostaglandin synthesis and their analgesic potencies is fairly low (Crook et al. 1976). For some

Table 1. Effective doses and time schedule of administration of non-narcotic analgesics for the control of cancer pain (after Gerbershagen 1979)

Generic name	Dose (mg)	Interval of administration during day
Acetylsalicylic acid	750–1,250	q. 3 h
Salicylamide	750–1,000	q. 3 h
Phenacetin	400– 600	q. 3 h
Paracetamol	600– 800	q. 3 h
Acetylaminosalol	400– 800	q. 3 h
Phenazon	500–1,000	q. 3 h
Propyphenazon	450– 800	q. 3 h
4-Aminophenazon	450– 800	q. 3 h
Aminophenazon	450– 800	q. 3 h
Noramidopyrin methansulfonate-sodium (metamizol)	750–1,000	q. 3 h
Mofebutazon		
monophenylbutazon	200– 400	q. 4 h
phenylbutazon	200– 400	q. 4 h
oxyphenbutazone	100– 200	q. 4 h
Mefenamic acid	500	q. 3 h
Flufenamic acid	200	q. 4 h
Indomethacin	50– 75	q. 4 h
Benzydamin	100	q. 4 h
Ibufenac		q. 4 h
Ibuprofen	200– 400	q. 3 h
Naproxen	250– 500	q. 3–4 h
Niflumic acid	250– 500	q. 3–4 h
Bumadizon	220	q. 4 h
Alclofenac	500–1,000	q. 4 h
Nefopam	60– 120	q. 3 h

peripherally acting analgesics, an anti-inflammatory effect is even lacking. It has, therefore, been suggested that additional factors other than prostaglandin synthesis might be relevant in the analgesic actions of these drugs, e.g., direct interference with the nervous mechanisms of nociceptor excitation.

Biochemical processes also contribute in some cases of carcinomatous pain. For example, bone tumors and metastases produce considerable amounts of prostaglandins which are involved in osteolysis. It is conceivable that these prostaglandins sensitize or excite nociceptors and, therefore, contribute to the bone pain in such cases. Similar mechanisms have also been suggested as determining the pain in other tumors. This is because the tissue surrounding a tumor often reveals signs of severe inflammation, indicating the production of algesic substances. These, in turn, might excite and sensitize the nociceptors in this region which effect can be blocked by anti-inflammatory analgesic drugs. Thus, consideration of the pathogenetic mechanisms suggests that these drugs can be of considerable therapeutic efficacy in many kinds of cancer pain.

As long as no controlled clinical studies exist that would allow one to predict which kinds of tumor-related pain might best be treated with the various types of the peripherally acting analgesics, it would seem wise to try their use when starting to treat any kind of cancer pain. If there is no sufficient analgesic efficacy initially, the dose might be increased. To prevent recurrence of the pain, the intervals of administration have to be short enough to account for the duration of analgesic effects after a single dose. For example, a total daily dose of 4 g or more of acetylsalicylic acid could be given and the intervals between administrations might be as short as 3 h. The usually recommended regimen of two or three administrations per day often is inappropriate for lasting pain relief. As is generally true for any analgesic therapy, it is an important principle that the next dose be given before pain recurs. Therefore, administration according to a fixed schedule rather than at the request of the patient has to be chosen. Recommended doses and intervals of administration have been compiled in Table 1.

Mixtures of non-narcotic analgesics with other drugs, e.g., barbiturates, caffeine, vitamins, cannot be recommended; their analgesic potency is not greater than that of the monosubstances. However, some drugs might be given simultaneously, e.g., codeine and an anti-inflammatory analgesic drug, or a neuroleptic and an anti-inflammatory analgesic drug. The rationale is that they activate complementary therapeutic mechanisms appropriate for a patient. For example, it is conceivable that the anxiolytic effect of a neuroleptic facilitates analgesia obtained with an anti-inflammatory analgesic drug.

The side effects of the anti-inflammatory drugs, e.g., the gastrointestinal hemorrhage induced by acetylsalicylic acid and related drugs, can be reduced or avoided by changing the drug from time to time, e.g., every month (drug rotation). It is commonly accepted that the analgesic drugs with a peripheral mechanism of action are similar in their analgesic efficacy, but exhibit major differences in their detrimental side effects.

Corticosteroids

The use of corticosteroids has an important place in the control of many symptoms of cancer, particularly in very advanced cases (Table 2). A major indication with regard to pain is edema, which might increase intracranial pressure (brain tumor) or potentiate compression of peripheral nerves, veins, and lymph vessels. Edema is reduced by corticosteroid therapy, and thus the total size of the tumor is reduced. The combined use of a non-narcotic analgesic and corticosteroids, therefore, appears promising in providing considerable pain relief in cases involving inflammatory as well as edematous processes. Apart from pain relief, patients might derive additional benefits from the effects on other symptoms of the disease (Table 2). The only significant side effect from corticosteroid therapy is the increased risk of peptic ulcer, which, however, may not be a serious factor in patients with a poor prognosis.

Psychotropic Drugs

Cancer patients are often depressive or anxious, or both, because they know about their disease and its prognosis. It is well established that these psychic situations might enhance the pain. Some functional concepts of pain even suggest that the supposed interaction between anxiety or depression and pain could give rise to a vicious circle potentiating both the pain and the psychic alteration (Kocher, this volume). In any case, it seems logical to apply psychotropic drugs to interfere with such adverse reactions and interactions.

Table 2. Indications and therapeutic benefits of the use of corticosteroids in terminal cancer (after Twycross 1980)

Nonspecific uses	Coanalgesic	Other specific uses
1. Improve appetite	1. Raised intracranial pressure[a]	1. Hypercalcemia
2. Reduce fever	2. Nerve compression	2. Carcinomatous neuromyopathy
3. Enhance sense of well-being	3. Hepatomegaly	3. Incipient paraplegia
4. Improve strength	4. Head and neck tumor[a]	4. Superior vena caval obstruction
	5. Intrapelvic tumor	5. Airways obstruction
	6. Abdominal tumor	6. Hemoptysis
	7. Retroperitoneal tumor	7. Leukoerythroblastic anemia
	8. Lymphoedema[a]	8. Malignant effusion[a]
	9. Metastatic arthralgia	9. Discharge from rectal tumor[b]
		10. Minimize radiation-induced reactive edema
		11. Minimize toxic effects of radiation or chemotherapy
		12. As an adjunct to chemotherapy

[a] May benefit by concurrent use of a diuretic
[b] Given rectally (Predsol enema)

Three kinds of psychotropic drugs are currently considered to support pain therapy by decreasing the psychic reaction to pain as well as to the supposed positive feedback mechanisms – neuroleptics (e.g., haloperidol), antidepressants (e.g., amitriptyline), and tranquilizers (e.g., diazepam). Their indication results from a consideration of the patient's type of adverse psychic reaction that is thought to enhance the pain. Thus, if a patient is depressive, an antidepressant should be applied in addition to the analgesic methods used. If he is overreacting to his situation of severe illness, a neuroleptic or an anxiolytic tranquilizer might be indicated. Since signs of both depression and anxiety might be simultaneously present in many cancer patients, it has been suggested that combinations of neuroleptics and antidepressants be used (Kocher, this volume; Halpern 1979). Thus, although psychotropic drugs normally do not have a direct analgesic effect, they may facilitate pain relief obtained by other measures. In many cases, a combination of a non-narcotic analgesic drug and a psychotropic drug has been found to give better pain relief than the analgesic alone. Most importantly, this combination has been claimed to delay the onset of use of narcotic drugs during the progress of the disease (Gerbershagen 1979). It is important to note that these supportive effects of psychotropic drugs occur at a fairly low dosage, below the threshold dosage for the antidepressant or antipsychotic effects in psychiatric patients.

Apart from their psychic effects, the psychotropic drugs can be of benefit in relation to other symptoms (Gerbershagen 1979; Twycross 1980). Thus, diazepam has a central nervous muscle-relaxant effect and, therefore, can help to relieve muscle spasms and the related pain. Chlorpromazine reduces rectal and bladder tenesmus. Phenothiazine is antiemetic; tricyclic antidepressants alleviate dysesthesia associated with partial nerve damage or postherpetic neuralgia. Sympathetic disturbances often respond to neuroleptics (Gerbershagen 1979).

Local Anesthetics for Treatment of Pain

Local anesthetics produce a block of nerve conduction or nociceptor excitation. Usually, their analgesic effect has the same duration as the anesthesia they produce, i.e., several hours. Therefore, local anesthesia does not seem to be an appropriate measure for the relief of the continuous pain in a cancer patient. However, there are some exceptions where the use of local anesthetics might be beneficial to the patient. The general practitioner should be encouraged to be familiar with at least some of the applications of local anesthesia – their usefulness is not just restricted to the field of pain in cancer! Since a major contribution to this topic will follow (Porges, this volume), we will just emphasize some of the more important cases indicating the use of local anesthetics.

A diagnostic block can unequivocally indicate whether a particular nerve is involved in the conduction of nociceptive impulses. This should be tested before a long-term nerve block is performed with alcohol or phenol (see Drechsel, this volume) or by local freezing.

Therapeutic Blocks. Local anesthesia of spinal nerves (paravertebral injection), peripheral nerves, or myofascial trigger points can give long-term pain relief. In these cases, the pain is thought to be enhanced and even sustained by efferent mechanisms of the motor system, thereby producing a reflex hypertonus or spasm of skeletal muscles. This might be a sequela of a minor primary irritation of a nerve or plexus by a tumor.

Sympathetic blocks will give pain relief when dysfunction of the (efferent) sympathetic system is involved in the pathomechanism of the pain. A self-sustained pain might ensue (sympathetic algodystrophy). This could be due to a Pancoast's tumor or a neuropathy from therapeutic X-irradiation.
Other applications such as spinal anesthesia are not detailed here since they usually will be beyond the technical capabilities of the practitioner.

Narcotic Analgesics

If the pain in a cancer patient cannot be sufficiently relieved by the methods reviewed in the preceding sections, the use of narcotic analgesic drugs has to be considered. Unfortunately, considerable prejudice has governed the realm of narcotics in analgesic therapy; doctors fear, for example, that patients could become addicted to the drug; there might be a risk of respiratory depression; mood alteration might occur, either sedation or euphoria; other unpleasant side effects, such as nausea, vomiting, allergic reactions, and constipation, might introduce additional problems. These fears have often caused appropriate pain therapy to be withheld from many patients. However, there is convincing evidence that by overcoming these myths even so-called intractable pain can be prevented or alleviated by the appropriate use of morphine or other narcotic drugs (Wörz, this volume; Mount 1980; Twycross 1983). Thus, it has been estimated that the analgesic measures described in the previous sections and including the oral administration of narcotics will provide pain relief in at least 90% of cancer patients with pain.
There are a few important principles that when followed make the narcotics the drugs of first choice when the other methods in the ladder of pain strategy are no longer effective. These principles are as follows:

- The narcotic should be administered orally
- It should be given at regular intervals (e.g., every 4 h) in order not to relieve the pain, but to prevent it
- The dosage should be adjusted carefully in order to yield the appropriate analgesia
- Dependence and respiratory depression should not be feared since they are usually not a problem
- The most serious side effects should be prevented or treated, i.e., constipation and nausea

What are the pharmacological mechanisms that render oral opioid therapy so superior? This superiority is mainly due to the fact that the plasma level of the analgesic is maintained above the concentration necessary for analgesia over a longer period of time than with parenteral administration. As shown in Fig. 2, the slow resorption from the gastrointestinal tract results in a slower rise and, more important, a slower decay of the drug plasma level. Time courses for parenteral administration are much faster and, also important, the peak level reached is considerably higher than with a comparable oral dose. Thus, with repeated oral administration at, e.g., 4-h intervals, the blood concentration of the drug can be maintained sufficiently high even though the maximum concentration is below the threshold of toxic effects, such as respiratory depression. With parenteral administration, it is difficult to keep the blood level of the drug within these limits. Of course, an orally administered drug must have sufficient resorption from the gastrointestinal tract. Thus, if the rate of absorption is fairly low, as with morphine, the amount ingested has to be appropriately increased to account for this deficiency. Practically, a dose increased to 1.5 or 2 times that of the parenteral route dose is appropriate for the oral administration of morphine.

The slow rise in blood concentration during absorption from the gastrointestinal tract is probably a major reason why no psychic dependence (or addiction) usually develops in

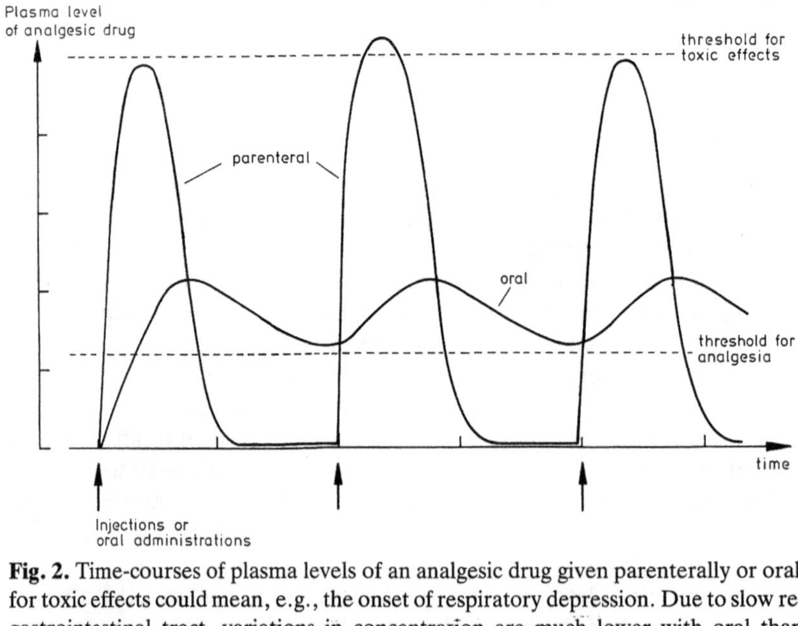

Fig. 2. Time-courses of plasma levels of an analgesic drug given parenterally or orally. The threshold for toxic effects could mean, e.g., the onset of respiratory depression. Due to slow resorption from the gastrointestinal tract, variations in concentration are much lower with oral than with parenteral administration, and analgesic levels can better be maintained

patients suffering from pain undergoing oral opiate therapy. Thus, prolonged therapy with morphine has been reported, e.g., of more than 1 year, and the dosage reached may be as high as 1,000 mg/day (Twycross 1983).

During prolonged administration of opioids, an increase in dosage is often required to maintain analgesia. This may be due to the development of tolerance or to an increase in nociceptor excitation during the progress of the cancer. However, this gradual increase in the dosage does not result in an increased risk of respiratory depression, since the plasma levels of opioids necessary for effects on the respiratory system are always higher than the plasma levels for analgesia. When tolerance develops, both thresholds are elevated.

Another major advantage of oral rather than parenteral administration of opioids is that the patient maintains self-control of the pain. He can administer the narcotic tablets or aqueous elixir of morphine sulfate himself at the prescribed intervals. In contrast, the frequent injections necessary during parenteral administration of opiates require the patient's dependence on a nurse or physician, and this normally entails the patient staying in the hospital. Many patients on oral morphine, however, can stay at home!

Palliative Procedures for Pain Relief

A considerable effect on pain and other symptoms of cancer can be obtained from palliative procedures such as tumor and metastasis surgery, including bone surgery, X-irradiation, chemotherapy and hormone therapy. It is important here that sometimes such measures are applied or continued only for the relief of symptoms, in cases where no curative effects can be expected. Thus, reduction of a tumor by surgery or irradiation could result in a period of life with less pain. In cases of hormone-dependent tumors (metastatic breast and prostate cancer), dramatic pain relief often occurs with estrogen treatment. This latter palliative measure may be a case for the practitioner.

The indications for palliative help should be carefully analyzed by the team outlined above, i.e., the oncologist, the pain specialist, and the family doctor. It is of the utmost importance that a compromise be found between the pain relief to be expected and the physical and psychic troubles inflicted upon the patient by the procedure.

Home Care Service for the (Terminal) Cancer Patient

Mainly for psychological reasons, it is better for the patient to stay at home as long as possible and even to die at home. Of course, this could raise considerable problems in the therapy of symptoms, above all of pain. Often, too much is demanded of the family doctor when there is a dramatic increase in pain in the terminally ill patient, since he usually does not know enough about how to treat such pain effectively.

To meet with these problems most efficiently, home care services (HCS) have been organized in Great Britain. These are teams usually of two physicians, several nurses, a social worker, and a physical therapist. The HCS is requested by the family doctor if he cannot provide sufficient help to the patient. However, the family doctor is still responsible for medical and psychological care of the patient; the HCS is a specialist team to fight the pain and other severe symptoms. Of course, the HCS must be familiar with the etiology, the careful assessment, and the therapy of pain. It is necessary to inform the patient that the purpose of the HCS is to provide effective treatment at home rather than necessitate transferring the patient to a hospital, and this knowledge is often a great help to the patient.

The HCS is available upon telephone request at any time day and night. This encourages the family and the home physician to continue caring for the patient at home.

Pain in the Dying Patient

The patient in a terminal state sometimes requires specific efforts for effective pain control. In many cases, narcotic analgesics provide satisfactory relief, again preferably by the oral route. If, however, systemic narcotic drugs fail to give adequate relief, other methods, such as peridural application of a local anesthetic or opiates, should be considered (see contributions by Porges and Zenz, this volume). However, the dying patient needs more than just analgesic therapy. It is most important to prevent his social isolation and to talk with him about the problems he is confronted with – his dying, his pain, the fate of his family. In Great Britain, a number of centres have been founded in recent years that aim at realizing the basic tenets of humanity for these patients (see Walsh and Saunders, this volume).

The utmost incentive of all these efforts is to maintain the quality of life for the cancer patient to the end and to allow him to die in dignity.

References

Bonica JJ (1980) Cancer pain. In: Bonica JJ (ed) Pain. Raven Press, New York, pp 335–362

Crook D, Collins AJ, Bacon PA, Chan R (1976) Effect of "aspirin-like" drug therapy. Prostaglandin synthetase activity from human rheumatoid synovial microsomes. Ann Rheum Dis 35:327–332

De Vita VT, Hellmann S, Rosenberg SA (eds) (1982) Cancer. Principles and Practice of Oncology. Lippincott, Philadelphia

Gerbershagen HU (1979) Nonnarcotic analgesics. In: Bonica JJ, Ventrafridda V (eds) Advances in pain research and therapy, vol 2. Raven, New York, pp 255–262

Halpern LM (1979) Psychotropics, ataractics, and related drugs. In: Bonica JJ, Ventafridda V (eds) Advances in pain research and therapy, vol 2. Raven, New York, pp 275–283

Mount BM (1980) Narcotic analgesics. In: Twycross RG, Ventrafridda V (eds) The continuing care of terminal cancer patients. Pergamon, Oxford, pp 97–116

Twycross RG (1980) Non-narcotic, corticosteroid and psychotropic drugs. In: Twycross RG, Ventrafridda V (eds) The continuing care of terminal cancer patients. Pergamon, Oxford, pp 117–134

Twycross RG (1983) Narcotic analgesics in clinical practice. In: Bonica JJ, Lindblom U, Iggo A (eds) Advances in pain research and therapy, vol 5. Raven, New York, pp 435–459

Management of Cancer Pain

J. J. Bonica

Multidisciplinary Pain Center, University of Washington, Seattle, WA 98195, USA

Introduction

Cancer pain has long been, and continues to be, one of the most important and pressing issues of modern society and the health care systems of many countries throughout the world. This importance stems from the following facts: (a) cancer pain afflicts millions of people throughout the world annually, and in addition to the severe physiologic, emotional, affective, and economic impact of pain in general, cancer pain has special attributes and significance to the patients and their families; and (b) for reasons given below, all too frequently cancer pain is inadequately managed and consequently many patients spend the last weeks and months or even years of their lives in great discomfort, suffering, and disability, which precludes a quality of life that is vital to these patients.

In this presentation I will give a brief overview of (a) the magnitude of the problem, including its importance and prevalence; (b) the physiologic, psychologic, affective, and sociologic effects of cancer pain; (c) the current status of its management and the reasons for deficiencies which exist in cancer pain therapy; (d) some recommendations for future activities in order to improve this serious health problem; and (e) a summary of the basic principles of management. This material is intended to serve as a framework or background for the presentations that follow. Following a long tradition throughout the world, I will use "cancer pain" generically to include pain caused by any malignant neoplasm or as a consequence of therapeutic intervention for the disease, or both.

Magnitude of the Problem

Importance

It deserves reemphasis that cancer pain is one of the most important health care problems in many countries. This importance stems from several interrelated factors. For one thing, pain is the most dreaded complication of cancer among the millions of persons worldwide who develop the disease. Once the patient accepts and somewhat adjusts to the shocking news that he or she has cancer, one of the greatest problems is the fear of excruciating pain and suffering that the patient believes will inevitably ensue. In a survey of public opinion on cancer, Aitkin-Swan (1959) found that pain ranked next to incurability in people's fear of cancer. In epidemiologic studies being carried out at the University of Wisconsin Pain Center and by our own group sponsored by the National Cancer Institute of the United States, it was found that the general public believes cancer to be much more painful than it

Recent Results in Cancer Research. Vol. 89

actually is. This fear has been generated in part by the fact that a significant percentage of patients with advanced cancer do develop moderate to severe pain and that in many patients the pain has been and continues to be inadequately managed. In recent years these facts have come to the attention of the general public, and this in turn has generated more fear and apprehension about cancer pain and the inability of many health professionals to relieve it effectively.

Prevalence

For reasons that will be given later, the prevalence of pain associated with cancer throughout the world cannot be defined with accuracy. However, one can gain some insight by citing statistics on the incidence of cancer and cancer deaths and from data derived from a number of local and regional surveys on the prevalence of pain among the general cancer population and among those with various specific neoplasms. On the basis of 1979 cancer statistics it is estimated that worldwide, annually cancer afflicts over 15 million persons and is responsible for more than 5 million deaths, which represents 10% of all deaths throughout the world. Moreover, in developed countries in Europe and North America and other parts of the world where major infectious diseases and nutritional problems are no longer significant causes of death, cancer is responsible for 20% of the total deaths. For example, based on 1977 data collected by the American Cancer Society (1981), it can be estimated that cancer was responsible for over 21% of the deaths in the United States in 1981. Table 1 lists the 1981 estimates of new cases diagnosed and the death rates from the most frequent cancers that occur among the American population. A study of the data published by the World Health Organization reveals that for selected cancer sites the age-adjusted death rates per 100,000 population in 39 countries including all of the Western European countries, Canada, most Central and South American countries, Australia, New Zealand, Japan, and Singapore were similar to those in the United States. Table 2 shows the close similarity in death rates consequent to the six most frequent cancers in Austria, Germany, Switzerland, and the United States.

Although accurate statistics from comprehensive national and international epidemiologic studies on the prevalence and impact of pain associated with cancer are not available, there are data from a number of surveys carried out in specific hospitals in the United Kingdom, the United States, Canada, Italy, and a few other countries which provide some indication of the prevalence of cancer pain. Those carried out in the United Kingdom include the one by Wilkes (1974), in which he reported that of nearly 300 patients admitted in an English provincial city to a 25-bed unit used for the care of dying cancer patients, pain was the major symptom in 58% of cases. It occurred in 82% of patients with cervical cancer, 75% of patients with gastric cancer, and 45–60% of patients with cancer of the lung, rectum, or breast. Twycross (1976) reviewed the records of consecutive admissions to St. Christopher's Hospice, where about 500 patients are admitted each year, and found that over 80% required diamorphine (heroin) for severe pain during their hospital stay. In another British survey of 276 cancer patients who received terminal care, Parkes (1978) found that among those given care in hospitals, 38% had moderate pain and 22% had severe or very severe pain, whereas among patients managed in the home the figures were 21% and 48%, respectively. Still other British reports include those of Aitkin-Swan (1959), who found an incidence of approximately 50%, and Cartwright and associates (1973), who found that 87% of patients who died from cancer had pain prior to death.

Table 1. Cancer statistics: 1981 estimates for the USA. (American Cancer Society, 1981)

Site	Estimated new cases diagnosed		Estimated deaths	
	Number	% of total[a]	Number	% of total
Lung	122,000	15.0	105,000	25.0
Colon/Rectum	120,000	14.7	56,000	13.3
Breast	111,000	13.6	37,000	8.8
Uterus (Cervix, Corpus)	72,000	8.8	21,700	5.2
Prostate	70,000	8.6	22,200	5.3
Leukemias and Lymphomas	63,000	7.7	37,500	8.9
Urinary (Bladder/Kidney)	54,600	6.7	18,700	4.5
Stomach/Esophagus	32,700	4.0	22,000	5.2
Oral Cavity and Pharynx	26,600	3.3	9,200	2.2
Pancreas	24,200	3.0	22,000	5.2
Bone/Connective tissue	20,900	2.6	10,000	2.4
Liver/Gallbladder	13,000	1.6	9,400	2.3
Central Nervous System	12,100	1.5	10,200	2.4
Larynx	10,700	1.3	3,700	0.9
All others	62,200	7.6	35,400	8.4
Total	815,000	100.0	420,000	100.0

[a] Percent rounded to nearest decimal

Table 2. Comparison of death rates from cancer (1974–1975) age-adjusted death rates/100 000 population

Lesion	Austria	Germany	Switzerland	USA
All Sites Male	189	182	175	159
Female	123	121	103	106
Lung Male	52	48	47	51
Female	7	5	4	12
Breast	19	20	24	22
Colon/Rectum Male	24	24	20	19
Female	17	18	12	15
Prostate	15	16	19	15
Uterus	19	11	10	22
Stomach Male	31	27	18	7
Female	16	14	10	4

Of the surveys done in the United States, those carried out by Foley, Houde, and their co-workers (Foley 1979) at the Memorial Sloan-Kettering Cancer Center are among the most comprehensive published to date. In one survey of 540 inpatients, pain was experienced by 85% of patients with primary bone tumors, 80% with cancer of the oral cavity, 75% of males and 70% of females with cancer of the genito-urinary system, 52% of patients with breast cancer, 45% of patients with cancer of the lung, 20% of patients with lymphoma, and only 5% of patients with leukemia. In a subsequent survey of 397 patients, about 38% had pain related to cancer, but the figure rose to 60% among the terminally ill patients in the hospital. Foley also reported that among cancer patients who had pain, in 75% it was caused by the neoplastic process, in 20% it was the result of anticancer therapy, and in 5% it was unrelated to the cancer. Norton and Lack (1980), associated with two American hospices, reported that pain was a significant symptom in 75% of 100 consecutive cancer patients managed in their own homes. Kornell (1980), a member of our cancer pain study group, noted that 86% of patients with advanced cancer reported pain, and these patients ranked pain as the most distressing symptom they experienced.

The two epidemiologic studies being carried out at the University of Wisconsin (Cleland and Daut 1982) and the University of Washington (Bonica et al. 1982) have already provided an even more comprehensive overview of the prevalance of pain and its impact on the patient. For one thing, these studies have revealed that contrary to the general belief that cancer is not painful at its onset, it was found that pain was an early symptom and was present when cancer was first diagnosed in 40%–50% of patients who had cancer of the breast, prostate, colon, rectum, ovary, or cervix, and it occurred as an early symptom in 60%–70% of patients with cancer of the lung or pancreas. These two studies also revealed that in patients with metastatic cancer or advanced lesion, the incidence of pain increased significantly to 65%–100% of patients.

Turnbull (1979) studied the prevalence and characteristics of pain in 280 patients with recurrent cancer of the lung who had been referred to the British Columbia (Canada) Cancer Control Agency (Institute) for Palliative Therapy. At the time the patients were first seen at the Institute and a diagnosis of an incurable lesion was made, 71% had pain which had the characteristics of five pain syndromes. At the end of palliative therapy, pain was still present in 45% of patients, and during the last 2 months of life, 65% of the patients had significant pain.

Table 3. Prevalence of cancer pain (average data)

Author	Number of patients	Stage	Percent with pain
Bonica et al. (1982)	310	All stages	47
Foley (1979)	397	All stages	38
Cleland et al. (1982)	667	All stages	43
Bonica et al. (1982)	125	Advanced	78
Cleland et al. (1982)	341	Advanced	70
Cartwright et al. (1973)	215	Advanced	87
Kornell (1980)	30	Advanced	86
Pannuti et al. (1980)	324	Advanced	87
Turnbull (1979)	280	Advanced	71
Foley (1979)	39	Terminal	60
Norton and Lack (1980)	100	Terminal	75
Parkes (1978)			
Hospital care	100	Terminal	70
Home care	65	Terminal	70
Twycross and Wald (1976)	500	Terminal	80
Wilkes (1974)	300	Terminal	38

Pannutti and associates (1980) of the Division of Oncology, Malpighi Hospital, Bologna, Italy, reported that of 324 patients with advanced cancer managed in their service during a $3^1/_2$-year period, 88% had moderate to severe pain. The incidence of pain in patients with specific tumors was as follows: 100% with cancer of the ovary or cancer of the cervix; 95% with cancer of the rectum or cancer of the breast; 85% with cancer of the lung or cancer of the colon; and 75% with stomach cancer. They reported that these patients averaged 3 months of survival time with pain, that various forms of chemotherapy resulted in remission of pain in only 23% of the patients, and that 15 days before death pain was present in 80% of patients with bone metastasis, 67% of patients with soft-tissue tumors,

Table 4. Prevalence of moderate to very severe pain with specific cancers ranges from intermediate to advanced stages

Site of cancer	Patients with pain (%)	Site of cancer	Patients with pain (%)
Bone (primary/ metastasis)	85–100	Breast	35–65
Ovary/Cervix	40–100	Prostate	40–75
Uterus	40– 70	Lung	45–85
Colon/Rectum	50– 95	Oral Cavity	60–80
Stomach	60– 75	Urinary Tract	45–75
Intestine	40– 60	Larynx	50–70
Pancreas	70–100	Lymphoma	15–20

Table 5. Prevalence of moderate to very severe cancer pain in the USA (1981 estimates)

Stage/type of cancer	Number of patients ($\times 10^3$)	Prevalence (% of patients)	Patients with moderate–very severe pain ($\times 10^3$)
A. Advanced			
Lung	105	75	78.8
Colon/Rectum	56	75	43.0
Breast	37	75	27.8
Stomach	22	73	16.1
Pancreas	22	75	16.5
Prostate	22	67	14.7
Lymphomas	22	20	4.4
Ovary/Cervix	19	90	17.1
Leukemia	15	5	0.8
Bone	10	90	9.0
Larynx	4	62	2.5
All other	86	20	17.2
Subtotal	420		248.0
B. Intermediate/ Therapy	800(?)	38	304.0
Total	1 220		552.0

and 50% of patients with visceral cancer. In another series of 291 patients with advanced solid tumors managed by Pannuti and associates (1979), moderate to severe pain was experienced by nearly 70% of those with cancer of the prostate and those with cancer of the stomach, about 60% of those with intestinal tumors and those with lung cancers, 55% of those with kidney tumors, and nearly half of those with head or neck cancer.

The foregoing data, which are summarized in Tables 3 and 4, indicate that moderate to severe pain is already present in about 40%–45% of patients when the lesion is diagnosed, in about 35%–40% of patients with intermediate stages of the disease, and in 60%–85% of patients with advanced cancer, depending on the type and site of the lesion. The data also suggest that the pain is severe or very severe in an overall average of 60% of patients with advanced cancer. Extrapolation of these data and those in Table 1 suggests that annually about a quarter million Americans with advanced cancer have moderate to severe pain and that another 300,000 have pain caused by the intermediate stages of the disease and/or by cancer therapy (Table 5). Moreover, on the basis of previously cited data, it can be speculated that the relative magnitude of the problem in Western European countries is similar to that in the United States.

Effects of Cancer Pain

Chronic persistent pain and suffering due to causes other than cancer produces a progressive physical deterioration due to disturbances in sleep and appetite and often also to excessive medication, all of which contribute to the general fatigue and debility of the patient. Moreover, many patients with chronic pain undergo serious emotional, affective, and behavioral changes including anxiety, depression, hypochondriasis, an increased level of neuroticism, somatic preoccupation with the disease, and somatic focussing (Pilowsky et al. 1977; Sternbach 1974). As a consequence, there is less contact with friends and a progressive reduction in social activities. Because of the prolonged disability it often causes, chronic pain is now generally considered a serious world health and economic problem (Bonica 1976).

Usually, the physiologic and psychologic impact of cancer pain on the patient is greater than that of nonmalignant chronic pain (Bond 1979; Bonica 1979). The physical deterioration is more severe because these patients have greater problems with sleep disturbance and with nausea, vomiting, and lack of appetite. Bonica and co-workers (1982) and Cleland and his associates (1982) noted that cancer patients with moderate to severe pain (Visual Analogue Scale [VAS] rating of 5 or more on a scale of 0–10) reported significant interference with their activity and enjoyment of life. In addition, 60%–65% of patients with advanced cancer pain reported that the pain disrupted their sleep. Moreover, the physiologic impact of cancer pain was greater than that produced by nonmalignant chronic pain syndromes.

Cancer patients also develop greater emotional reactions (i.e., anxiety, depression, hypochondriasis, somatic focussing, and neuroticism) to the pain when it develops than do patients with nonmalignant chronic pain (Bond and Pearson 1969; Bond 1971; Woodforde and Fielding 1975). Woodforde and Fielding (1975) examined cancer patients with and without pain using the Cornell Medical Index and demonstrated that the former group was significantly more emotionally disturbed than the latter and that they responded less well to treatment of their cancer and died sooner. The causes of emotional morbidity were depression, hypochondriasis, and psychosomatic symptoms, which together with intractable pain represent symptomatology indicative of a state of helplessness or inability to cope with disease, damage to the body, and the threat to life – responses to having a progressive and potentially fatal illness. Bond (1979) found that cancer patients with pain had raised levels of hypochondriasis and neuroticism, whereas pain-free cancer patients had low levels. He further noted that the scores of patients with high levels of emotionality fell reduced after the pain was relieved by percutaneous cordotomy. This led Bond to conclude that personality factors are distorted by severe pain, and that its relief results in restoration in the direction of normality.

Many patients with cancer pain, knowing that the causative factors are unremovable, cannot give meaningful purpose to the pain and develop feelings of hopelessness and despair. These feelings, like the sleeplessness, spiral to greater proportion as the patient is subjected to surgical operations, chemotherapy, or radiation therapy, and other anticancer modalities. Each time therapy is undertaken the patient experiences hopefulness, and if the therapy fails, this is followed by disappointment and gradually increasing bitterness, anger, and resentment. Many of these patients become more and more preoccupied with the pain and lose interest in social activities: the pain becomes the central focus of their lives and the lives of their family members.

The social effects of uncontrolled cancer pain are equally devastating. Many patients develop interpersonal problems with members of their family, friends, and the community. The fact that most patients with advanced cancer have to stop working poses not only an economic, but also an emotional stress and a feeling of dependency and uselessness. The physical appearance and behavior produced by the patient's pain and suffering stresses the family emotionally, which is, in turn, perceived by the patient and consequently aggravates the pain and suffering. Some patients with severe intractable pain become so discouraged and desperate as to contemplate suicide.

Current Status of Cancer Pain Control

Various sources of information suggest that like chronic pain in general, cancer pain all too frequently is improperly managed. A study carried out by Marks and Sachar (1973) of Montefiore Hospital in New York revealed that physicians prescribed amounts of narcotic analgesic for patients with moderate to severe pain due to cancer (and other medical disorders) which were about 50%–65% of the established effective doses of such drugs, and that the nurses administered as little as 20%–30% of the (inadequate) amount prescribed by physicians. For example, for patients with severe pain due to abdominal cancer, cancer of the pancreas, or lymphosarcoma, 50 mg meperidine every 4 h was prescribed; however, they received only 25–75 mg of the drug per day. Consequently, in most patients moderate to severe pain persisted after the narcotic therapy.

In his survey, Parkes (1978) found that among patients with severe or very severe pain cared for in hospital, the pain remained unrelieved during the terminal stage of the disease. Moreover, of patients managed in their homes, the incidence of unrelieved severe to very severe pain during the terminal phase increased nearly sixfold over that experienced prior to the terminal phase of the disease. These figures suggest that pain control was inadequate in the hospital and even worse in the home. Parkes noted this was in contrast to what happened to patients managed in St. Christopher's Hospice, where pain control is effectively carried out: the incidence of severe and unrelieved pain was 36% during the preterminal period, but this dropped to 8% during the terminal phase of the disease.

Aitkin-Swan (1959) interviewed the relatives of 200 cancer patients who had died and noted that of the 52% who had significant pain over a continuous period of time, in 18% the pain was relieved "to a certain extent" and in 20% the "distressing pain" remained unrelieved until death. She cited an earlier survey of public opinion on cancer which revealed that pain ranked next to incurability as reasons for their fear of cancer. Hinton (1963) reported that of 82 patients interviewed prior to their dying from cancer, 67% had pain and in 31% it remained unrelieved. Other British clinicians who have reported on unrelieved cancer pain include Cartwright and associates (1973) and Rees (1972), and this problem was the subject of an editorial comment by Cicely Saunders (1978).
Similar reports of inadequate cancer pain therapy were made by many participants of the International Symposium on Advanced Cancer Pain that was held in Venice, Italy, in May 1978 (Bonica and Ventafridda 1979). Moreover, as already mentioned, Turnbull (1979) reported that at the end of palliative therapy, pain was present in 45% of patients, and that two-thirds of patients died with unrelieved pain. A study at the University of Washington (Bonica et al. 1982) has shown that patients during and after anticancer therapy continue to have significant pain as follows: pain was present after surgical therapy in 85% of patients with cancer of the lung, 100% of patients with cancer of the pancreas, 57% of patients with cancer of the prostate, and 70% of patients with cancer of the cervix. The figures for those receiving chemotherapy and suffering pain were 60% with lung cancer and 50% with prostate cancer; after radiation therapy pain was present in 50% of patients with lung cancer, 75% with prostate cancer, and 60% with cervical cancer.

Reasons for Therapeutic Deficiencies

In view of the great advances in biomedical scientific knowledge and technology and, especially, the great amount of interest in, and effort devoted to, cancer research and therapy, why is cancer *pain* inadequately relieved? Serious consideration of this important question by the author in the course of the past quarter century has repeatedly suggested that it is due to an inadequate appreciation or outright neglect of the problem of pain (in contrast to the problem of cancer) by oncologists, medical educators, investigators, research institutions, and national and international cancer agencies (Bonica 1953, 1976, 1978, 1979, 1980). Consequently, there are great voids in our knowledge of various clinically relevant aspects of cancer pain, and whatever knowledge is currently available is often improperly applied (Bonica 1979).

Lack of Knowledge

Great voids exist in our knowledge of the mechanisms and physiopathology of acute and chronic pain in general and cancer pain in particular. This is due to the fact that until recently pain research was neglected by the biomedical scientific community, and only a few basic and clinical scientists devoted efforts to this field (Bonica 1980). Moreover, of those basic scientists who studied pain, most did so in the isolation of the animal laboratory and most were not concerned with pathologic pain. Until recently the scientific community failed to take advantage of the great advances in medical science and technology and to apply these to pain research. This was especially true of the investigation of the mechanisms and physiopathology of chronic pain states. Perhaps this was due in part to the fact that most scientists, like most clinicians, did not appreciate differences between acute and chronic pain.

These comments are especially true of cancer-related pain. To date there are no published reports of studies on the anatomic, physiologic, and biochemical substrates of cancer pain. Consequently we have no data on the basic mechanisms of the excruciating pain experienced by patients with cancer of the bone, pancreas, and other types of advanced neoplastic processes. We have no information on the neuropathologic changes in the brachial plexus that may be the substrates of the severe pain found in patients with Pancoast's tumor and those who have had radiation therapy. What are the biochemical events that produce the severe pain of mucositis? Why do some patients with various types of cancers have severe pain whereas others with the very same type of cancer and similar pathology do not have pain? Answers to these questions are not available.

A very important reason for the voids in our knowledge of pain in general and cancer pain in particular has been the lack of sufficient numbers of scientifically trained persons devoting their time to pain research. Related to this has been the meager amount of funds for research and training in this field. For example, in the United States over $ 2 billion will be spent this year for cancer research by the National Cancer Institute (NCI) and other federal, state, and municipal agencies, and by the American Cancer Society and other private agencies, private institutions, and the pharmaceutical industry. These funds will support the research of tens of thousands of scientists, technicians, physicians, and other health professionals who are investigating the cause, prevention, and treatment modalities of every form of cancer. However, until recently, research on cancer pain per se, which from the viewpoint of the patient and his family is one of the most important aspects of this dreadful disease, was virtually nonexistent. Analysis of a computer printout for the period 1971–1975 revealed that the NCI spent a total of nearly $ 2.5 billion to support its programs, and of this amount, only $ 560,000 was spent for cancer pain research. This total for the 5-year period represented 0.022% of the NCI budget for those years (Bonica 1979).

Moreover, although the NCI has carried out very comprehensive epidemiologic studies on the incidence of every kind of cancer and has the most sophisticated computer system for the storage and easy retrieval of data, it has no data on the prevalence, magnitude, and cost of the pain associated with cancer. This neglect of epidemilogic studies pervades the entire network of cancer hospitals, cancer centers, and cancer agencies (Bonica 1979).

Fortunately, things have begun to improve during the past few years, and the NCI has initiated support for a number of cancer pain research programs and studies of evaluation of the various therapeutic modalities that may be effective in relieving cancer pain.

Improper Application of Current Knowledge and Therapeutic Modalities

Improper application of current knowledge and therapeutic modalities is definetely the most important reason for inadequate cancer pain control. This, in turn, is due to a number of interrelated factors, including lack of organized teaching of medical students, physicians, and other health professionals, and the meager amount of published information on the proper treatment of cancer pain. Review of the curricula of medical schools reveals that few, if any, teach students the basic principles of the use of narcotics and other therapeutic modalities that effectively relieve cancer pain. Moreover, many physicians in residency training for specialization in surgical, medical, and radiation oncology receive little or no teaching about the proper management of cancer pain.

Usually, the senior house officer, who has vague and scanty information about cancer pain and its proper control, teaches the junior house officer how to deal with the problem in a rather empirical way and so passes on some of the misconceptions that will be mentioned below.

Inadequate or total lack of interest or concern about the problem of pain by oncologists is further attested by the fact that very little, if any, information about the proper management of the pain problem is found in the oncology literature, voluminous as it is. Of the many textbooks on various aspects of cancer, only a few deal with the problem of pain management, and they do so in a totally inadequate manner. For example, a review of ten important textbooks and monographs on the clinical management of cancer published in the United States reveals the startling fact that of a total of 9,300 pages, only 18 pages are devoted to the treatment of cancer pain (Ackerman and Del Regato 1970; American Cancer Society 1968; Becker 1975–1977; Union International Contre la Cancer 1973, 1978; Holland and Frei 1973; Horton and Hill 1977; Najerian and Delaney 1976; Raven 1977; Rubin and Bakemeier 1971). I'm informed that the same situation exists in Germany (see Wagner, this volume). Moreover, review of the current literature reveals that of the thousands of articles written on aspects of cancer each year, only a miniscule number, less than 0.1% are concerned with pain diagnosis and therapy. Finally, of the hundreds of local, regional, national, and international meetings on cancer research and therapy, less than 1%, include pain as a subject for consideration. From these data, the only conclusion that can be drawn is that pain has not been considered important by oncologic scientists and clinicans.

As the result of this lack of education of students, graduate physicians, and other health professionals, cancer pain has been and continues to be treated in an empirical manner. Most practitioners rely on narcotic analgesics which, although they are very useful and have their definite role in the control of cancer pain, for a variety of reasons are often misused. In a small percent of patients, potent narcotics are used initially for mild pain which could be relieved by nonnarcotic analgesics alone or combined with psychotropic drugs. At the other end of the spectrum, many, if not most, patients with moderate to severe pain from advanced cancer are given inadequate amounts of narcotics. The very high incidence of undertreatment of cancer pain with narcotics is due to inadequate knowledge of the pharmacology of these drugs and, particularly, to serious misconceptions among physicians and nurses about the risk of addiction and narcotic-induced respiratory depression. As part of the study previously mentioned, Marks and Sachar (1973) surveyed 102 physicians in training in two major hospitals and found that because of inadequate knowledge, most physicians underestimated the effective dose range of narcotics, overestimated the duration of their action, and had an exaggerated opinion of the dangers of addiction.

Apparently, this problem of inadequate knowledge and misconception about the risk of addiction and narcotic-induced depression is widespread, because many others have reported similar findings, including Bond (1979), Saunders (1979), Twycross (1979), and other participants in the aforementioned International Symposium on Pain of Advanced Cancer. Moreover, the National Committee on the Treatment of Intractable Pain (Quattelbaum, personal communication 1981), an American nonprofit organization concerned with the proper therapy of pain in cancer care, has received thousands of reports from relatives of patients who died with severe unrelieved cancer pain because they either received insufficient amounts of potent narcotics or were managed with ineffective drugs. Apparently, many physicians do not appreciate the fact that since severe pain is a powerful respiratory stimulant and can antagonize the depressant effects of narcotics, a physician can achieve good pain relief without hypoventilation by carefully titrating the drug administration to the needs of the patient. Moreover, addiction and physiologic dependence should not be considered an important problem in patients with recurrent or metastatic advanced cancer.

In some patients, even properly administered narcotics and other systemic drugs do not produce sufficient relief, and other modalities need to be used alone or in combination with drugs. These include chemical interruption of pain pathway with nerve blocks or with neurosurgical operations, or the use of neurostimulating techniques, hypnosis, and other psychologic procedures which have been shown to be effective in decreasing or totally relieving cancer pain. Unfortunately, for the aforementioned reasons, the role of these therapeutic modalities is not known by most practitioners and even many oncologists. Consequently, for most patients who could be more effectively relieved by one or a combination of these procedures, they are not considered or, if they are considered, this is done too late. Related to this is the lack of personnel with interest and expertise in the proper application of these other therapeutic modalities. Moreover, in some of these patients the cancer pain problem is such a complex array of sensory, perceptual, emotional, and affective events that it requires the concerted and well-coordinated efforts of specialists from different disciplines working as a team.

Recent Trends

Fortunately, during the past decade or so, several developments have taken place which, if sustained and expanded, hold the promise of helping to rectify some of the above deficiencies. One such development has been an impressive surge of interest among some basic scientists concerning the mechanisms of acute and chronic pain syndromes, and in collaborating with clinical investigators and practitioners to begin to solve some of the major clinical problems of pain management. These have included numerous studies which have provided more comprehensive information on the neurophysiologic, biochemical, and psychologic substrates of acute pain, and some new information about chronic pain syndromes.

Some progress has been made in certain areas of pain diagnosis and therapy. An impressive number of physicians have manifested an interest in acquiring more knowledge about pain and its treatment as reflected in part by the large attendance at numerous postgraduate seminars, and international, national, and regional meetings. Moreover, during the past several years, the concept of the multidisciplinary team approach to the diagnosis and therapy of complex chronic pain problems, first proposed by the author over three decades ago (Bonica 1953), has been adopted in a progressively larger number of medical centers in the United States and other countries.

In recent years, there has also been some progress with regard to communication and transfer of information. In addition to postgraduate courses, there have been a number of international symposia, and three World Congresses on Pain, and numerous monographs and books containing new and clinically relevant information have been published. The founding of the International Association for the Study of Pain (IASP) in 1974 must be considered one of the most important developments in the field of pain research and therapy. Through the scientific programs of these congresses and the publication of PAIN and the proceedings of the congresses, IASP has done much to enhance the dissemination of basic and clinical information of multidisciplinary interest and has further improved communication. I also wish to take this occasion to congratulate the German-speaking chapter of IASP for being one of the most active and productive of all our chapters. In addition to the magnificent scientific contribution, this chapter has done more in initiating educational programs for students, specialists in training, and practitioners than virtually any other chapter of IASP. Moreover, through its national congresses, it has had a significant impact on improving communication among pain researchers and therapists at the national and regional levels.

Future Needs and Goals

Recent developments in research, patient care, and communication are encouraging, but we are very far from our goal of understanding pain sufficiently and applying the information rapidly and effectively to prevent or to promptly eliminate pain without side effects or complications. This is especially true of cancer pain, which obviously has been so badly neglected by oncologic investigators and practitioners. The challenge to the biomedical scientific community, health professions, and society as a whole is to organize, mount, and support a multipronged program consisting of (a) greatly expanded pain research and research training programs, (b) activation of highly effective teaching programs for students and practitioners, and (c) improved systems of communications.

The overview in the previous section makes it obvious that there remains an urgent need for much greater research on cancer-related pain. Of course, the support for studies on the causes, prevention, and treatment of cancer must be sustained and expanded. However, until this dreadful disease can be effectively prevented, it is also essential to find better and more effective means to relieve cancer-related pain. Future research should provide much new information on the precise biochemical, neurophysiologic, and psychologic substrates of chronic pain in general and cancer pain in particular. Once such information is available, we can use the vast amount of knowledge and technology now available in chemistry, pharmacology, and biochemistry to develop agents that can act in an exquisitely specific way to inhibit or eliminate the various biochemical and neurologic factors that act at the molecular and cellular levels and in neural systems to produce pain in cancer patients. Such new agents would produce complete relief without any side effects.

Studies should also be carried out to permit refinement of current techniques of blocking nociceptive pathways in peripheral nerves and the neuraxis and to develop entirely new approaches to chemical interruption of nociceptive pathways. Moreover, future studies should permit more specific definition of the impact of various emotional, psychologic, sociologic, and environmental factors on patients with cancer-related pain and how this information could be applied more effectively in its relief. Recent studies suggest that using such information as a basis in the application of cognitive and behavioral methods should prove not only effective in relieving pain and suffering, but it has the added advantage of being noninvasive, without inherent risk of serious physical complications.

Until we acquire new information, we should be able to effectively use the knowledge and therapeutic modalities currently available to do a much better job in relieving the suffering and pain of cancer. To achieve this goal, it is necessary to mount intensive educational and training programs for medical students and other health professionals as well as physicians in practice. These programs should impart knowledge about (a) the causes and pathophysiology of cancer-related pain; (b) the efficacy, indications, limitations, and complications of current methods of pain relief; and (c) specific guidelines concerning proper management of the patients. In addition to such courses, it is essential to provide better sources of information through the oncologic literature, including books and special articles as well as brochures on cancer pain and its management. Moreover, because cancer pain problems are often too complex for one health professional to manage, it is highly desirable to have multidisciplinary cancer pain diagnostic and therapy teams, especially in the larger comprehensive cancer centers. Finally, it is also important to develop active programs for the information and education of the public about cancer-related pain in order to place it in proper perspective. This will not only decrease or eliminate the unnecessary fear and apprehension about cancer-related pain but will also enhance the cooperation and collaboration of those patients who do have pain to help the efforts of the practitioner in its relief.

To achieve all of these goals, it is desirable and indeed necessary to develop a type of broad-based multi- and interdisciplinary program in research and training. Such programs should evolve into cancer pain centers as part of large comprehensive cancer centers. The centers should include a critical mass of basic and clinical scientists and clinical oncologists who have special interest and expertise in cancer pain research and therapy. The basic science group should include anatomists, biochemists, neurochemists, neurophysiologists, neuropathologists, behavioral scientists, computer specialists, biostatisticians, and others that may be needed to study specific aspects of cancer-related pain. The aforementioned multidisciplinary cancer pain diagnostic and therapy team must include medical, surgical, and radiation oncologists, pain specialists (who may be anesthesiologists, neurosurgeons, psychiatrists, or psychologists), and should also include clinical pharmacologists, nurses, sociologists, social workers, and others with special interest, knowledge, and expertise in cancer and cancer pain. In addition to having sufficient skilled personnel for research and patient care, the centers should greatly enhance interaction among investigators and pain clinicians and encourage communication, exchange of information, collaboration, and cross-fertilization of ideas.

Basic Principles of Management

In determining the best therapeutic modality or combination of therapies to relieve the pain effectively, it is essential to consider the characteristics of the pain, the chronology of the disease and of previous therapy, and various other aspects which can only be ascertained by a very detailed history and comprehensive general physical, neurologic, orthopedic, and other appropriate examinations (Bonica 1953, 1979). Since most patients with cancer pain present a complex array of physical, psychologic, behavioral, and affective manifestations, a total psychologic and social evaluation is mandatory to develop the most appropriate therapeutic strategy.

A careful history of the pain complaint is an essential first step in determining a therapy. It is important to consider the location and distribution of the pain and its possible spread, quality, severity, and time-characteristics (i.e., whether it is continuous or occurs in bouts), and what factors aggravate and relieve the pain. It is also important to elicit information about associated phenomena including sensory deficits, muscle weakness, and visceral dysfunction. It is also important to obtain a history of the oncologic process in order to determine which of the major etiologic factors is responsible for the pain. If the pain is directly due to the neoplasm, it is essential to know the type and grade of differentiation and site of spread or metastasis. If the pain is the result of therapy, an attempt should be made to predict its timecourse.

Careful examination of the painful region and general physical, neurologic, and orthopedic examinations are also essential to acquire objective data and substantiate the clinical history. A detailed neurologic examination is particularly useful in differentiating local pain from referred pain, and in differentiating pain due to peripheral-nerve involvement from pain due to plexus or cord involvement. For example, in a patient with low back pain and radicular symptomatology in L5–S1 distribution, together with an absent ankle jerk, nerve root rather than plexus involvement is suggested.

A comprehensive psychologic and social evaluation is essential in order to develop the most effective therapeutic strategy. This should include a general psychologic and behavioral assessment and the application of appropriate psychometric tests. Psychosocial evaluation should include determination of cultural background, religious beliefs, interaction with spouse and family unit, social activities, and the impact of these on the pain. *Various diagnostic tools* may be essential to determine the mechanisms of pain. Since ordinary X-rays have limitations, it may be necessary to supplement them with bone scan and tomography (CT scan). In addition to the usual laboratory examination, special biochemical procedures may be necessary. Cisternal and lumbar myography and cerebrospinal fluid cytology are sometimes necessary to determine the etiology of the pain. The part which appropriate nerve blocks can play in ascertaining the mechanisms and pathways of cancer pain will be discussed in a subsequent paper.

Evaluation of all therapeutic modalities currently available for the relief of cancer pain is crucial to the selection of the most effective therapy. It is essential to know not only the analgesic efficacy and advantages, but also the limitations and disadvantages of each procedure. Only with such knowledge integrated with the information obtained from the history and physical examinations will it be possible to determine which is the best method (or methods) of relieving cancer pain. It deserves reemphasis that complex cancer pain problems require a multidisciplinary team effort in evaluating the patient and in developing the most appropriate therapeutic strategy.

References

Ackerman LV, Del Regato JAW (eds) (1970) Cancer diagnosis, treatment and prognosis, 4th edn. Mosby, St. Louis

Aitken-Swan J (1959) Nursing the late cancer patient at home. Practitioner 183: 64–69

American Cancer Society (1981) Cancer facts and figures. American Cancer Society, New York

American Cancer Society – Massachusetts Division (1968) Cancer: a manual for practitioners. American Cancer Society, Boston

Becker F (ed) (1975–1977) Cancer: a comprehensive treatise. Plenum, New York

Bond MR (1971) The relation of pain to the Eysenck personality inventory, Cornell medical index and Whitely index of hypochondriasis. Br J Psychiatr 119: 671–678

Bond MR (1979) Psychologic and emotional aspects of cancer pain. In: Bonica JJ, Ventafridda V (eds) Proceedings of the international symposium on pain of advanced cancer. Raven, New York, pp 81–88 (Advances in pain research and therapy, vol 2)

Bond MR, Pearson IB (1969) Psychologic aspects of pain in women with advanced cancer of the cervix. J Psychosom Res 13: 13–19

Bonica JJ (1953) The management of pain. Lea and Febiger, Philadelphia

Bonica JJ (1976) Cancer pain – a national health problem. Presented to the cancer control grant review committee of the National Cancer Institute, June 28, 1976

Bonica JJ (1978) Cancer pain: a major national health problem. Cancer Nur J 4: 313–316

Bonica JJ (1979) Cancer pain: importance of the problem. In: Bonica JJ, Ventafridda V (eds) Proceedings of the international symposium on pain of advanced cancer. Raven, New York, pp 1–12 (Advances in pain research and therapy, vol 2)

Bonica JJ (1980) Pain research and therapy: past and current status and future needs. In: Ng LKY, Bonica JJ (eds) Pain, discomfort and humanitarian care. Proceedings of the national conference on pain, discomfort and humanitarian care. Elsevier, Amsterdam, pp 1–46

Bonica JJ, Ventafridda V (eds) (1979) Proceedings of the international symposium on pain of advanced cancer. Raven, New York (Advances in pain research and therapy, vol 2)

Bonica JJ, Greenwald H, Francis A, Bergner M (1982) Report on epidemiology of cancer pain. Meeting of the National Cancer Institute, USA

Cartwright A, Hockey L, Anderson ABM (eds) (1973) Life before death. Routledge and Kegan Paul, London

Cleland CS, Daut RL (1982) The prevalence and severity of cancer. Meeting of the National Cancer Institute, USA

Foley KM (1979) Pain syndromes in patients with cancer. In: Bonica JJ, Ventafridda V (eds) Proceedings of the international symposium on pain of advanced cancer. Raven, New York, pp 59–78 (Advances in pain research and therapy, vol 2)

Hinton JM (1963) The physical and mental distress of the dying. Q J Med 32: 1–21

Holland JF, Frei E III (eds) (1973) Cancer medicine. Lea and Febiger, Philadelphia

Horton J, Hill GJ (eds) (1977) Clinical oncology. Saunders, Philadelphia

International Union Against Cancer (1978) Clinical oncology: a manual for students and doctors, 2nd edn. Springer, Berlin, Heidelberg, New York

Kornell JA (1980) Pain in advanced cancer patients. M.A. thesis, School of Nursing, University of Washington

Marks RM, Sachar EJ (1973) Undertreatment of medical inpatients with narcotic analgesics. Ann Intern Med 78: 173–181

Najerian JS, Delaney P (eds) (1976) Advances in cancer surgery. Stratton Intercontinental Medical, New York, p 608

Norton WS, Lack SA (1980) Control of symptoms other than pain. In: Twycross RG, Ventafridda V (eds) The Continuing care of terminal patients. Pergamon, New York, pp 167–178

Pannuti E, Martoni A, Rossi AP, Piana E (1979) The role of endocrine therapy for relief of pain due to advanced cancer. In: Bonica JJ, Ventafridda V (eds) Proceedings of the international symposium on pain of advanced cancer. Raven, New York, pp 145–166 (Advances in pain research and therapy, vol 2)

Pannutti F, Rossi AP, Marraro D, Strocchi E, Cricca A, Piana A, Pollutri E (1980) Natural history of cancer pain. In: Twycross RG, Ventafridda V (eds) The continuing care of terminal patients. Pergamon, New York, pp 75–79

Parkes CM (1978) Home or hospital? Terminal care as seen by surviving spouse. J R Coll Gen Pract 28: 19–30

Pilowsky I, Chapman CR, Bonica JJ (1977) Pain, depression and illness behavior in a pain clinic population. Pain 4: 183–192

Raven RW (ed) (1977) Principles of surgical oncology. Plenum, New York

Rees WD (1972) The distress of dying. Br Med J 2: 105–108

Rubin P, Bakemeier R (eds) (1971) Clinical oncology for medical students and physicians. A multidisciplinary approach, 3rd edn. American Cancer Society, New York

Saunders CM (1978) Editorial note to relief of pain. In: Saunders CM (ed) The management of terminal disease. Year Book Publishers, Chicago, pp 65–66

Sternbach RH (1974) Pain patients, traits and treatments. Academic, New York

Turnbull F (1979) The nature of pain that may accompany cancer of the lung. Pain 7: 371–375

Twycross RG, Wald SJ (1976) Long-term use of diamorphine in advanced cancer. In: Bonica JJ, Albe-Fessard D (eds) Proceeding of the First World Congress on Pain. Raven, New York, pp 653–661 (Advances in pain research and therapy, vol 1)

Wilkes F (1974) Some problems in cancer management. Proc R Soc Med 67: 23–27

Woodforde JM, Fielding JR (1975) Pain and cancer. In: Weisenburg M (ed) Pain, clinical and experimental perspectives. Mosby, St. Louis, pp 332–336

The Telos and Ethos of Pain and Suffering

H. Pompey

Falkenstrasse 8, 8700 Würzburg 25, FRG

The Genesis and Telos of Suffering and Pain

The following considerations not only examine pain and suffering from a different point of view, they also examine them – in part at least – in a manner not customarily practised in natural science: the following scientific analysis does not proceed inductively-empirically, but rather synductively-speculatively with the inclusion of deduction. Among other things, knowledge can also be derived from religious tradition. Suffering, the fact and its Christian interpretation, are the subject of the discourse on the telos and ethos of pain and suffering. In this context suffering is understood as the experience and consciousness (embracing the human being in his entirety) of pain in all its suffered and experienced spiritual, psychological, social, and somatic dimensions (Pompey 1974).

The experience of pain and suffering and the coping with pain and suffering are to be seen in a greater context, anthropologically and theologically, and always represent – at least theologically – the experience of the disastrous situation of mankind in general as well (Pompey 1981). From the Christian viewpoint, every disaster – sickness, pain, etc. – is the fact or symptom of a disturbed and broken relation, that is:

1. A disturbance in the relation of man to himself, to his somatic-materialistic reality as well as to his psychological-spiritual reality.
2. A disturbance in the relation to his contemporaries and his environment, to his interpersonal-social as well as to his economic-natural world. In the Judeo-Christian conception of man and the world, but in the conception of other religions as well, the ultimate cause for this relation disturbance is the break in man's relation to God. The original causality of this relation disturbance is traditionally described by the term *Ursünde* (original sin), because mankind bears the responsibility for this original break in relations (Pompey 1981). This does not mean, however, that every individual disturbed relation of man to himself, his neighbors, and his nature results in somatic illnesses and definite pains, although this factor cannot be ruled out. Mankind as a whole bears responsibility and continuously effects disturbances in its relation to the natural foundations of life and to interpersonal life-reality within its respective societies. Consequently, in the eyes of the early church (*Urkirche*), illness, the suffering of and the coping with pain are the tasks of the Christian community and not of the individual alone (Pompey 1982b).

According to Christian belief, God aspires, through the incarnation of Jesus Christ, to make possible again the *Ur*-relation, the fundamental contact of man to God, and that means in the last analysis every relation, retaining at the same time man's freedom of decision and his self-responsibility. God's belief in the goodness of mankind, His loving devotion to mankind, should overcome us and motivate us to believe in the good in

Recent Results in Cancer Research. Vol. 89

ourselves and in the world and to approach ourselves and the world with love; that is not to overtax, exploit or abuse ourselves, but to live together in a benevolent, beneficial relationship. God wishes to rouse mankind through Jesus Christ for and through this spirit of faith and love (cf. the mission of the Spirit). Christ's death and resurrection are the verifications of the message. In accepting pain and suffering as an expression of the manifold broken relations of mankind, Christ makes evident the creative power of suffering and death in the mystery of salvation, which extends from his incarnation to the resurrection and makes suffering as well as death principally surmountable.

For the practical-theological reflection the anthropological reality of illness, pain, and suffering is also a decisive premise: the experience of and coping with pain and suffering are dependent variables of the psychological and spiritual as well as the physical reality of the individual and of the material-economical as well as the interpersonal life situation. Here the individual affective, cognitive, somatic, as well as the social and material factors are interdependent. Body, soul, spirit, as well as the contemporaries and the environment do not represent self-contained monad systems. Principally, all dependent and interdependent relations are either disturbable or disturbed.

This is also the fundamental cause of cancer and cancer pain. Cancerous diseases represent a disorder of the interdependent relations, above all, of the material-physical substrates but also of the spiritual-psychological life reality. On the other hand, cancer pain as a warning signal and tormentor is dependent upon these disturbed interpendences.

Theology and ministry attempt through religious reorganization and support of the spiritual-psychological reality of man to ease the experience of and the coping with pain and suffering which, due to the interdependence between the spiritual-psychological and the material-physical can, by all means have physically noticeable results. The individual cancerous disease, like the extraordinary spreading of cancer among mankind – according to Bonica (1979), 5 million people die annually of cancer –, is not only a result of man's disturbed relations to his spiritual, psychological, social, and material nature, but in itself a cause for new disorders in these relation areas. Thus the causality of evil, in a process of continuous self-procreation, becomes evident as a relation disturbance for which man searches the fundamental cause (*Urgrund*) or origin (*Ursprung*).

In a comprehensive sense Christ's salvation seeks to confront the disastrous situation, the no longer intact relations. The telos of the Christian vanquishment of pain and suffering is man's reconciliation with his psychological, spiritual, social, and physical reality, which finds its ultimate orientation in the restoration of a positive relationship to God. Man bears responsibility for obtaining this global or these partial goals, from which an ethos for the actualization of successful relation variables ensues.

The Practice and Ethos of Dealing with Pain and Suffering

According to Christian theological tradition, pain disturbances and the suffering of the human being in his entirety as a result are caused by not wanting or not being able to face up to one's own reality and to the reality of the relationship partner (Pompey 1980). Man, represented by the *Gestalt* Adam, wanted to be like God, his *Ur*-relationship partner. He did not want to accept the relation to God in its given existence. Each and every inter- and intra-individual relation disturbance is based on this *Ur-Nein*. The refusal to accept the truth – a rejection of concrete reality – finds its practical expression in the overestimation of oneself and others, in the overtaxing of one's strength, in the making of ideals and the creation of idols of reality etc., all of which find their ominous expression in the rampant growth of cells. It is undisputed, that the intra-individual disturbances of man's spiritual, psychological, and social relation reality can also materialize, can become physical, and finally – although for the single individual neither evident nor provable – are the cause of disturbances in man's somatic-material substrates. Pain and suffering as warning signals and tormentors of the relation disturbances can only be overcome when the single individual and mankind attain self-acceptance and become motivated to seek reconciliation with themselves and nature. This acceptance of the truth of life as the reality of life (Pompey 1980) means, in other words, facing up frankly and honestly to the experience of one's own, admittedly always broken reality, and thus recognizing one's own possibilities and limits. Not resistance, but loving acceptance is the way. Religious identification with the suffering Christ can bring about the psychically necessary distance to one's own situation of suffering.

According to the basic therapeutic model of Christus medicus, the practice of Christian salvation, which includes coping with pain, presupposes the archetype of the healing professions of the early Middle Ages (Schipperges 1965):

1. The formation of a helping relation to the sufferer. One who is suffering due to a relation disturbance can only accept himself and his reality when someone is there to accept his disturbances.
2. The willingness of the sufferer to face the painful appeal and challenge of a somatic, spiritual, psychological, or social relation disturbance and to listen to his inner self (Pompey 1980, 1982a) and hear, for example, what his body says about these disturbances. (This can also be seen as an equivalent to the voice of God speaking in man.)

Christ called Himself the Way and the Truth. Therefore, the requirements for salvation and healing shall be derived from His reality: for the radical vanquishment of suffering and its causes, God appears to us as a concrete person in Jesus Christ. In Him is manifest God's greatest possible nearness, which is characterized by faith. Faith and nearness are expressed in the Lord's Covenant. The Covenant personalizes the factor of space of finite realities through nearness and the factor of time through faith. Accordingly, a personal, tangible relation in faith and nearness forms the structural basis of every therapeutic accompaniment. The healing variables – as the functional elements of the healing relation – are likewise analogously given in the reality of God's Covenant with man:

1. The revelation of the reality of God in Jesus Christ, that is, the openness and transparentness of His doing and His purpose.
2. The belief in the goodness of man and nature despite the original break in relations.
3. The loving acceptance of man, which is not based on advance commitments and stipulations, and the goodness and mercy of God.
4. The hope that goodness shall prevail and – strengthened through His grace – shall finally achieve perfection (Pompey 1981).

These virtues as well as this spiritualness are the foundation of a successful, that means in the end a therapeutic healing relation, which can lead to the overcoming of the fundamental causes of illness and, consequently, of the suffering involved. As a result of the consonance and analogy of creation with the revelation, it is theologically acceptable that comparative psychotherapeutic research has come up with similar basic criteria known as the common factors of every positive therapeutic relation such as openness, congruence, esteem, and understanding nearness (Pompey 1982a). If a doctor, nurse, or minister actualizes these lines of basic behavior, he is most likely to make the person suffering believe in the possibility of relations despite his given suffering and present life situation and thus help him overcome his fear of life; furthermore, to help him hope for a positive relation to himself and to nature and thus to reduce depressive and resignative tendencies; moreover to help him lovingly accept himself and the actual given choices in life and, in doing so, to give up aggression toward others and himself, to free himself from his responsibility for others and to see the truth as a reality, which also means consciously accepting the fact of illness and furthermore perceiving and accepting the possibility of death and giving up all denials. In this way, a desensibilization of the typical psychic side effects caused by cancer pain or suffering from cancer is possible. If this "No" to reality can be converted into acceptance by this method, even when this acceptance is burdensome, then this *conversio* or *metanoia* sets a vitality free which is no longer occupied with maintaining the "No". Furthermore, new perspectives to life enter the picture, perspectives which were in part formerly never taken into consideration. A new way of life becomes possible, even if it has its limitations. In this pastoral-medical (cf. Pompey 1968) and pastoral-psychological (cf. Pompey 1976) teleology, one dare not forget that totally successful relations and a truly happy life always also represent a not yet fulfilled eschatological dimension and reality (Pompey 1981).

Special Ethic Perspectives in Dealing with Cancer and Cancer Pain

A number of solutions to special ethical problems arise from this fundamental ethos of a healing relation: If a person is confronted with pain and suffering as a warning signal of psychosomatic or psychosocial relation disturbances in himself, then he should not ignore the warning but instead follow up this call in order to forge ahead to his own truth and to come to terms again with his own reality. This is possible in cases of acute pain as well as in the beginning phases of chronic pain. However, if a person is confronted with suffering as a tormentor which obstructs his relations to himself and to his contemporaries and his environment, then it may and should be eliminated with the help of analgesics. Furthermore, it is legitimate according to Christian tradition to obviate meaningless pain during surgery. There is also no obligation to extend human life at all costs, that is, at the cost of bearing interminable and extraordinary pain (Pius XII 1954, Pius 1961); moreover, the possibility of the abuse of euphoric agents does not forbid their positive use, for example, in fighting chronic pain. In the case of irrevocably approaching death, it may even be ethically permissible to carry out treatment against pain, although bodily damage results as a side effect of this treatment, that is, in the case of a process of irreversible deterioration or excrescence, treatment against pain with the effect of shortening the life of the patient can be risked when the measure serves the purpose of improving his life quality or the relation to himself, his contemporaries, and his environment (Pompey 1974). Furthermore, a sick person may refuse extraordinarily painful treatment or a corresponding measure of treatment as he is only obligated to accept the application of measures which actually offer him a real chance of being cured. *Lege artis,* and thus ethically, it certainly would not be justifiable to fight pain with the aid of biochemical substrates, surgery, electrophysiological methods, etc. alone. Instead, all the psychic and psychological strength, that is, the religious also, should be activated. Severe and chronic pain always causes a reality of suffering which affects the entire human being and for that reason, in pain therapy, one must also think and act comprehensively. The availability and use of *every* possible type of method is especially necessary in fighting cancer pain during the final phase of suffering, as at this stage the classical analgesics and euphorica generally become increasingly less effective.

As the aim of the Christian message of salvation is to overcome all relation disturbances and blockages as well as their painful and distressful consequences, every cure of pain is in accordance with the Christian perspective of salvation. Christus medicus has come to vanquish the illness, pain, and suffering of the individual as well as mankind. Yet the message of His own earthly-bodily existence shows that in this aeon the confrontation with and the overcoming of unavoidable and unalterable pain also exists. Only the belief in the nearness and faithfulness of God in this situation, the grappling with this terrible reality – for Christ also, the most difficult events of His life took place between Gethsemane and Golgatha – as well as the hope of the transformation of all suffering into immeasurable joy (Romans 8: 18) give mankind in its endless suffering and boundless pain the chance to live, to experience, to survive at all.

References

Bonica JJ (1979) Importance of the problem. In: Bonica JJ, Ventafridda V (eds) Advances in pain research and therapy, vol 2. Raven, New York, pp 1–12

Pius XII (1954) Die Aufgabe des christlichen Arztes. In: Utz AF, Groner JF (eds) Aufbau und Entfaltung des Gesellschaftlichen Lebens, vol 1. Paulusverlag, Freiburg, pp 1116–1118

Pius XII (1961) Drei religiöse und moralische Fragen bezüglich der Anästhesie. In: Utz AF, Groner JF (eds) Aufbau und Entfaltung des Gesellschaftlichen Lebens, vol 3. Paulusverlag, Freiburg, pp 3242–3265

Pompey H (1968) Die Bedeutung der Medizin für die kirchliche Seelsorge im Selbstverständnis der sogenannten Pastoralmedizin. Herder, Freiburg

Pompey H (1974) Fortschritt der Medizin und christliche Humanität – Der Dienst der Praktischen Theologie an einer Medizin im Umbruch. Echter, Würzburg

Pompey H (1976) Seelsorge in den Krisen des Lebens. Tendenzen und Möglichkeiten beratender seelsorglicher Hilfe in Geschichte und Gegenwart. In: Henrich F (ed) Seelsorge ohne Priester? Zur Problematik von Beratung und Psychotherapie in der Pastoral. Patmos, Düsseldorf, pp 29–72

Pompey H (1980) Wahrheit und Wahrhaftigkeit. Arzt und Christ 26: 5–13

Pompey H (1981) Beziehungstheologische Gesichtspunkte des Gelingens ehelicher Partnerschaft. Lebendige Katechese 3: 95–105

Pompey H (1982a) Technik im Krankenhaus – Chance oder Gefahr? In: Caritasverband Hildesheim (ed) 15. Norddeutscher Krankenhaustag Hildesheim – "Technik im Krankenhaus – Chance oder Gefahr". Caritas, Hildesheim, pp E1–26

Pompey H (1982b) Die theologisch-psychologische Begründung der geistlichen Barmherzigkeit in der gemeindlichen Krankenpflegepraxis. Seminar für Gemeindekrankenpflege, Koblenz-Arenberg

Schipperges H (1965) Zur Tradition des "Christus Medicus" im frühen Christentum und in der älteren Heilkunde. Arzt und Christ 11: 12–19

Pathological Anatomy of Cancer Pain

K. Hill

Institut für Pathologie, Evangelisches Krankenhaus Hamm,
Werler Strasse 110, 4700 Hamm, FRG

Introduction

Since pain is a functional and multifactorial phenomenon (cf. Bonica 1979, Rolf and Brune 1982, Strempel 1981), it is not usually accessible to morphological methods. In particular, the study of cancer pain by the pathological anatomist is hampered by the lack of information as to whether or not pain symptoms have been present clinically in his cases. Therefore, I should like first of all to thank my clinical colleagues who have provided information to make possible the following review of painful organ and tissue changes (cf. also Bonadonna and Molinari 1979; Bonica 1979; Foley 1979; Schlegel 1982; Twycross 1978).

In principle, pain sensations are elicited by stimulation of peripheral nociceptors or by a lesion of afferent nerve fibers (Zimmermann 1979, 1981). Physical influences such as pressure, traction, compression, and tumor infiltration, as well as metabolic or chemical disturbances can give rise to pain impulses. The latter may involve bradykinin, serotonin, or prostaglandins. The sensitivity of peripheral nerves to pain-eliciting influences probably depends on their content of afferent nociceptive fibers. Finally, the superordinate organ of pain perception, the central nervous system, contains pain receptors only in its membranes. Unfortunately, neither the nociceptors nor the nociceptive nerve fibers can be distinguished from other modalities by conventional anatomical methods.

The following synopsis does not follow the usual principles of special or general pathology but is arranged according to the anatomical structures in which clinical experience shows that lesions lead to pain.

Tumor Affection of Encapsulated Organs

Primary or secondary tumors of the liver are the most frequent examples of tumors of encapsulated organs. These can lead to enlargement of the organ of up to several times the normal size. Since the organ capsule of connective tissue grows less rapidly than the tumor, the intracapsular pressure rises and capsular distension develops. In addition, the capsule is focally infiltrated by the tumor. In such cases, dull and rarely also stabbing pains are reported. In a corresponding observation (our case S. 55/81), the latter have clinically indicated rapid growth of a primary angiosarcoma of the liver with underlying thorotrastosis. The massive and rapid growth of the organ probably does not only lead to stimulation of the nociceptors of the capsule alone, but to irritation of larger nerves, namely by pressure or traction on the tissue suspending the organ. Similar organ-enlarging processes in the spleen and kidneys do not lead to pain to the same extent as in the liver.

Recent Results in Cancer Research. Vol. 89

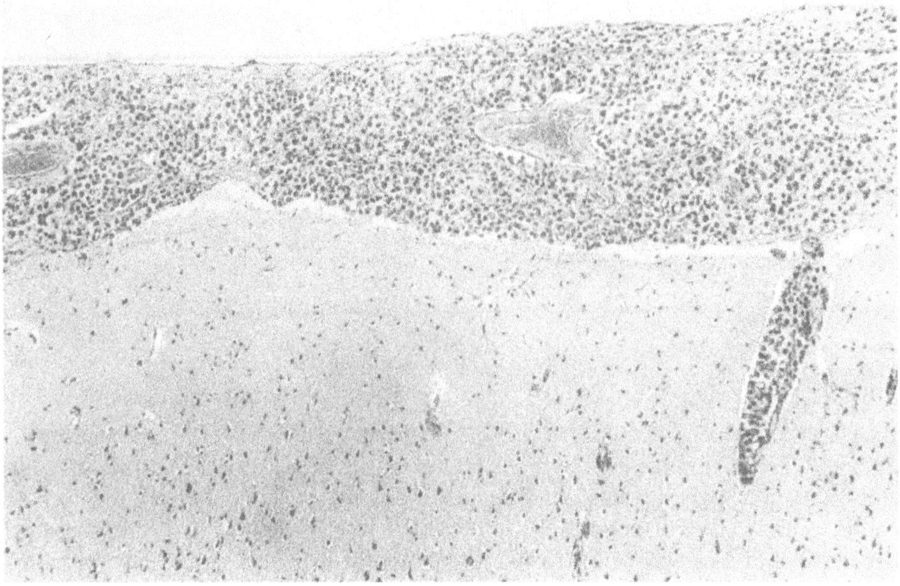

Fig. 1. Diffuse metastatic carcinosis of the subarachnoid space in gallbladder carcinoma. HE, × 100

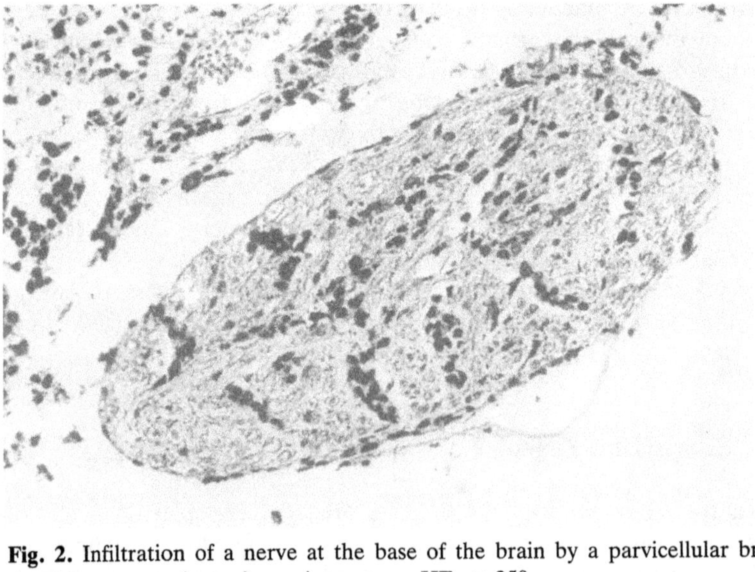

Fig. 2. Infiltration of a nerve at the base of the brain by a parvicellular bronchial carcinoma in simultaneous meningeosis carcinomatosa. HE, × 250

This might be explained by the more stable suspension or embedding of these organs, which are farther away from the midline with its abundant nerve pathways. In kidney tumors, pain is only reported at all when the kidney has been almost completely destroyed and the tumor has invaded the pararenal tissue or when it destroys the renal pelvis. The brain is also an encapsulated organ. Its special feature is that its bony skull capsule prevents any enlargement. Pain arises here not by destruction of parenchyma, but by the

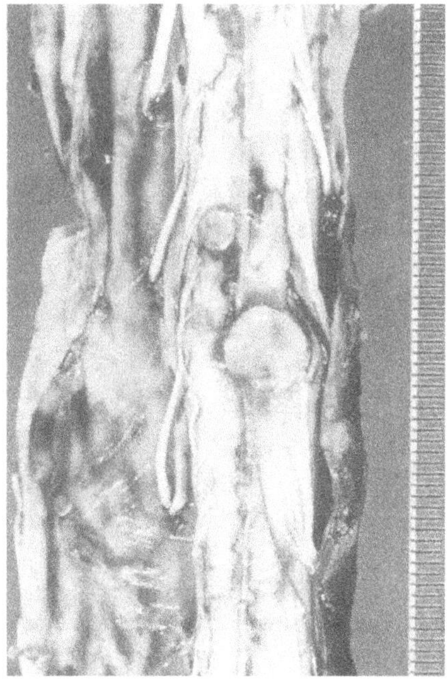

Fig. 3. Nodular subdural metastases of a malignant melanoma on the spinal cord. Compression of a nerve root by the larger nodule

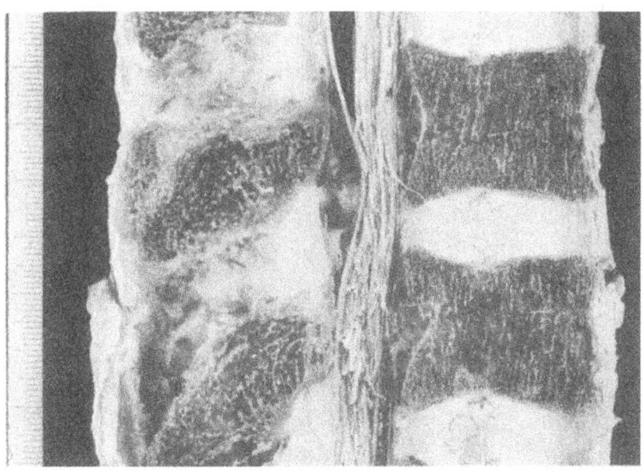

Fig. 4. Epidural metastasis of a bronchial carcinoma with compression of the cauda equina. Clinical manifestations: cauda equina syndrome with pain in the legs

increase of the intracranial pressure with stimulation of the meningeal nociceptors. Such an increase of intracranial pressure occurs in space-occupying tumor growth or in focal or generalized brain edema. Focally, an edema can arise around isolated tumors, e.g., around a meningeoma. A generalized edema arises especially in diffuse metastatic invasion of the meninges (Fig. 1) due to a disturbance of the circulation of the cerebrospinal fluid. Such a tumor invasion of the leptomeninges is especially frequent in malignant lymphomas (Mackintosh et al. 1982). However, metastatic invasion of the leptomeninges is also observed in patients with solid tumors, e.g., mammary carcinoma, bronchial carcinoma, and malignant melanoma (Sondak et al. 1981; Wasserstrom et al. 1982). Its leading symptom is headache. However, in such cases the cranial nerves can also be infiltrated by the tumor (Fig. 2). This is a process which possibly gives the pain a different character.

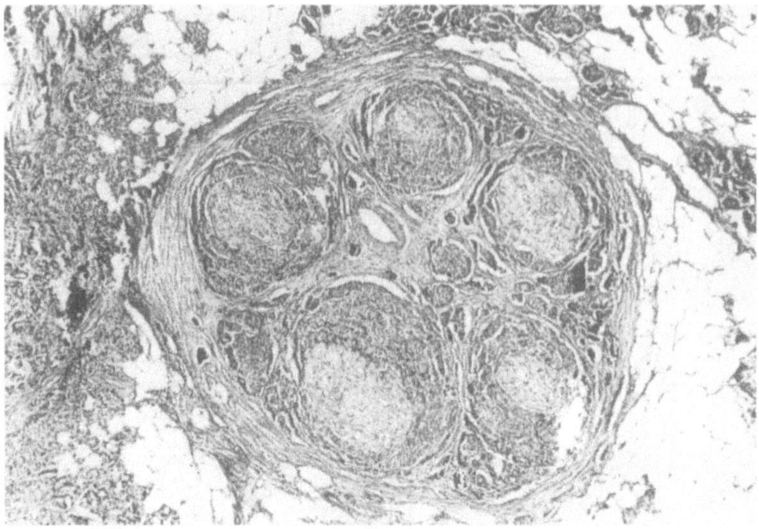

Fig. 5. Entrapment of all nerves of a plexus by a local recurrence of a mammary carcinoma (epineural and endoneural infiltration). Clinical manifestations: pain which cannot be influenced. HE, × 40

When nodular meningeal metastases do not press directly on cranial nerves (as in acoustic neurinoma; Payten 1972), they act in the cranial cavity-like tumors of the brain, that is via a focal, pressure-raising edema. On the other hand, a direct compression of nerve roots (Fig. 3) or of the cauda equina (Fig. 4) is more likely to occur in the spinal canal because of the topographical preconditions. This applies both to subdural and epidural metastases.

Tumor Infiltration of Peripheral Nerves

Since peripheral nerves can usually evade pressure from a tumor on one side, infiltration by tumor tissue is the essential pain stimulus (Asbury and Johnson 1978; McLeod 1975; McLeod and Walsh 1975; Sunderland 1978; Swerdlow 1979). In addition, indirect damage of unknown pathogenesis might also occur to peripheral nerves in the context of tumor conditions (i.e., paraneoplastic conditions). It may present clinically as a sensory neuropathy (Brain and Adams 1965; Denny-Brown 1948; Kashef and Das Gupta 1968; Thomas et al. 1972). This type of damage will not be considered here.

Infiltration of tumor tissue into the perineural cleft is seen fairly often. As we know in particular from prostate carcinomas, it does not regularly lead to pain. A massive and then painful entrapment of the nerve plexus or individual nerves occurs especially in extensive mammary carcinomas and their recurrences (Fig. 5) or in chest wall metastases of bronchial carcinomas (Fig. 6). The perineural cleft is widened by the infiltration and an infiltration of the tumor into the nerve itself is not uncommonly found. Degenerative changes of the axis cylinders can occasionally be visualized even using conventional screening methods. Primary tumors of the peripheral nerves themselves likewise lead to painful destruction.

A compression regularly elicits pain when the affected nerve cannot give way, e.g., a spinal nerve (Schölmerich et al. 1980). In a corresponding observation of our own (our case S.

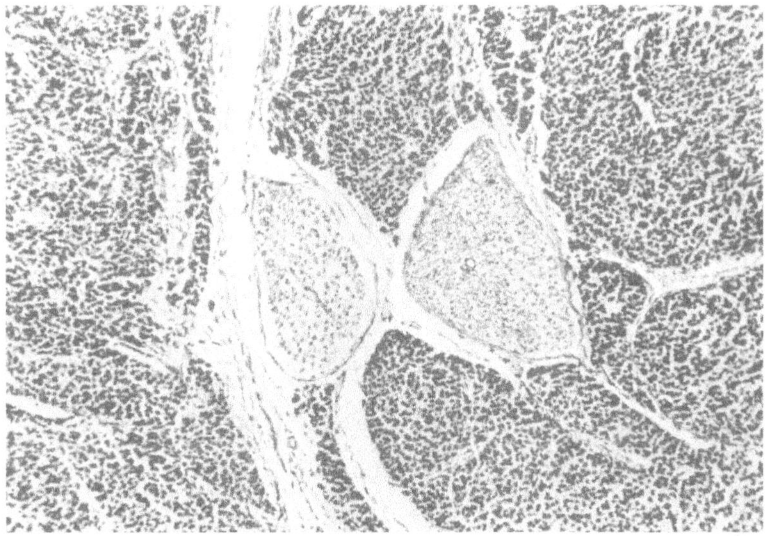

Fig. 6. Entrapment of the intercostal nerves in chest wall metastases of a parvicellular bronchial carcinoma (perineural infiltration). Clinical manifestations: pain in the chest wall. HE, × 100

79/82), the base of the skull on the left side was infiltrated by a meningeoma originating from the tentorium cerebelli. The intraosseous region of the trigeminal nerve was thereby entrapped. The patient had suffered from a trigeminal neuralgia of the left side.

Tumor Infiltration of Soft Tissues

On the one hand, an infiltration of soft tissues can elicit pain by the same kind of changes in the neural structures as have been described above. This is to be assumed especially for massive infiltrations of the retroperitoneum (Flowers 1968). On the other hand, infiltration and destruction of mobile structures, e.g., of the skeletal musculature, can lead to pain via disturbance of the function. Here, the tumor spreads in the interstitium and destroys blood vessels, lymphatics, and nerves. However, the muscle fibers themselves can be infiltrated and destroyed by the tumor.

Tumor Infiltration of Bone

The most frequent cause of pain in tumor patients is infiltration of bone (Bonica 1979; Foley 1979). This applies to primary (Campbell et al. 1975) and secondary neoplasias originating from the bone marrow as well as to neoplasias of the bone itself. Such tumors always cause pain when they lead to an elevation of the intraosseous pressure, to loss of stability, or to a lesion of the periosteum. The neural structures responsible for the pain are situated in the bone marrow, in the bone, and in the periosteum. An example of a primary bone tumor is a chordoma of the clivus, which in one of our cases led to intractable pain in the neck and shoulder girdle (our case S. 30/81).

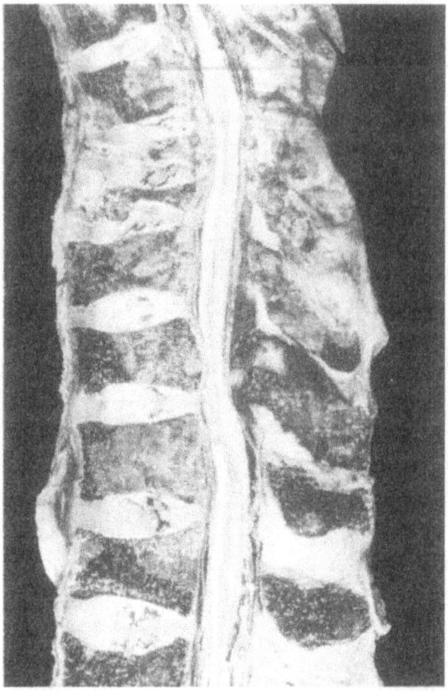

Fig. 7. Metastases of a bronchial carcinoma in the vertebral column with compression fracture of two vertebral bodies and with compressions of the spinal cord

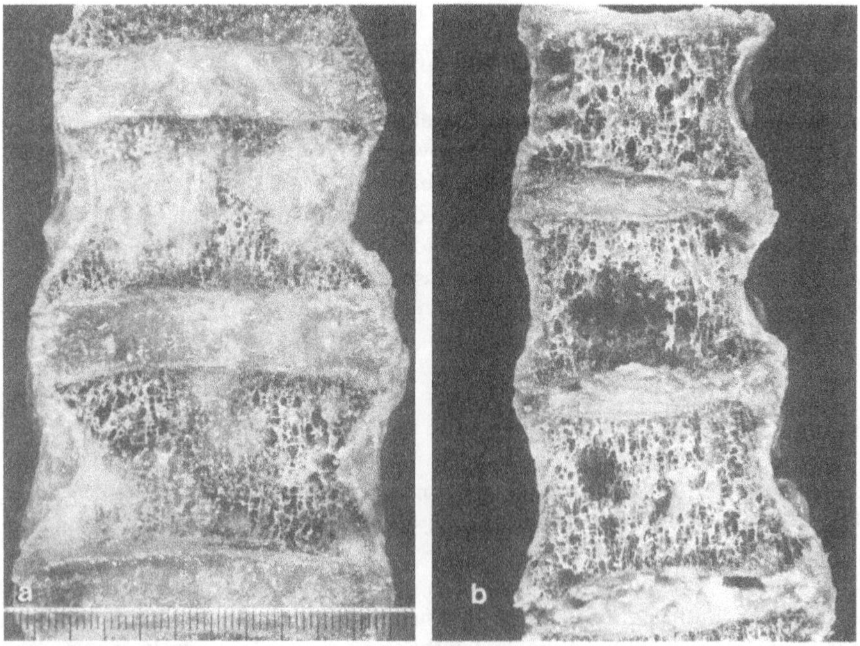

Fig. 8. a Compact foci which cannot be flushed out in osteoblastic vertebral metastases. **b** Spongiosa defects after flushing out osteolytic vertebral body metastases

In metastatic processes, the degree of bone destruction is often extensive. Thus, for example in Pancoast carcinomas, whole ribs are completely destroyed. Such carcinomas can also infiltrate vertebrae and the intervertebral foramina, where they then compress the nerve roots. A further spread in this direction leads to envelopment of the spinal cord and the spinal nerves. Clinical manifestations are pain in the shoulders and back. An example of a metastasizing bronchial carcinoma shows the extent to which a vertebral column can be destroyed by metastases (Fig. 7). In this case, all vertebrae contain tumor tissue and two of the vertebrae have collapsed. The patient suffered from severe back pain. The penetration of the metastases into the epidural space led to kinking of the spinal cord resulting in paraplegia. The pain symptoms were thereby abolished.

In bone, the metastases primarily localized in the bone marrow result in osteolysis (Fig. 8b) or osteosclerosis (Fig. 8a). These various reactions are based pathogenetically on irritation of the endosteum. In the former case, osteoclastic bone degradation, and in the second case osteoblastic or connective tissue bone regeneration predominate (Cramer et al. 1981). As a rule, these mechanisms occur simultaneously with the quantitative differences mentioned. Necroses and hemorrhages are frequently observed in bone metastases and doubtless play a role in the etiology of pain. The hemorrhages probably result from microfractures. Both processes are thought to elicit pain via prostaglandins.

Tumor Infiltration of Abdominal Hollow Organs

As a rule, tumors and their sequelae in the bronchial tree are indolent, whereas those in abdominal hollow organs lead to pain (Bonadonna and Molinari 1979; Bonica 1979). This applies to all primary and secondary intestinal tumors. However, their pain-eliciting potency differs widely from individual to individual. The pain results from ulcerations, motility disorders, dilatations, and disorders of blood flow. In accordance with the extent of the lymphatic tissue, large tumors with extensive ulceration and hemorrhage are found especially in malignant lymphomas of the gastrointestinal tract. In particular, the high frequency of pain in malignant lymphomas of the stomach (Fig. 9) has been pointed out

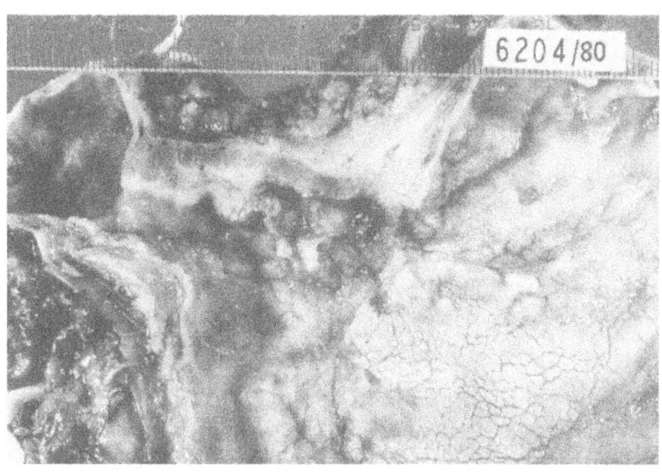

Fig. 9. Malignant lymphoma in the gastric antrum with extensive mucosal infiltration and ulceration

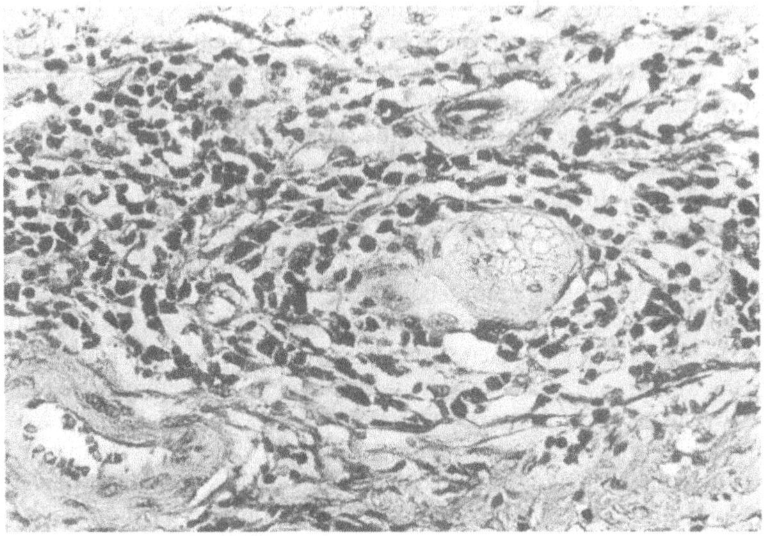

Fig. 10. Lymphoplasmacellular infiltration around a small nerve in urinary bladder carcinoma. HE, × 400

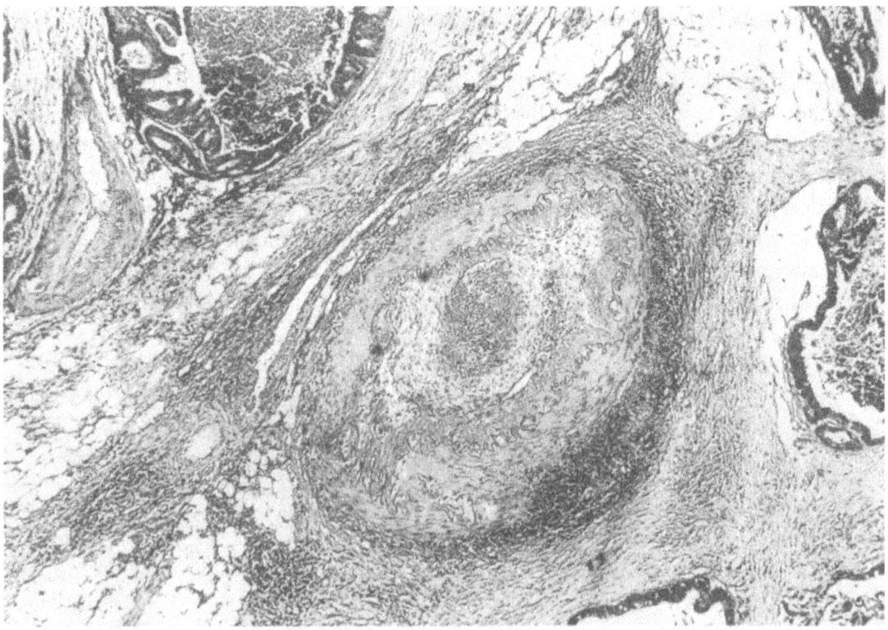

Fig. 11. Obliterative arteritis in colon carcinoma with tumor envelopment of a mesenteric artery. Clinical manifestations: pain as the first symptom of the carcinoma. HE, × 40

(Saraga et al. 1981). In one of our cases (S. 183/80) a massive hemorrhage in the urinary bladder from a carcinoma, with coagulation of the blood, led to a painful motility disorder. A perineural tumor infiltration, an arteritis (Fig. 11), or a perineural inflammatory reaction (Fig. 10) are found not at all uncommonly in tumors of the abdominal and urinogenital hollow organs.

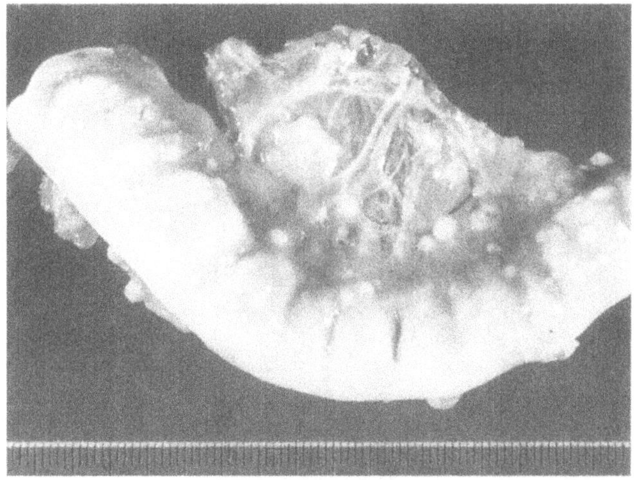

Fig. 12. Peritoneal carcinosis. One of the nodules of a mesenteric nerve directly apposed

Tumor Infiltration and Inflammation of Serous Mucosa

As a rule, pleural carcinosis does not result in pain, probably because of the development of pleural effusion, which prevents the pleurae from rubbing together. In peritoneal carcinosis, pain is reported more frequently, and it may indeed be the first symptom of the tumor disease. This is caused either by direct contact of the metastases with peripheral nerves (Fig. 12) or by an inflammatory reaction elicited by the carcinosis with disorders of visceral motility. Acute inflammatory reactions of the peritoneum with the clinical picture of "acute abdomen" and possibly with empyema are found after tumor-induced perforation or penetration of hollow viscera.

Tumor-Induced Necroses in Solid Organs

An organ in which the specific (namely tryptic) necroses lead to typical pain symptoms is the pancreas. Such necroses, with the clinical picture of autodigestive pancreatitis, can be elicited by pancreatic metastases of a bronchial carcinoma (Matthews 1976; Reinhard and Hill 1977). The autodigestion probably results from tumorous destruction of the parenchyma together with tumor infiltration and stenoses of the excretory ducts.

Tumor-Induced Occlusions of Blood Vessels

Invasion of the lymphatics and blood vessels is part of the biology of malignant neoplasias and is the precondition for metastasis. As a rule, small and peripheral vessels are involved, obstruction of which does not result in any appreciable disorder of the circulation. However, larger veins are occasionally also infiltrated and occluded. On the other hand, an infiltration of larger arteries is rarely observed. Here, stenotic and obliterative arteritis occurs as a reaction to tumor envelopment (Fig. 11). Presumably the pain is due to excitation of the vascular nerves, which are themselves included in the process of inflammation, or to the disorders of blood flow due to the vascular changes.

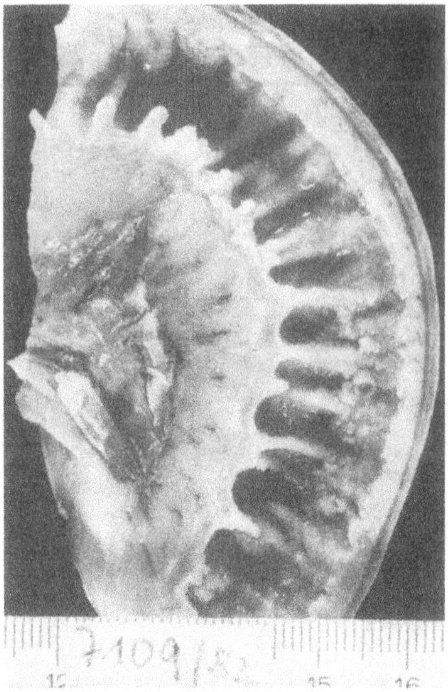

Fig. 13. Radiation enteritis with atrophy and ulceration of the mucosa after radiation treatment of an ovarian carcinoma. Clinical manifestations: increasing abdominal pains because of perforation and peritonitis

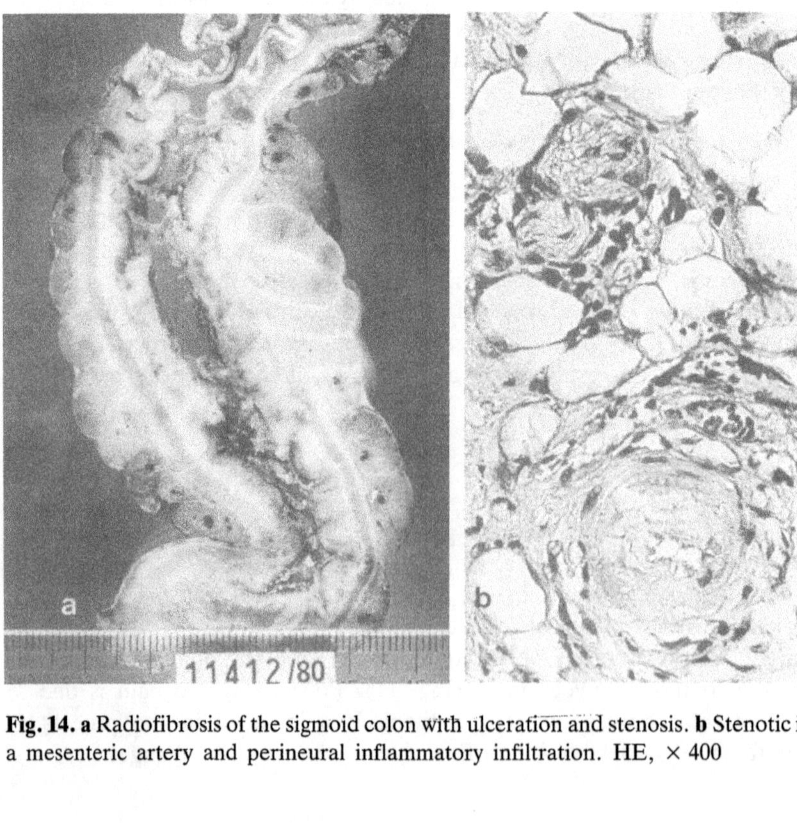

Fig. 14. a Radiofibrosis of the sigmoid colon with ulceration and stenosis. **b** Stenotic intimal fibrosis of a mesenteric artery and perineural inflammatory infiltration. HE, × 400

Complications of Cancer Therapy

Vascular occlusions such as radiovasculitis are also elicited by therapy. A well-known example is the obliteration of the lymphatic tracts of the axilla with ectasia of the peripheral lymphatics resulting in elephantiasis of the affected limb and tension pain. In the intestine, ionizing radiation can lead to radioenteritis (Fig. 13), in which there is threat of perforation or fibrosis as a complication (Fig. 14a). Apart from the typical vascular changes, a perineural inflammation is occasionally found (Fig. 14b).

After systemic cytostatic therapy, degenerative alterations of the central and peripheral nervous system have been described (among others, Mena et al. 1981). They lead to pain only in exceptional cases. Local misapplication (for example, paravenous injection) of cytostatics results in painful necroses. The inclusion of a subcutaneous nerve in the necrosis can occasionally be observed in such cases. Misinjections of other drugs (into the adipose tissue instead of into the skeletal musculature) are not uncommonly the cause of painful adipose tissue necroses.

Tumor surgery itself can also be the cause of persistent pain occurring later. Thus, a traumatic neuroma in which the pain arises by abnormal ongoing discharge can develop from a nerve lesion (Zimmermann 1981). Another complication of surgical therapy is nodular cicatricial fibrosis, e.g., after breast amputation. In these nodules, the foreign bodies maintaining the fibrosis can occasionally be demonstrated. Excruciating pain may necessitate secondary excision.

No claim is made to completeness with regard to the results described. They are intended merely to show some of the presumed pain-inducing mechanisms in tumor diseases. Overlaps cannot be avoided. The morphologist has no direct access to the neural mechanisms which are important to explain the phenomenon of pain. His results must therefore be interpreted with the help of the neurophysiologist.

References

Asbury AK, Johnson PC (1978) Pathology of peripheral nerve. Saunders, Philadelphia

Bonadonna G, Molinari R (1979) Role and limits of anticancer drugs in the treatment of advanced cancer pain. In: Bonica JJ, Ventafridda V (eds) Advances in pain research and therapy, vol 2. Raven, New York, pp 131–138

Bonica JJ (1979) Introduction to management of pain of advanced cancer. In: Bonica JJ, Ventafridda V (eds) Advances in pain research and therapy, vol 2. Raven, New York, pp 115–130

Brain L, Adams RD (1965) A guide to the classification and investigation of neurological disorders associated with neoplasms. In: Brain L, Norris FH (eds) The remote effects of cancer on the nervous system. Grune and Stratton, New York

Campbell E, Maldonado W, Suhrland G (1975) Painful lytic bone lesion in an adult with chronic myelogenous leukemia. Cancer 35: 1354–1356

Cramer StF, Fried L, Carter KJ (1981) The cellular basis of metastatic bone disease in patients with lung cancer. Cancer 48: 2649–2660

Denny-Brown D (1948) Primary sensory neuropathy with muscular changes associated with carcinoma. J Neurol Neurosurg Psychiat 11: 73

Flowers RS (1968) Meralgia paresthetica. A clue to retroperitoneal malignant tumor. Am J Surg 116: 89–92

Foley KM (1979) Pain syndromes in patients with cancer. In: Bonica JJ, Ventafridda V (eds) Advances in pain research and therapy, vol 2. Raven, New York, pp 59–75

Kashef R, Das Gupta TK (1968) Segmental demyelination of peripheral nerves in the presence of malignant tumors. Br J Cancer 21: 411–417

Mackintosh FR, Colby TV, Podolsky WJ, Burke JS, Hoppe RT, Rosenfelt FP, Rosenberg SA, Kaplan HS (1982) Central nervous system involvement in non-Hodgkin's lymphoma: an analysis of 105 cases. Cancer 49: 586–595

Matthews MJ (1976) Problems in morphology and behavior of bronchopulmonary malignant disease. In: Israel L, Chahinian APh (eds) Lung cancer. Natural history, prognosis and therapy. Academic, New York, pp 23–62

McLeod JG (1975) Carcinomatous neuropathy. In: Dyck PG, Thomas PK, Lambert EH (eds) Peripheral neuropathy, vol 2. Saunders, Philadelphia

McLeod JG, Walsh JC (1975) Peripheral neuropathy associated with lymphomas and other reticuloses. In: Dyck PJ, Thomas PK, Lambert EH (eds) Peripheral neuropathy, vol 2. Saunders, Philadelphia

Mena H, Garcia JH, Velandia F (1981) Central and peripheral myelinopathy associated with systemic neoplasia and chemotherapy. Cancer 48: 1724–1737

Payten RJ (1972) Facial pain as the first symptom in acoustic neuroma. J Laryngol 86: 523–534

Reinhard H, Hill K (1977) Tryptische Pankreatitis bei kleinzelligem Bronchialkarzinom. Dtsch Med Wochenschr 102: 797–799

Rolf LH, Brune GG (1982) Placebo-Analgesie. Dtsch Med Wochenschr 107: 283–284

Saraga P, Hurliman J, Ozello L (1981) Lymphomas and pseudolymphomas of the alimentary tract. An immunohistochemical study with clinicopathologic correlations. Human Pathol 12: 713–723

Schlegel G (1982) Die Therapie des Tumorschmerzes. Tumor-Diagnostik 3: 10–16

Schölmerich J, Guzman J, Bauer G, Walter K, Gerok W (1980) Neurologische Primärsymptomatik eines Pankreaskarzinoms. Inn Med 7: 91–94

Sondak V, Deckers PJ, Feller JH, Mozden PJ (1981) Leptomeningeal spread of breast cancer: report of case and review of the literature. Cancer 48: 395–399

Strempel H (1981) Der duale Charakter des Schmerzerlebnisses. Dtsch Ärztebl 43: 2017–2024

Sunderland S (1978) Nerves and nerve injuries, 2nd edn. Churchill Livingstone, Edinburgh

Swerdlow M (1979) Role of nerve blocks in pain involving the chest and brachial plexus. In: Bonica JJ, Ventafridda V (eds) Advances in pain research and therapy, vol 2. Raven, New York, pp 325–337

Thomas C, Zengerling W, Noetzel H (1972) Neurologische Formen des paraneoplastischen Syndroms. Schattauer, Stuttgart

Twycross RG (1978) Relief of pain. In: Saunders CM (ed) The management of terminal disease. Arnold, London, pp 65–92

Wasserstrom WR, Glass JP, Posner JB (1982) Diagnosis and treatment of leptomeningeal metastases from solid tumors: experience with 90 patients. Cancer 49: 759–772

Zimmermann M (1979) Peripheral and central nervous mechanisms of nociception, pain, and pain therapy: facts and hypotheses. In: Bonica JJ, Liebeskind JC, Albe-Fessard DG (eds) Advances in pain research and therapy, vol 3. Raven, New York, pp 3–32

Zimmermann M (1981) Physiological mechanisms of pain and pain therapy. Triangle 20: 7–18

*Neurophysiological Mechanisms of Cancer Pain**

W. Jänig

Physiologisches Institut, Universität Kiel, Olshausenstrasse 40–60, 2300 Kiel, FRG

Introduction

The clinical symptomatology of cancer pain and its treatment (Bonica 1953, 1979; Foley 1979; see contributions in this volume) show that pain due to cancer is largely produced by processes which affect primary afferent fibers and their receptors over extended periods of time. This pathophysiological pain is, therefore, very similar to chronic and recurrent pain states which are initiated by processes other than cancer.

A variety of mechanisms may contribute to the generation of cancer pain (Bonica 1953, 1979). Figure 1 and Table 1 illustrate how cancer may lead to pain. The possible pathophysiological changes which occur at different sites along the afferent neurons, in the dorsal horn, and in the reflex actions of efferent (motor and sympathetic) pathways and which can contribute to pain due to cancer in humans are abundant. The primary events are mostly the stimulation of nociceptors in different tissues (visceral organs, capsules of organs, vessels, periost, fascia, ligaments, skeletal muscle) and the irritation of the afferent axons.

Particularly the latter events may entail secondary processes which are due to the disturbance of the continuity between the afferent neuron and its target tissue in the periphery. These are, e.g., degenerative and regenerative processes at the afferent neuron, changes of the axoplasmic flow in the axons, depletion of the neuropeptide content of the afferent terminals in the spinal cord, changes of receptor properties and therefore of discharge characteristics of the afferent neuron, and changes of synaptic transmission in the spinal cord (Sunderland 1978, Wall 1979, Knyihar-Csillik and Csillik 1981). At present we do not comprehend the functional implications of these reactive changes and their interactions in detail and cannot put them together into a unifying concept which explains the neuronal mechanisms of the pathological pain states in patients. It seems quite obvious that particularly the understanding of the pathobiological processes occurring at the primary afferent neurons is essential for a deeper insight into the mechanisms of pain states produced by cancer and probably also for a more successful treatment of them.

We have experienced considerable progress during the past 10 years in research on the peripheral and central mechanisms of nociception. This research has largely been confined to the cutaneous system and to acute pain (Brown and Réthelyi 1981; Burgess and Perl 1973; Zimmermann 1979; Zotterman 1976; Willis and Coggeshall 1978). Our knowledge of nociceptors from deep somatic structures and from visceral organs and about the processing of the information from these nociceptors in the central nervous system is less well developed (Cervero 1980). Yet these nociceptive afferents, and not those from the

* Supported by the Deutsche Forschungsgemeinschaft

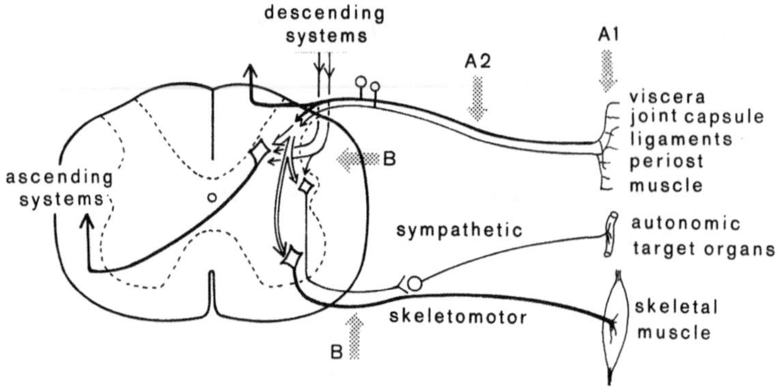

Fig. 1. Neuronal structures possibly involved in the generation of cancer pain. The *shaded arrows* labeled *A1, A2* and *B* refer to section headings in Table 1

Table 1. Peripheral and central mechanisms which may contribute to generation of pain due to cancer. (After Wall and Devor 1978)

A. Peripheral afferent neuron

1. Stimulation of receptors
   a) Continuous excitation (e.g., viscera, periost)
   b) Change of receptive properties by change of micromilieu (ischemia, release of algesic chemicals, inflammation)
   Sensitization of receptors (lowering of threshold)
2. Lesion of axons in nerves
   a) Retrograde cell reactions: biochemical changes in whole neuron for reparation; decrease in peptide content (substance P, fluoride-resistant phosphatase); atrophy and degeneration of axon and soma
   b) Anterograde cell reactions: sprouting of fibers with axon-receptor mismatch and development of abnormal membrane properties of sprouts
   c) Generation of resting activity by sprouting fibers
   d) Development of abnormal chemosensitivity of sprouting fibers
   e) Ephaptic transmission ("cross-talk") among afferent fibers and between afferent and postganglionic sympathetic fibers

B. Secondary changes in spinal cord

1. Changes in distribution of axon terminals in the spinal cord (degeneration, sprouting)
2. Unmasking and changes in the efficacy of synapses from primary afferents on secondary sensory neurones; formation of new aberrant synaptic connections
3. Biochemical changes of secondary neurones (decrease of peptide content); development of supersensitivity to neurotransmitters and neuromodulators due to deafferentation
4. Change in receptive fields of dorsal horn neurons; change in inhibitory mechanisms in dorsal horn (e.g., decrease of primary afferent depolarization)
5. Development of abnormal skeletomotor and sympathetic reflexes which may lead directly or indirectly to excitation of nociceptors; establishment of vicious circles (positive-feedback mechanism)

skin, are mainly involved in the generation of cancer pain. Furthermore, animal models in which these afferents can be studied neurobiologically during chronic pathological conditions (e.g., nerve lesions, chronic inflammation) are either absent or just being developed.

This chapter focusses chiefly on the discharge properties of afferents from deep somatic and visceral structures which most likely have a nociceptive function and on the discharge properties of afferent fibers in a chronically lesioned nerve. It is intended to make clear (a) that experimental work on the mechanisms of "cancer pain" is largely identical with the experimental approach to chronic (pathological) pain of various origins and (b) that the neurobiological techniques (neurophysiological, morphological, pharmacological, biochemical, behavioral) are available for the investigation of the mechanisms of this type of pain.

Methodological Considerations

Nociceptive afferent fibers are unmyelinated Group-IV or C fibers or thin myelinated Group-III or Aδ fibers. For quantitative experimental work on the encoding of stimuli which excite these fibers it is necessary to isolate single afferents for recording (rec fiber, Fig. 2). Figure 3A shows profiles of unmyelinated fibers in part of a section through the superficial peroneal nerve. Figures 3B and C illustrate the recording from two unmyelinated afferent fibers in a bundle which has been isolated from a nerve to the colon. The signals were recorded by a bare platinum wire electrode and amplified by a low-noise AC amplifier. Stimulation of the colonic nerve (stim fiber, Fig. 2) excites the axons at stable latency (Fig. 3B). One fiber exhibited resting activity (Fig. 3C).

Strands with a single or a few thin afferent fibers can be isolated from practically all nerves to deep somatic and visceral structures of the cat (provided the nerves have sufficient length), but also from nerves of smaller and larger animals. The receptive endings of the fibers can be stimulated by mechanical, thermal, or chemical stimuli (applied intra-arterially or locally, see Fig. 2). In humans, it is also possible to record from single unmyelinated afferent fibers using the microneurographical technique (Gybels et al. 1979; Vallbo et al. 1979). Necessary details of methodological procedures will be supplied as results are presented.

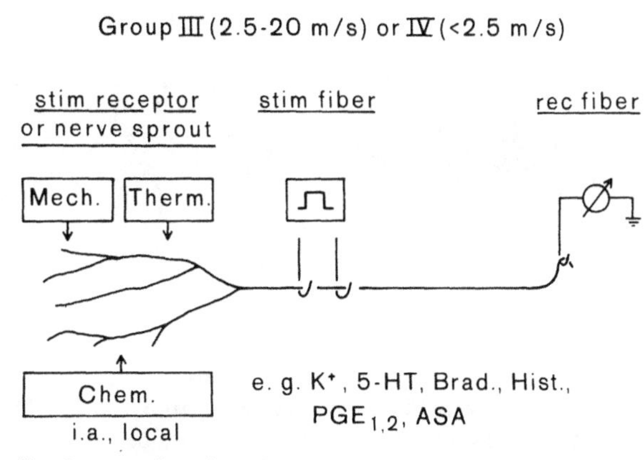

Fig. 2. Methodological approach to recording from nociceptive afferents. *5-HT*, 5-hydroxytryptamine or serotonin; *Brad.*, bradykinin; *Hist.*, histamine; *PGE*, prostaglandin; *ASA*, acetylsalicylic acid; *Mech.*, mechanical stimulation; *Therm.*, thermal stimulation; *Chem.*, chemical stimulation

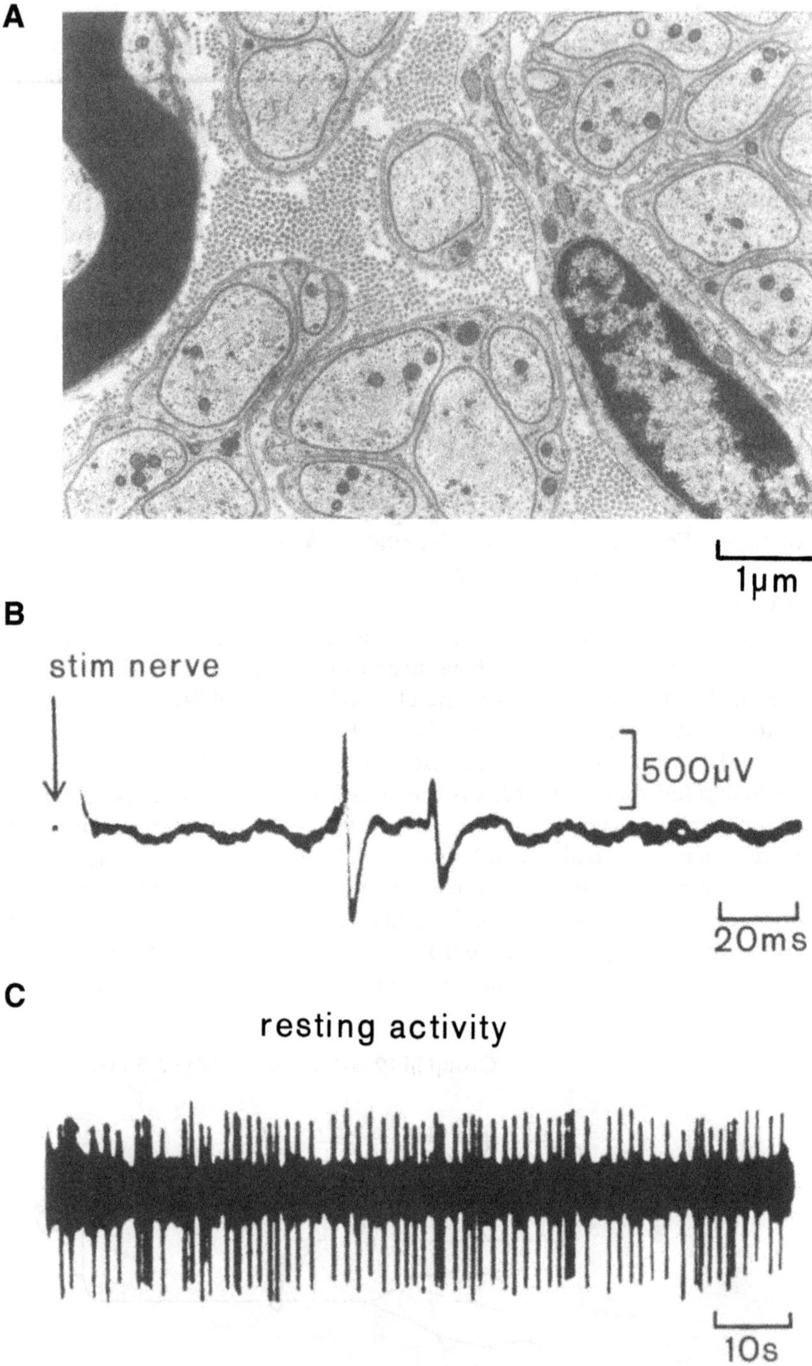

Fig. 3A–C. Neurophysiological identification of afferent fibers. **A** Electronmicrograph of cross-sectioned unmyelinated fibers in a superficial peroneal nerve. Modified from Blumberg and Jänig (1981). **B, C** Recordings from unmyelinated afferent fibers in a bundle isolated from one inferior splanchnic nerve. **B** Electrical stimulation of the colonic nerve (10 V, 0.5 ms pulse duration). The fibers conducted at 0.75 and 0.58 m/s, respectively. **C** Resting activity in the faster-conducting afferent fiber (large signal in **B**)

Stimulation of Receptors

Cancer tumors and their metastases may lead to direct stimulation of afferent receptors. This occurs mechanically by increase in volume of encapsulated organs (e.g., liver), by mechanical irritation of organs, by mechanical occlusion of organs (viscera, vessels), or by invasive penetration of organs. In all these cases visceral or deep somatic nociceptors are affected. The ensuing pain is complex: it consists of direct pain, referred pain, and – more rarely – pain elicited indirectly via excitation of the motor system and the sympathetic nervous system (Lewis 1942; Cervero 1980). Our knowledge of the discharge properties of these nociceptors is incomplete. For most organs we cannot give a consistent answer as to the typical discharge properties of the respective nociceptors. One may even question the existence of specific nociceptive afferents from deep structures similar to those in the skin (Cervero 1980). Cutaneous nociceptive afferent fibers have high thresholds to natural stimuli and respond either to all tissue damaging stimuli (polymodal cutaneous nociceptive afferent fibers) or preferentially to only one of these stimuli (e.g., mechanical, heat). Visceral and deep somatic afferent fibers which have – inter alia – a nociceptive function may also respond to stimuli which do not elicit pain in man or the equivalent sensation in animals. Thus, the events of "visceral pain" and "deep somatic pain" may depend on the degree of excitation of these afferents (Goldscheider 1920; Jänig 1982; Malliani and Lombardi 1982).

For the deep structures the most solid knowledge we have so far concerns the thin afferents from skeletal muscle, joint capsule, some viscera, and the testis (Franz and Mense 1975; Kumazawa and Mizumura 1977, 1980a, b; Mense 1977, 1981b; Haupt et al. 1981, 1983; Schaible and Schmidt 1983a, b; Blumberg et al. 1983). The difficulty faced by the investigators when examining afferents from various organs in animals in the Group III and IV range (A δ and C fibers) is how to recognize a nociceptive afferent fiber from fibers having other sensory functions. It is obvious from experiments on humans and from everyday experience which types of stimuli and conditions produce deep somatic and visceral pain; however, it is difficult to find and define afferent fibers which unequivocally meet the criteria of nociceptive afferents from the respective organs. For example, isometric contractions of *skeletal muscle* under ischemic conditions elicit excruciating pain in humans (Lewis 1942); yet Mense (Mense and Stahnke 1978; Kniffki et al. 1981) found only very few afferent Group-IV fibers (10%) from the gastrocnemius-soleus muscle of the cat which could be activated under these conditions. He found many other thin fibers which could be excited by mechanical and/or chemical stimuli which also produce pain in man (Mense 1977, 1981b). Figure 4A illustrates one example.

Forceful distension of a *joint* capsule is very painful. The pain may considerably outlast the stimulus, and any minor event thereafter which changes the position of the affected joint elicits similar painful sensations and protective reactions, thus leading to immobilization of the respective joint. Thin (myelinated and unmyelinated) afferents from the knee joint capsule of the cat have only recently been studied by Schaible and Schmidt (1983a, b). These afferents react mostly to forceful lateral (outward) or medial (inward) rotation of the lower leg and not to flexion and extension. They have well-defined receptive fields and are excited upon application of firm pressure to the knee joint capsule or by chemical stimuli with algesic substances. Figure 4B illustrates the excitation of a knee joint afferent by forceful inward rotation and by bradykinin injected close intra-arterially (see Schaible and Schmidt 1983a, b).

A third example is from the *colon*. From clinical experience we would predict that afferent nociceptive fibers from the gastrointestinal tract, which run in sympathetic nerves to the

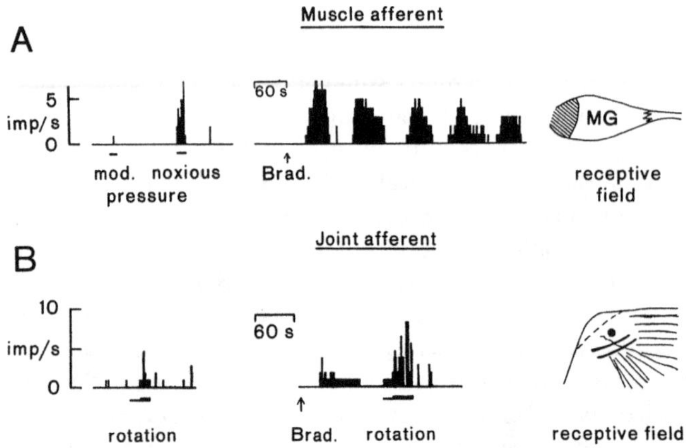

Fig. 4. A Responses of a Group III (6.2 m/s) muscle afferent fiber to moderate and noxious pressure on the muscle (*MG*, m. gastrocnemius-soleus of the cat) and to injection of 6.5 μg bradykinin (*Brad*) into the receptive field. **B** Responses of a Group IV afferent (0.9 m/s) from the knee joint of the cat hindlimb to forceful (noxious) rotation and to close intra-arterial injection of 2.5 μg bradykinin. Note the sensitization of the afferent fiber by bradykinin (increased response to rotation). **A** from S. Mense (unpublished); **B** from H.-G. Schaible and R.F. Schmidt, with permission (unpublished)

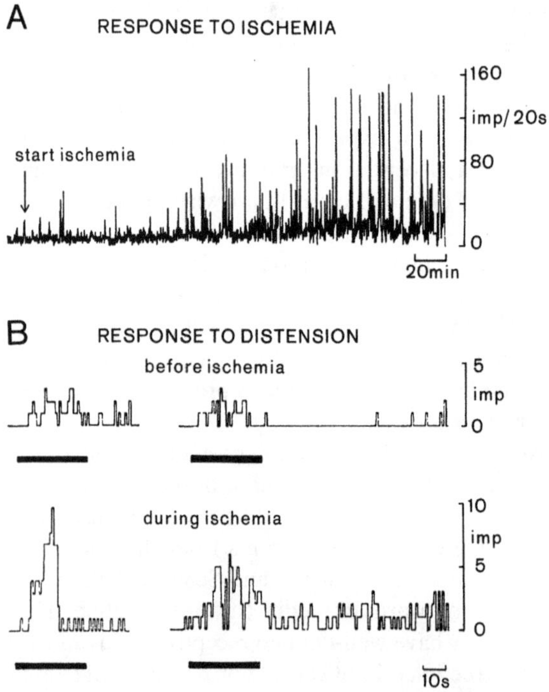

Fig. 5. Response of nociceptive visceral afferent fibers from the colon (cat) **A** to ischemia of the colon (occlusion of inferior mesenteric artery) and **B** to distension of the colon (50 mmHG intraluminal pressure for 30 s, *black bars*) before and during ischemia. Bin width of histograms is 1 s. The fibers were isolated from the inferior splanchnic nerves, conduction velocities in **A** 0.9 m/s and **B** 0.8 m/s. Haupt, Jänig, and Kohler (unpublished)

thoracic and lumbar spinal cord, are excited by distension and contraction of the organs and by traction of their mesenteries. These stimuli cause visceral pain and vigorous autonomic reactions. Our investigations on cats show that the afferents from the colon in the inferior splanchnic nerves are excited by these stimuli and by algesic substances (Fig. 5B). The receptive sites of these afferents are located at the insertion of the mesentery of the colon and in the mesentery close to the colon along the vessels, but most likely not in the colon wall or at the antimesenteric side of the colon (Lewis 1942; Morrison 1977; Haupt et al. 1981; Blumberg et al. 1983). In the sacral ventral roots there are other unmyelinated and thin myelinated fibers which have their receptive fields in the wall of the colon, rectum, and anus, and which probably have nociceptive function (Clifton et al. 1976).

Sensitization of Receptors

Several questions arise concerning these primary afferent neurons and similar primary afferent neurons which have not yet been studied.

First, many of them have low resting activity which originates in the periphery. Is this resting activity an experimental artifact or do these afferents also display it normally? We believe that the latter is the case. Thus, we must assume that the neurons in the spinal cord normally "ignore" this resting activity so that it is not relayed to higher structures of the central nervous system. Neurons in the dorsal horn are controlled by local and descending inhibitory mechanisms (Zimmermann 1979) which might determine their discharge threshold ("central threshold"; see below).

Second, how do the deep somatic and visceral receptor populations react when the organs are permanently displaced, distended, or infiltrated by a tumor? When judged by the success of neurosurgical procedures (e.g., rhizotomy, anterolateral cordotomy; see this volume) or the peripheral application of neurolytics (e.g., in the visceral domain; see this volume) it is likely that these afferents are continuously excited by the tumor. This continuous stimulation may lead to enhanced responses of the nociceptors and to a decrease of their threshold; thus they may be sensitized in the same way as cutaneous nociceptors by repeated noxious stimulation (hyperalgesia, see Perl et al. 1976; Lynn 1977, 1979; Fitzgerald and Lynn 1977; Fitzgerald 1979).

Third, nociceptive afferents are excited by chemical substances which elicit pain in humans and pseudo-affective reactions in animals (algesic substances; Fig. 4) (Keele and Armstrong 1964, Lim 1970, Handwerker 1980). The excitation by these algesic substances is fairly selective, though not exclusive (Beck and Handwerker 1974, Handwerker 1980). Algesic substances, and substances which modulate the excitability of nociceptors (e.g., prostaglandins, substance P, and noradrenaline), may be released in the tissues which have been invaded by the cancer. Additionally, the microenvironment of the nociceptors in the tissue invaded by the cancer may change by local decrease of pH and PO_2 and by accumulation of metabolic substances (e.g., lactic acid) (see Zimmermann 1979, 1980). This may be induced by the high metabolic activity of the cancer cells. Local chemical changes may also follow occlusion of blood vessels by the cancer (ischemia) and inflammation of the cancerous tissue. The chemical changes may lead to changes of the chemosensibility, and to sensitization of afferent nociceptive fibers with consequent increase of resting activity, decrease in threshold, and increase in response to mechanical and chemical stimuli. Figure 6A illustrates the sensitization of a nociceptive afferent fiber from the cat knee joint by prostaglandin E_1 (injected close intra-arterially). The response to a small dose of bradykinin (injected i.a.) was strongly enhanced for up to 12 min after

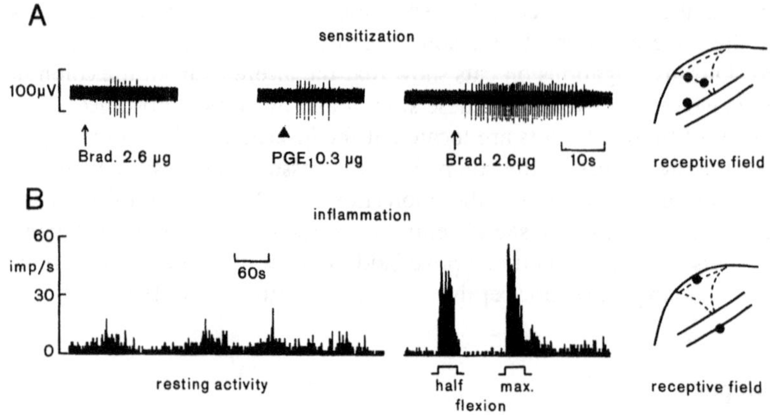

Fig. 6. A Sensitization of the response of a joint afferent fiber to bradykinin (*Brad.;* 2.6 µg, injected close intra-arterially) by prostaglandin E_1 (*PGE*$_1$; 0.3 µg i.a.). **B** Resting activity and response of a joint afferent fiber to non-noxious flexion during inflammation of the joint. The inflammation was produced by kaolin and carrageenan injected into the joint cavity 12 h before the measurements. Compare resting activity and response to flexion with the response of joint afferent fiber from normal noninflamed joint in Fig. 4B. Conduction velocity of afferents: **A** 0.9 m/s and **B** 1.1 m/s. The afferents had **A** three and **B** two mechanoreceptive sites in the knee joint capsula, respectively. From Schaible and Schmidt, with permission (unpublished)

application of prostaglandin. Prostaglandin itself excited the receptive terminals weakly. Preliminary experiments from Schaible and Schmidt show that also responses to mechanical stimuli (pressure, rotation, flexion) are sensitized by prostaglandins. Comparable sensitizations have been reported by Mense for Group IV afferents from skeletal muscle (Mense 1981a, b). Figure 6B illustrates the discharges of a Group IV afferent fiber with a receptive field in an inflamed capsule of the cat knee joint (induced by kaolin and carrageenan injected into the joint cavity 12 h before the measurements; inflammation histologically verified). The fiber had an unusually high resting activity (Fig. 6B left; compare with Fig. 4B) and responded to flexions of the knee joint which never excited these afferent fibers when the knee joint was not inflamed (Fig. 6B right; Coggeshall et al. 1982).

Figure 5 illustrates the activity of a nociceptive visceral afferent fiber from the colon before and after occlusion of the inferior mesenteric artery (with consequent partial ischemia of the colon). Resting activity as well as responses to intraluminal pressure (50 mm Hg) in the colon increased after the arterial occlusion. This increase was observed when the colon contracted as well as when it was quiet.

Irritation of Nerve Axons

Compression and invasion of nerves by a tumor results in the destruction of myelinated and unmyelinated fibers and of their supporting tissue (see Hill, this volume). This process entails several degenerative, regenerative, and other pathophysiological processes which are listed in Table 1 (see also Fig. 1). The whole afferent neuron is affected and goes through reactive, presumably reparative, biochemical changes. The neuron loses its neuropeptides (e.g., substance P: see Lembeck, this volume; Jessel et al. 1979;

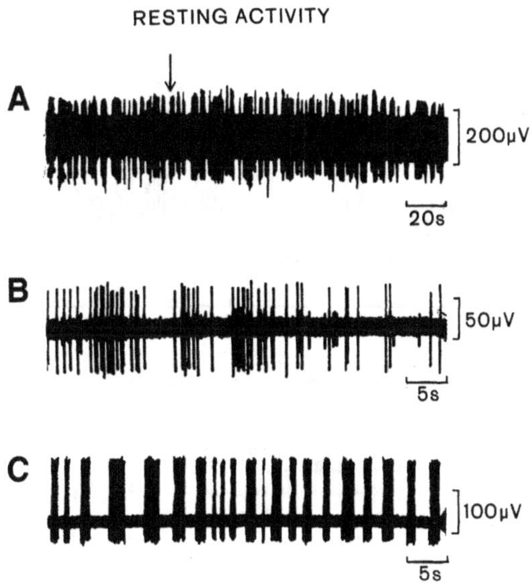

Fig. 7 A–C. Resting activity in afferent fibers from neuromata of the superficial peroneal nerve of the cat. **A, B** Multiunit bundles. **C** Single-unit bundle. At *arrow* in **A** the common peroneal nerve was cut proximal to the recording electrode in order to show that the resting activity derives from the neuroma. The neuromata were produced by ligating, cutting, and encapsulating the superficial personeal nerve **A** 63 days, **B** 108 days and **C** 6 days before the experiments. Blumberg and Jänig (unpublished)

Knyihar-Csillik and Csillik 1981); it atrophies and may finally degenerate. This applies particularly to afferent neurons with unmyelinated fibers. Knowledge of the circumstances of these changes is unsatisfactory (for review see Liebermann 1974). The conditions in a nerve when invaded or compressed by cancerous tissue are probably similar to those after lesions of nerves induced by mechanical or other events (Sunderland 1978).

Models for studying afferent fibers under these conditions are the experimentally produced stump neuroma, partial nerve lesions, or inadequate nerve connections in animals (Blumberg and Jänig 1981).

Afferent fibers which have been lesioned and prevented from regenerating to their normal target tissue may develop resting activity. This can have various patterns (bursting, continuous, etc.) and has been observed in myelinated and unmyelinated fibers in cats (Fig. 7). Resting activity may temporarily increase to 10 impulses/s in afferents from neuromata of the superficial peroneal nerve of cats and to 50 impulses/s in afferents from neuromata of the sciatic nerve of rats and mice (Govrin-Lippmann and Devor 1978; Scadding 1981). The resting activity has its origin largely in the lesioned part of the nerve (stump neuroma or neuroma-in-continuity). Also, in humans with neuromata, resting activity has been measured microneurographically in myelinated and unmyelinated fibers in the neuroma nerves (Nyström and Hagbarth 1981). This resting activity persists when the conduction of the nerve fibers is blocked central to the recording electrode (see also Fig. 7A). Thus the resting activity originates in the lesioned part of the nerve in the periphery.

Afferent fibers from a neuroma acquire other abnormal properties as compared with afferent fibers connected to the peripheral target tissue: they react to light and strong pressure applied to the neuroma and commonly exhibit long-lasting afterdischarges following mechanical stimulation (Fig. 8A). The sprouting fibers develop abnormal chemosensitivity: they may be excited by noradrenalin released by postganglionic axons (Fig. 8B) (Devor and Jänig 1981). In the neuromata, part of the myelinated and unmyelinated fibers can be excited from other afferent fibers by ephaptic transmission (Blumberg and Jänig 1981, 1982a). This type of pathological "cross-talk" between afferent fibers, which does not occur in normal intact nerves and which we did not find from

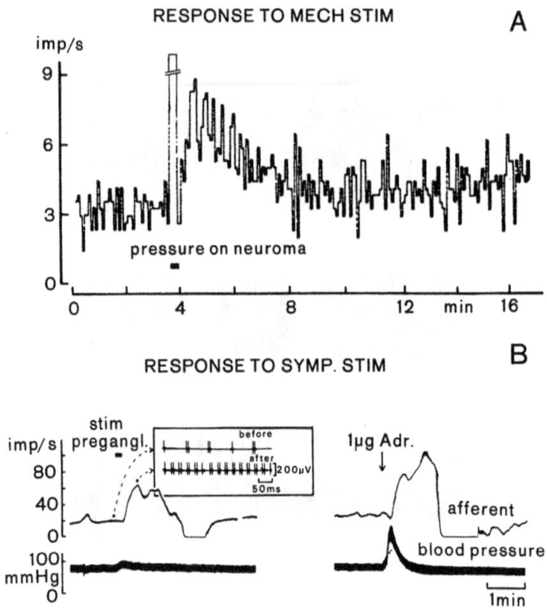

Fig. 8 A, B. Responses of afferent fibers from neuromata to mechanical stimulation and to excitation of postganglionic sympathetic fibers supplying the neuroma. **A** Multifiber bundle; gentle pressure on neuroma (*black bar*); response during pressure truncated; note long-lasting after-discharge. Neuroma of the superficial peroneal nerve of cat 6 days after cutting and ligating the nerve. Modified from Blumberg and Jänig (1981). **B** Single-fiber bundle from the sciatic nerve of a rat 10 days after cutting and ligating the nerve. Stimulation of all preganglionic axons in the lumbar sympathetic chain (*stim pregangl.* at 25 Hz for 10 s) and i.v. injection of 1 μg adrenaline (*Adr.*). *Inset:* activity of the fiber before stimulation and after stimulation of the preganglionic axons (see *dots*). Modified from Devor and Jänig (1981)

postganglionic sympathetic to afferent fibers in the cat, may enable the spread of excitation from fiber to fiber in a neuroma when only a few fibers are stimulated mechanically. It is possible that ephaptic transmission occurs between fibers in parts of a nerve which is demyelinated and otherwise damaged by tumor compression (Rasminsky 1980).

Development of resting activity, of chemosensibility, and of low thresholds to mechanical stimulation in afferent nerve fibers after their lesion might be due to abnormal membrane properties of the sprouts of these fibers. Existing ionic channels may change their properties; calcium channels may become prominent in the membrane (Meiri et al. 1981). However, we do not know whether the fibers which display these properties were originally nociceptive fibers or not, i.e., whether nociceptive fibers with high mechanical and thermal thresholds have changed in their membrane properties relative to low-threshold mechanosensitive fibers.

Changes in the Spinal Cord

Chronic lesions of primary afferent fibers do not only lead to chronic changes in the afferent neurons (see Table 1, A. 2) but also to considerable changes in the spinal cord (Devor and Wall 1978, 1981; Barbut et al. 1981, Horch et al. 1981, Wall and Devor 1981).

Some of the changes which may be important with respect to chronic pain are listed in Table 1 B. It is possible that these changes in the spinal cord are additional factors in the production of persistent pain in patients with cancer. There is evidence that the fine fibers which have nociceptive functions are involved in these changes (Knyihar-Csillik and Csillik 1981).

Without going into detail it must be admitted that we are not able to relate these complex neurochemical, morphological, and physiological changes to distorted function. Even normal processing of impulses from deep somatic and visceral nociceptors in the dorsal horn of the spinal cord is only marginally understood (Cervero 1980). The most consistent, though still very incomplete, knowledge we have so far is of the cutaneous nociceptive system (Willis and Coggeshall 1978; Zimmermann 1979; Brown and Réthelyi 1981).

Despite this deficiency in knowledge we must not ignore the fact that the neuronal machinery in the spinal cord is probably very important for the generation of many types of pain due to cancer. This neuronal network does not just relay impulses from the primary afferent nociceptive fibers to the thalamocortical system. It is probably the neuronal network which gives the afferent information from the peripheral nociceptors its typical spatiotemporal pattern. Deeply involved in this shaping of incoming nociceptive information are various descending inhibitory control systems from the brain stem, i.e., afferent (forward) inhibition and presynaptic inhibition in the dorsal horn (Zimmermann 1979; Duggan 1982). The impairment of the efficacy of these inhibitory mechanisms at the spinal cord level may lead to a distortion of the discharge patterns of the dorsal horn neurons. It is possible that these neurons lower their discharge thresholds ("central threshold") to excitation of nociceptive and other afferents.

Furthermore, we must be aware that different types of pain can be experienced when different types of organs (skin, viscera, skeletal muscle, etc.) are stimulated. At present, we do not know the neuronal correlates for this difference. However, it is conceivable that also in this regard the neuronal processes in the spinal cord are most important. Is it then very surprising that the dramatic changes which may occur in the spinal cord after chronic affection of nociceptive nerve fibers (and of nociceptors?) lead to serious distortions of encoding of nociceptive impulses in the spinal cord, and that various types of cancer pain therapy, such as peridural application of opiates (Zenz, this volume), and pain therapy by focal lesions in the dorsal horn of the spinal cord (Krainick, this volume) are successful?

Future Perspectives

When seen from the standpoint of neurobiological mechanisms there exists, with some possible exceptions, no cancer pain per se. Research on the mechanisms of cancer pain should concentrate on animal models in which the peripheral conditions generated by growing cancer tissue are simulated (see Table 1). This does not necessarily require the production of cancerous tissue in an animal. It does, however, require the development of several types of chronic animal models for studying the peripheral as well as the central mechanisms: animals with various types of nerve lesions, chronic stimulation of nociceptors, chronic inflammation of deep tissue, etc. Research in this field, which has its major impetus from practical medicine, requires collaboration between the experimental working scientist, the clinically oriented scientist, and the clinician. Without this collaboration all three groups tend to ask less valid questions and, consequently, receive incomplete answers. Pertinent to the understanding of the pathophysiological mechanisms of cancer pain is the understanding of the neuronal mechanisms of deep somatic and of visceral pain under normal, healthy conditions. We have all the techniques (neurophysiological, morphological, pharmacological, biochemical, and behavioral) available for studying the mechanisms which lead to cancer pain and are able to use these techniques. However, it would be naive to assume that the problems involved can be solved in a few years.

Summary

According to the mechanisms, pain due to cancer can be divided into two categories:

1. Cancer and its metastases chronically affect sensory receptors from deep somatic structures and visceral organs. This permanent stimulation of nociceptors probably additionally involves chemical components (due to inflammation, release of toxic compounds, change in pH and PO_2 concentration) with sensitization of the receptors.
2. Cancer directly affecting nerves leads to the destruction of the integrity of afferent nerve fibers and their supporting tissues. This process induces regenerative and degenerative changes in the afferent nociceptive neurons with subsequent changes in their discharge properties (resting activity, response to mechanical and chemical stimulation).

Chronic irritation of afferent nociceptive neurons, and possibly chronic stimulation of nociceptors, entails considerable biochemical, morphological, and physiological reactions in the spinal cord. This leads to distortions of the neuronal processing of information from nociceptive afferents.

Research on cancer pain, which is essentially research on mechanisms of chronic and recurrent pain in different domains of the body, requires a multidisciplinary approach. It is largely clear what types of questions we have to ask; the techniques for approaching these questions experimentally are available.

References

Barbut D, Polak JM, Wall PD (1981) Substance P in spinal cord dorsal horn decreases following peripheral nerve injury. Brain Res 205: 289–298

Beck PW, Handwerker HO (1974) Bradykinin and serotonin effects on various types of cutaneous nerve fibres. Pflügers Arch 347: 209–222

Blumberg H, Jänig W (1981) Neurophysiological analysis of efferent sympathetic and afferent fibers in skin nerves with experimentally produced neuromata. In: Siegfried J, Zimmermann M (eds) Phantom and stump pain. Springer Berlin Heidelberg New York, pp 15–31

Blumberg H, Jänig W (1982a) Activation of fibers via experimentally produced stump neuromas of skin nerves: ephaptic transmission or retrograde sprouting. Exp Neurol 76: 468–482

Blumberg H, Jänig W (1982b) Changes in unmyelinated fibers including sympathetic postganglionic fibers of a skin nerve after peripheral neuroma formation. J Auton Nerve Syst 6: 173–183

Blumberg H, Haupt P, Jänig W, Kohler W (1983) Encoding of visceral noxious stimuli in the discharge patterns of visceral afferent fibres from the colon. Pflügers Arch 398: 33–40

Bonica JJ (1953) The management of pain. Lea & Febiger, Philadelphia (Honji Shoji Reprint, Tokyo, 1980)

Bonica JJ (1979) Introduction to management of pain of advanced cancer. In: Bonica JJ, Ventafridda V (eds) Advances in pain research and therapy, vol 2. Raven, New York, pp 115–130

Brown AG, Réthelyi M (1981) Spinal cord sensation. Scottish Academic, Edinburgh

Burgess PR, Perl ER (1973) Cutaneous mechanoreceptors and nociceptors. In: Iggo A (ed) Somatosensory system. Springer, Berlin Heidelberg New York, pp 29–78 (Handbook of sensory physiology, vol 2)

Cervero F (1980) Deep and visceral pain. In: Kosterlitz HW, Terenius LY (eds) Pain and society. Dahlem Konferenzen. Verlag Chemie, Weinheim pp 263–282

Clifton GL, Coggeshall RE, Vance WH, Willis WD (1976) Receptive fields of unmyelinated ventral root afferent fibres in the cat. J Physiol 256: 573–600

Coggeshall RE, Hong KA, Langford LA, Schaible H-G, Schmidt RF (1982) Fine afferent unit discharge characteristics of inflamed knee joints in the cat. Soc Neurosci Abstr 8: 263

Devor M, Jänig W (1981) Activation of myelinated afferents ending in a neuroma by stimulation of the sympathetic supply in the rat. Neurosci Lett 24: 43–47

Devor M, Wall PD (1978) Reorganisation of spinal cord sensory map after peripheral nerve injury. Nature 276: 75–76

Devor M, Wall PD (1981) Plasticity in the spinal cord sensory map following peripheral nerve injury in rats. J Neurosci 1: 679–684

Duggan AW (1982) Brain stem control of the responses of spinal neurones to painful skin stimuli. Trends Neurosci 5: 127–130

Fitzgerald M (1979) The spread of sensitization of polymodal nociceptors in the rabbit from nearby injury and by antidromic nerve stimulation. J Physiol 297: 207–216

Fitzgerald M, Lynn B (1977) The sensitization of high threshold mechanoreceptors with myelinated axons by repeated heating. J Physiol 265: 549–563

Foley KM (1979) Pain syndromes in patients with cancer. In: Bonica JJ, Ventafridda V (eds) Advances in pain research and therapy, vol 2. Raven, New York, pp 59–75

Franz M, Mense S (1975) Muscle receptors with group IV afferent fibres responding to application of bradykinin. Brain Res 92: 369–383

Goldscheider A (1920) Das Schmerzproblem. Springer-Verlag Berlin

Govrin-Lippmann R, Devor M (1978) Ongoing activity in severed nerves. Brain Res 159: 406–410

Gybels J, Handwerker HO, van Hees J (1979) A comparison between the discharges of human nociceptive nerve fibres and the subject's ratings of his sensation. J Physiol 292: 193–206

Handwerker HO (1980) Pain producing substances. In: Kosterlitz HW, Terenius LY (eds) Pain and society. Dahlem Konferenzen. Verlag Chemie, Weinheim, pp 325–338

Haupt P, Jänig W, Kohler W (1981) How are stimuli which are harmful to the colon and elicit pain in man encoded in the discharge pattern of visceral thoracolumbar afferents? Pain [Suppl] 1: 88

Haupt P, Jänig W, Kohler W (1983) Response pattern of visceral afferent fibres, supplying colon, upon chemical and mechanical stimuli. Pflügers Arch 398: 41–47

Horch KW, Lisney SJW (1981) Changes in primary afferent depolarization of sensory neurones during peripheral nerve regeneration in the cat. J Physiol 313: 287–299

Jänig W (1982) Viszeraler Schmerz – Sympathisches Nervensystem und Schmerz. Diagnostik 15: 1123–1134

Jessel T, Tsunoo A, Kanazawa I, Otsuka M (1979) Substance P depletion in the dorsal horn of rat spinal cord after section of the peripheral processes of primary sensory neurones. Brain Res 168: 247–259

Keele CA, Armstrong D (1964) Substances producing pain and itch. Arnold, London

Kniffki K-D, Mense S, Schmidt RF (1981) Muscle receptors with fine afferent fibers which may evoke circulatory reflexes. Circ Res 48 [Suppl I] 25–31

Knyihar-Csillik E, Csillik B (1981) FRAP: histochemistry of the primary nociceptive neuron. Progr Histochem Cytochem 14: 1–137

Kumazawa T, Mizumura K (1977) Thin-fibre receptors responding to mechanical, chemical and thermal stimulation in the skeletal muscle of the dog. J Physiol 273: 179–194

Kumazawa T, Mizumura K (1980a) Chemical responses of polymodal receptors of the scrotal contents in dogs. J Physiol 299: 219–231

Kumazawa T, Mizumura K (1980b) Mechanical and thermal responses of polymodal receptors recorded from the superior spermatic nerve of dogs. J Physiol 299: 233–245

Lewis T (1942) Pain. Macmillan, New York

Liebermann AR (1974) Some factors affecting retrograde neuronal responses to axonal lesions. In: Bellairs R, Gray EG (eds) Essays on the nervous system. A Festschrift for Prof. JZ Young, Clarendon, Oxford, pp 71–105

Lim RKS (1970) Pain. Ann Rev Physiol 32:269–288

Lynn B (1977) Cutaneous hyperalgesia. Br Med Bull 33:103–108

Lynn B (1979) The heat sensitization of polymodal nociceptors in the rabbit and its independence of the local blood flow. J Physiol 287:493–507

Malliani A, Lombardi F (1982) Consideration of the fundamental mechanisms eliciting cardiac pain. Am Heart J 103:575–578

Meiri H, Spira ME, Parnas J (1981) Membrane conductance and action potential of a regenerating axonal tip. Science 211:709–712

Mense S (1977) Nervous outflow from skeletal muscle following chemical noxious stimulation. J Physiol 267:75–88

Mense S (1981a) Sensitization of group IV muscle receptors to bradykinin by 5-hydroxytryptamine and prostaglandin E_2. Brain Res 225:95–105

Mense S (1981b) Neurophysiologische Grundlagen der Schmerzentstehung in der Muskulatur und Möglichkeiten ihrer Beeinflussung. Verh. Dtsch Ges Rheumatol 7:36–44

Mense S, Stahnke M (1978) The possible role of group III and IV muscle afferents in the mediation of the pain of intermittent claudication. Pain 1:54 (abstract)

Morrison JFB (1977) The afferent innervation of the gastrointestinal tract. In: Brooks FP, Evers PW (eds) Nerves and the gut. Thorofare, Slack

Nyström B, Hagbarth KE (1981) Microelectrode recordings from transected nerves in amputees with phantom limb pain. Neurosci Lett 27:211–216

Perl ER, Kumazawa T, Lynn B, Kenins P (1976) Sensitization of high threshold receptors with unmyelinated (C) afferent fibres. Prog Brain Res 43:263–276

Rasminsky M (1980) Ephaptic transmission between single nerve fibres in the spinal nerve roots of "dystrophic" mice. J Physiol 305:151–169

Scadding JW (1981) Development of ongoing activity, mechanosensitivity, and adrenaline sensitivity in severed peripheral nerve axons. Exp Neurol 73:345–364

Schaible H-G, Schmidt RF (1983a) Activation of group III and IV sensory units in medial articular nerve by local mechanical stimulation of knee joint. J Neurophysiol 49:35–44

Schaible H-G, Schmidt RF (1983b) Responses of fine medial articular nerve afferents to passive movements of the knee joint. J Neurophysiol (in press)

Sunderland S (1978) Nerves and nerve injuries, 2nd edn. Churchill Livingstone, Edinburgh

Vallbo AB, Hagbarth KE, Torebjörk HE, Wallin BG (1979) Somatosensory proprioceptive, and sympathetic activity in human peripheral nerves. Physiol Rev 59:919–957

Wall PD (1979) Changes in damaged nerve and their sensory consequences. In: Bonica JJ, Liebeskind JC, Albe-Fessard DG (eds) Advances in pain research and therapy, vol 3. Raven, New York, pp 39–52

Wall PD (1981) On the origin of pain associated with amputation. In: Siegfried J, Zimmermann M (eds) Phantom and stump pain. Springer, Berlin Heidelberg New York, pp 2–14

Wall PD, Devor M (1978) Physiology of sensation after peripheral nerve injury, regeneration and neuroma formation. In: Waxman SG (ed) Physiology and pathophysiology of axons. Raven, New York, pp 377–388

Wall PD, Devor M (1981) The effect of peripheral nerve injury on dorsal root potentials and on transmission of afferent signals into the spinal cord. Brain Res 209:95–111

Willis WD, Coggeshall RE (1978) Sensory mechanisms of the spinal cord. Plenum, New York

Zimmermann M (1979) Peripheral and central nervous mechanisms of nociception, pain, and pain therapy: facts and hypotheses. In: Bonica JJ, Liebeskind JC, Albe-Fessard DG (eds) Advances in pain research and therapy, vol 3. Raven, New York, pp 3–32

Zimmermann M (1980) Physiological mechanisms of chronic pain. In: Kosterlitz HW, Terenius LY (eds) Pain and society. Dahlem Konferenzen. Verlag Chemie, Weinheim, pp 283–297

Zotterman Y (1976) Sensory functions of the skin in primates, with special reference to man. Pergamon, New York

Pharmacology of the Primary Nociceptive Neuron

F. Lembeck

Institut für experimentelle und klinische Pharmakologie, Karl-Franzens-Universität Graz, Universitätsplatz 4, 8010 Graz, Austria

Introduction

Pain is mediated by nociceptors. Morphologically, nociceptors are free nerve endings which are activated by various forms of injury, such as strong mechanical stimulation, heat greater than 45° C, or certain chemicals. The nociceptors begin firing above the threshold for the particular injuring influence. The intensity of the stimulus is encoded by the frequency of discharge and by the number of fibers firing; thus, an increase in the level of stimulation results in a greater total number of action potentials.

Nerve fibers convey the information of an injury not only as a quantified message, but also differentiated according to the type of injury. The information of an abrupt and sharp injury to the skin is carried by Aδ-fibers and recognized as a sharp pain originating in the skin. The other type of pain, a sickening burning sensation, results from a prolonged injury to the skin; such pain can also originate from visceral organs. It is mediated by C-fibers in the skin or in the deeper tissues. The responses to these two types of pain are different: the sharp pain initiates quick protective reflexes and quick movements accompanied by a rise in pulse rate; the slow burning sensation leads, e.g., to quiescence, anxiety, slowing of the pulse rate, and nausea. The C-fiber system is delayed in its response. The fibers conduct at about one-tenth the speed of Aδ-fibers, which means that an impulse in a toe, for example, reaches the spinal cord after a latency of 2 s.

The nociceptive information is furthermore dependent on the density of innervation, which is high in the skin, around vessels, and in mesentery, low in the gut and liver, and almost absent in the brain.

Substance P in Nociceptive Neurons

Recently, progress has been made in research toward a better understanding of the function of C-fibers. The perikarya of these nerves are the small cells in the dorsal root ganglion or in the trigeminal ganglion. Most of them are polymodal, which means that they respond to mechanical, thermal, and chemical injury at their peripheral terminals. Neurochemical studies have revealed that some of these neurons contain substance P, which is synthesized in the perikaryon and transported in a particle-bound form to the peripheral and central endings, where it is released in a Ca^{2+}-dependent fashion by depolarization of the fiber.

Other populations of C-fibers contain the putative transmitters somatostatin and fluoride-resistant acid phosphatase. The functional significance of these neurons awaits experimental elucidation.

Recent Results in Cancer Research. Vol. 89

The central terminals of the substance-P-containing primary afferents are located in the dorsal horn of the spinal cord. Substance P is presumably an excitatory transmitter active at the first synapse of a certain population of small-diameter afferents. At this synapse the incoming impulses are not simply transmitted to the next neuron, but rather they are submitted to a kind of tuner. Here the message can be modulated by spatial and temporal summation, by other afferent and descending inhibitory neurons, or by enkephalinergic interneurons. The second sensory neuron then carries the modulated information to higher levels of the central nervous system.

The second neuron of the nociceptive system is a unipolar nerve cell with its cell body in the dorsal horn, sending its fiber further up in the anterolateral system after crossing to the other side of the spinal cord. These fibers end (a) in the brain stem, where circulatory reflexes are mediated which are closely linked to all nociceptive responses (Duggan 1982); (b) in the midbrain, where descending inhibitory mechanisms are initiated and, via connection to the limbic system, emotional pain responses are mediated; and (c) in the thalamus, the relay station from which primary and secondary somatosensory areas of the cortex are reached, enabling the perception and localization of pain (see Kandel and Schwartz 1981; Yaksh and Hammond 1982).

Chemical Stimulation of Nociceptors

What finally ends up as a sensation of pain, always originates in the periphery through the stimulation of nociceptors. Besides mechanical and thermal stimulation, chemical stimulation by endogenous compounds released into the extracellular space of damaged or inflamed tissue plays a major role. Potassium may be released in large amounts from injured cells, kallikrein may be activated to release bradykinin from plasma constituents, and histamine may be released from mast cells. Low pH and anoxia may be two additional excitatory factors. All these substances directly stimulate nociceptors and also increase the formation and release of prostaglandins. Prostaglandins, which themselves do not stimulate nociceptors, powerfully potentiate the effects of all these noxious agents by a factor of 20–50 (see Juan 1978).

Peripheral Analgesia

The formation of prostaglandins can be pharmacologically inhibited by acetylsalicylic acid and its many more recent congeners, which are summarized under the term "nonsteroid anti-inflammatory agents" because they possess not only analgesic but also anti-inflammatory properties. Their effect is never a complete analgesia because they remove only the facilitatory effect of the prostaglandins but do not influence the direct effect of bradykinin or other compounds on the nociceptor. Nevertheless, their action leads to a considerable diminution of pain. They can be administered orally, and the incidence of adverse effects of most of these compounds is usually very low. Aspirin still seems to be superior to most of the other compounds because it is often tolerated in very large doses for long periods of time; the limit of the dosage is indicated by the onset of gastric distress and tinnitus. The main point is that treatment of chronic pain such as that from advanced cancer has to be performed at regular dose intervals of 4–6 h. Cancer pain does not basically differ from other types of chronic pain resulting from tissue damage, e.g., in rheumatic disorders. Therefore, the use of acetylsalicylic acid or similar drugs for pain caused by cancer exactly follows the therapeutic regimen for, e.g., chronic rheumatism. This should be the first step in the analgesic treatment of the cancer patient, followed by the second step, which is the use of morphine.

Pharmacology of Substance P Neurons

Small-diameter primary afferents contain substance P, which is assumed to function as a neurotransmitter in the dorsal horn. The content of substance P in these neurons, its axonal flow, and its release can be pharmacologically influenced by capsaicin, the pungent principle constituent of pepper, chilli, and paprika. These findings form the basis of the considerable new knowledge which has emerged concerning these neurons in recent years.

Substance P is an undecapeptide first described by von Euler and Gaddum in 1931 from observation of its smooth muscle stimulating and vasodilatatory properties. Its afferent neurotransmitter role was first postulated by Lembeck in 1953, but not before its isolation and synthesis was further progress achieved (see Leeman and Carraway 1976). Radioimmunological and immunohistochemical determinations in tissues allowed the detailed mapping of its distribution. Substance P is present in more than 30 different regions of the central nervous system, in afferent peripheral nerves, in the intrinsic nerve plexus of the intestine, together with serotonin in certain enterochromaffin cells of the intestinal mucosa, and again together with serotonin and other neuropeptides in the descending fibers of the spinal cord (see Hökfelt et al. 1982).

If primary afferent fibers are stimulated at their peripheral endings by an injury to the skin, substance P is also released from the peripheral terminal. The released substance P causes (a) vasodilatation, (b) plasma extravasation, and (c) release of histamine from closely adjacent mast cells. Vasodilatation and plasma extravasation may be regarded as a rinsing of the tissue by which noxious agents are removed via increased vascular and lymphatic flow.

Stimulation of a sufficient number of nociceptors generates orthodromic afferent volleys of impulses which submit the information to the first relay in the dorsal horn, where substance P is also released. Intraspinal injections of minute amounts of substance P cause a pain reaction in mice, and microinjections of substance P into the dorsal horn cause an increase of impulses in the dorsal horn nociceptive neuron (Lembeck et al. 1981a, b; Piercey et al. 1981). Morphine and enkephalin released from interneurons may inhibit the dorsal horn neurons. The mechanism of this inhibition by morphine is controversial at present, although at least part of its action may be due to inhibition of substance P released from primary afferent terminals.

Capsaicin Affects Substance P Neurons

Treatment of rats with high doses of capsaicin causes a depletion of substance P which lasts for months and may even be irreversible. Substance P is, however, depleted only in the primary afferent fibers, not in substance P-containing neurons of the central nervous system or in the gut. These observations provided the additional knowledge that the vagus and splanchnic nerves include many afferent fibers, although these nerves are still regarded mainly with reference to their efferent cholinergic mechanisms.

The depletion of substance P in the primary afferents has functional consequences. The sensitivity to pain is decreased in various experimental animals. After capsaicin treatment the antidromic vasodilatation, the reactive cutaneous hyperemia, and the flare due to the axon reflex are abolished, suggesting that the substance P-depleted nerve has lost the neurotransmitter released not only from its central, but also from its peripheral terminals. Vasodilatation and increased permeability of the capillaries are indeed the fastest mechanisms available to the skin for counteracting damage of any origin, e.g., violent stroking, heating by irradiation, administration of chemical irritants, or following an ischemic period. These studies have also led to a new concept of the axon reflex (Lembeck and Holzer 1979; Lembeck and Donnerer 1981 a, b; Erjavec et al. 1981).

The release of substance P from primary afferents was measured at their central and peripheral terminals. The release can be evoked by electrical stimulation of the nerve, by depolarization with increased K^+, and by capsaicin used as a chemical stimulus. A very small dose of capsaicin causes an immediate release of substance P from both the central and the peripheral terminals of only those neurons that can also be depleted of substance P by very large doses of capsaicin.

A third effect of capsaicin is the blocking of the axonal transport of substance P and the interruption of the conduction of nerve impulses, again specific for small-diameter afferent fibers containing substance P. Short-term local application of capsaicin was shown to have an effect on these afferents similar to that caused by their ligation or surgical interruption; not only does the peripheral part degenerate, but also the whole proximal part of the neuron undergoes a retrograde degeneration.

The stimulating, blocking, and depleting actions of capsaicin have different time courses and different sensitivities. The stimulation occurs within seconds with very small doses, whereas large doses induce depletion within hours and lasting for weeks. These effects have been valuable for functional studies on primary afferent C-fibers and have indicated a peripheral as well as a central physiological role for substance P in these neurons.

After depletion of substance P in rats by capsaicin, a decreased sensitivity to various but not all types of somatic pain has been reported. Almost complete analgesia is obtained to chemical irritants, whereas pain induced by pin prick to the skin is hardly affected. This can be explained by a more pronounced effect of capsaicin on the function of C-fibers than on Aδ-fibers. Another experimental model uses visceral pain induced by distension of the gut, simulating an episode of intestinal colic. The resulting reflex fall in blood pressure allows a quantification of this type of pain response in a fully anesthetized rat. This reflex hypotension can be inhibited by morphine and is completely absent in capsaicin-pretreated rats, indicating that this type of nociceptive stimulation is exclusively mediated by capsaicin-sensitive C-fibers (see Lembeck and Gamse 1982).

Conclusions

The afferent system in which substance P functions as a neurotransmitter is slow in the conduction of impulses as well as in its transmitter mechanism. These slow and sustained effects are seen in electrophysiological recordings at the central synapse of these neurons and in the long-lasting vasodilatation caused by neurogenic release of substance P at the peripheral terminal. Compared with cholinergic or adrenergic transmitters, which hit the receptor only briefly, the peptidergic transmitter substance P behaves slowly. The central nervous system obtains and delivers fast as well as slow and sustained messages; the most distressing forms of pain may be associated with the latter type.

From the practical point of view, in the therapeutic suppression of pain neither substance P nor capsaicin can be used as therapeutic tools. They do serve, however, as a new basis in pain research from which new therapeutic possibilities can be explored. Substance P analogues with central and peripheral antagonistic action have been found; the search for more specific capsaicin analogues is another challenge. Other neuropeptides, like somatostatin, which are distributed similarly to substance P, should be explored with regard to their physiological functions. The peripheral function of substance P-containing fibers is open to clinical research. The central neurotransmission opens the way to the study of the molecular basis of the action of morphine. There is no doubt that essential new developments in the management of pain, especially chronic pain, will emerge during the coming years.

References

Duggan AW (1982) Brain stem control of the responses of spinal neurones to painful skin stimuli. Trends Neurosci 5: 127–130

Erjavec F, Lembeck F, Florjanc-Irman T, Skofitsch G, Donnerer J, Saria A, Holzer P (1981) Release of histamine by substance P. Naunyn Schmiedebergs Arch Pharmacol 317: 67–70

Euler US von, Gaddum JH (1931) An unidentified depressor substance in certain tissue extracts. J Physiol 72: 181–197

Hökfelt T, Vincent S, Dalsgaard CJ, Skirboll L, Johansson O, Schultzberg M, Lundberg JM, Rosell S, Pernow B, Jancsó G (1982) Distribution of substance P in brain and periphery and its possible role as a co-transmitter. In: Porter R, O'Connor M (eds) Substance P in the nervous system. Ciba Foundation Symposium 91. Pitman, London, pp 84–106

Juan H (1978) Prostaglandins as modulators of pain. Gen Pharmacol 9: 403–409

Kandel ER, Schwartz JH (1981) Principles of neural science. Elsevier North Holland, Amsterdam

Leeman SE, Carraway RE (1976) The discovery of a sialogogic peptide in bovine hypothalamic extracts: its isolation, characterization as substance P, structure, and synthesis. In: von Euler US, Pernow B (eds) Substance P, Nobel symposium 37. Raven, New York, pp 5–14

Lembeck F (1953) Zur Frage der zentralen Übertragung afferenter Impulse. II. Mitteilung: Das Vorkommen und die Bedeutung von Substanz P in den dorsalen Wurzeln des Rückenmarks. Naunyn Schmiedebergs Arch Pharmacol 219: 197–213

Lembeck F, Donnerer J (1981a) Postocclusive cutaneous vasodilatation mediated by substance P. Naunyn Schmiedebergs Arch Pharmacol 316: 165–171

Lembeck F, Donnerer J (1981b) Time course of capsaicin-induced functional impairments in comparison with changes in neuronal substance P content. Naunyn Schmiedebergs Arch Pharmacol 316: 240–243

Lembeck F, Holzer P (1979) Substance P as neurogenic mediator of antidromic vasodilation and neurogenic plasma extravasation. Naunyn Schmiedebergs Arch Pharmacol 310: 175–183

Lembeck F, Gamse R (1982) Substance P in peripheral sensory processes. In: Porter R, O'Connor M (eds) Substance P in the nervous system. Ciba Foundation Symposium 91. Pitman, London, pp 34–54

Lembeck F, Folkers K, Donnerer J (1981a) Analgesic effect of antagonists of substance P. Biochem Biophys Res Commun 103: 1318–1321

Lembeck F, Donnerer J, Colpaert FC (1981b) Increase of substance P in primary afferent nerves during chronic pain. Neuropeptides 1: 175–180

Piercey MF, Dobry PJK, Schroeder LA, Einspahr FJ (1981) Behavioral evidence that substance P may be a spinal cord sensory transmitter. Brain Res 210: 407–413

Yaksh TL, Hammond DL (1982) Peripheral and central substrates involved in the rostrad transmission of nociceptive information. Pain 13: 1–85

Frequency of Pain in Patients with Cancer

G. Wagner

Deutsches Krebsforschungszentrum, Im Neuenheimer Feld 280, 6900 Heidelberg 1, FRG

Although more than 5 million people die of cancer every year throughout the world and although by now finely differentiated morbidity and mortality statistics exist on most forms of cancer, there is still practically no reliable information on the frequency and intensity of cancer pain, detailed by sex, age, form of cancer, and stage.

In the historical standard work by Jacob Wolff (1911), *Die Lehre von der Krebskrankheit von den ältesten Zeiten bis zur Gegenwart* (The Theory of Cancer from the Oldest Times up to the Present Day), cancer pain is dealt with on $1^1/_2$ of a total of 2,014 pages. We are told that von Swieten and Lorenz Heister considered pain to be the diagnostic criterion to differentiate between "scirrhus" and "cancer" (a scirrhus should always be painless whereas a cancer causes pain), and that Virchow believed that pain was a consequence rather than a cause or an early symptom of a carcinoma, but no more.

In K. H. Bauer's (1963) standard work *Das Krebsproblem* (The Cancer Problem) a few sentences are devoted to pain and its meaning as a diagnostic criterion within the framework of clinical symptoms of disease. He says (p. 11):

Pain is not constant and mostly does not exist at all in the beginning. However, when it occurs, it yields important diagnostic clues. If a "lump in the breast" of a woman is painful at the same time, this immediately increases the probability of malignity. Some organ cancers within the peritoneal cavity, e.g., the stomach or the colon are felt by the patient to be causing pain and, for this reason, are often localized surprisingly well. In infantile bone sarcomas, too, pain often precedes palpability. . . . The diagnosis of bone metastases is . . . suspected when "rheumatism-like" constant pain, particularly in the "small of the back", points to the skeletal system, even in cases where the bone metastases cannot yet be radiologically discovered, partly because of their small size, partly because they have not as yet destroyed any of the bone substance.

On 1,099 pages not a word is said about the frequency of pain with the various forms of cancer.

Intensive literature searches in all relevant databases such as Cancernet, Cancerlit, and Cancerproj yielded rather disappointing results. Whereas the searches in the first two special cancer literature databases yielded a few hundred titles, these almost exclusively represent clinical surveys or therapeutic contributions to the subject. Among 81 projects on cancer pain contained in the Cancerproj database, only one – namely that by Bonica and co-workers (1981) – deals with the question of the frequency of pain with four forms of cancer (lung, pancreas, uterus, and prostate gland) with regard to epidemiologically interesting parameters such as intensity of pain and course of the disease, stage of the disease, age, psychological and social factors, etc.

The Special Listings of the International Cancer Research Data Bank (ICRDB) do list some projects on "Pain Control in Cancer" in their issue SL-352 of 26 March 1980;

Recent Results in Cancer Research. Vol. 89

Table 1. The frequency of cancer pain (no differentiation according to forms of cancer and intensity of pain)

Authors	Number of patients	Percentage of patients with pain in various stages of cancer				Remarks
		Early	Middle	Late	No differentiation	
Dodd and Livingstone (1976)	NA				50	Cancer pain most frequently with cancer of the cervix, lungs, rectum and prostate gland
Baily et al. (1979)	117			83		Especially with urogenital, breast, and lung cancer in the last 3 months of life
Bonica (1979, 1981)	387		40	60–80		Estimated values from literature
Rosomoff et al. (1980)	NA		62	95		95% in the terminal phase
Wilkes (1974)	296			58		Patients in a hospice
Oster et al. (1978)	43				68	Without bone metastases
					80	With bone metastases
Twycross (1974)	~ 500			75		Patients in the terminal stage
Aitken–Swan (1959)	200			50		Answers from 200 relatives of patients who died from cancer
Foley (1979)	540				29	Inpatients of the Sloan-Kettering Cancer Center
Foley et al. (1978)	397				38	
Schreml et al. (1981)	195				29	Mostly hematologial cases
Senn-Glaus (1982)	400			34		Mostly patients in advanced stages

Table 2. Percentage of patients with pain among 540 consecutive cancer patients of the Sloan-Kettering Cancer Center (Foley et al 1978)

Type	No. of patients	Percentage[a]
Breast	46	52
Lung	30	45
Bone	6	85
Oral cavity	12	80
GI	20	40
GU–Male	10	75
Female	14	70
Lymphoma	4	20
Leukemia	1	5

[a] % patients admitted with tumor type

however, information on the frequency of pain is found only in a project by H.L. Rosomoff et al. (1981). Overall figures from the literature, not differentiated by forms of cancer and rarely by stage, are listed in Table 1. They range between 29% and 95% and merely serve to illustrate the poor state of the art.

According to information from the Interagency Committee on Pain and Discomfort of the National Cancer Institute of the USA (1981), about 33% of all cancer patients suffer severe pain, making treatment against pain necessary. The figures given by Wilkes (1974) from an English hospice for terminal cancer patients are almost twice as high (58%).

One of the very few attempts to establish the frequency of pain according to different tumor forms is the paper by Foley et al. (1978) based on 540 cancer patients admitted to the Memorial Sloan-Kettering Cancer Center in the course of a week. Of these patients, 156 (29%) needed analgesics against pain in the course of their treatment as inpatients, the proportion of patients treated for pain ranging between 85% of those with bone tumors and only 5% of those with leukemias (Table 2).

Lloyd et al. (1978) attempted to establish the frequency of pain with various organ cancers by relating the overall number of cancer patients admitted to an English hospital for pain relief from 1970 to 1974 – subdivided according to tumor localization – to the total number of cases reported to the Oxford cancer registry in the years 1968–1972. In their material (Table 3) the proportion of patients admitted to the pain relief unit per thousand cases reported to the registry was highest (38.2%) for cervical cancer and strikingly low (1.3%) for cancer of the ovary. The figures of Lloyd et al. can at best give a rough indication, since admission to a pain relief unit probably depends on numerous external factors and not solely on the frequency and intensity of pain.

Table 4 was compiled from numerous clinical data from the literature of the last few years. It shows considerable fluctuations not only among the various organ cancers but also within the same form of cancer; as a rule, there is no differentiation according to stage. This table, too, illustrates the fact that our present knowledge is merely based on roughly estimated values.

Under these circumstances, it is remarkable that in the imagination of laymen "pain" next to "incurability" is considered among the most typical characteristics of malignant tumors (e.g., Paterson and Aitken-Swan 1954), a deep-rooted belief which contributes to a large extent to the widespread fear of cancer.

Table 3. Referrals to the Regional Pain Relief Unit (Lloyd et al. 1978)

Types of carcinoma	No. admitted from Oct. 1970 to Oct. 1974	No of cases reported to ORHA 1968–1972[a]	Incidence of pain referral per 1,000 cases diagnosed in the region
Lung	67	5,285	12.7
Breast	46	3,760	12.2
Cervix uteri	27	707	38.2
Rectum	25	1,515	16.5
Bladder	23	1,255	18.3
Prostate	15	1,276	11.8
Pancreas	13	942	13.8
Colon	12	2,203	5.4
Stomach	7	2,069	3.4
Kidneys	5	421	11.9
Corpus uteri	3	670	4.5
Ovary	1	788	1.3

[a] Oxford Regional Health Authority; 1972 is the most recent complete year from which information is available at the Regional Cancer Registry, and there has been no significant alteration in the incidence of these tumors since 1966

Contrary to this widerspread belief, it is – apart from a few exceptions (e.g., certain brain tumors in which pain may occur as an early symptom) – almost characteristic for cancerous diseases that they develop unnoticed and without causing pain over long periods. Cancer creeps in through the back door; only when it has formed metastases or involved important organs and it is mostly too late for a cure, does pain occur – particularly frequently with metastases in the bones. In such cases, however, pain has long since lost its physiological function as a warning; it is senseless and merely hostile to life and thus is a difficult medical and social problem for hundreds of thousands or even millions of cancer patients a year in the terminal stages of their disease.

An important cause of our rather poor knowledge of cancer pain is probably the fact that it is impossible to measure the intensity of pain objectively and exactly. Pain is a highly individual experience which cannot be reconstructed by any other person in any way. Today, scientists in various places are working on so-called intensity of pain scales in order to define the intensity of pain as objectively as possible; nevertheless, we will continue to depend on subjective information. In this connection, the remark of a physician at a London cancer hospital within the framework of a questionnaire on analgesics for cancer pain may be of interest. He writes: "I am surprised how often patients complain of severe pain but stop their analgesics because they have been made constipated. To me this means that many patients overstate their degree of pain" (Robbie and Mennie, 1974).

The scientific treatment of our problem must be based on as exact a definition of the term "cancer pain" as possible. According to Bonica (1979) it is "... pain caused by any neoplastic disease or occurring as a consequence of therapeutic intervention for neoplastic disease or both." Pain may occur (Table 5) as a direct consequence of the tumor (e.g., by the involvement of bones or nerves, or by the obstruction of hollow organs); as a consequence of tumor therapy (e.g., surgical intervention, radiation therapy, or chemotherapy); as an indirect consequence of the tumor (e.g., due to infections or as a consequence of metabolic imbalances); or without any relation to the cancer.

Table 4. Frequency of pain in different forms of cancer

Form of Cancer	Percentage of patients with pain in various stages of cancer				Remarks	Sources
	Early	Middle	Late	No differentiation		
Hypopharynx				54	Pain in the throat in 87/162 cases	Carpenter et al. 1976
Oesophagus				2	Epigastric pain	Inberg et al. 1974
Stomach			67,5	39–77	Early cancer 39% later stages 77%	Fiore et al. 1978; Lempinen, 1971; Olearchyk 1978
Colon				32–58	Mostly stage III or IV, respectively	Basset and Goulston 1978; Hamann et al. 1978; Najem et al. 1977; Pheils et al. 1976
Liver				74	People of Taiwan!	(49) Sung et al. 1967
Gallbladder and ducts				39–86	Moderate to severe epigastric pain	Ertl 1976; Fuhse and Schreiber 1980; Kramer 1960; Palacio and Bedoya 1980; Ross et al. 1974
Pancreas				32–65	Mostly minor pain	Cornée et al.1974; Gulló et al. 1978; Ito 1979; Weingarten et al. 1978
Kidney				10–32	Pain in the small of the back	
Urinary bladder				10	Pain when urinating	Bladder Tumor Study Group 1977
Prostate gland				17–40	Dragging pain in the pelvis	Andersen 1959; Oliveux et al. 1977; Tjaden et al. 1965
Testis				27	Pain occasionally early symptom	Arvola and Lilius 1972
Mamma				35	Upon bone metastases	Hernandez 1978
Uterus				30–70	Pain in the final stage only	Foley et al. 1978
Ovary				40–60	Pain in lower abdomen	Persaud 1977; Reid 1981
Brain tumors	30				Headache frequently early symptom	Herrschaft 1977

Table 5. Causes of pain in cancer patients

I. Pain as a direct consequence of tumors
  A. Involvement of bones
     (e.g., metastases in the cranial fissa and the spine)
  B. Compression of nerves
     (e.g., peripheral neuropathies, involvement of the meninges, compression of the spinal cord)
  C. Obstruction of hollow organs
     (e.g., ileus, obstructive jaundice, atelectases)

II. Pain as a consequence of tumor therapy
  A. Following surgical intervention
     (e.g., phantom pains, postmastectomy syndrome, postthoracotomy syndrome)
  B. Following radiation
     (e.g., radiation fibrosis of the plexus brachialis, radiation myelopathy, neuralgias following radiation shingles)
  C. Following chemotherapy
     (e.g., neuritis, allergic dermatoses, cystitis, aseptic bone necrosis, hyperuricemia)

III. Pain as an indirect consequence of tumors
  A. By infections
     (e.g., mycoses, virus infections)
  B. By metabolic imbalances
     (e.g., hypercalcemia with bone metastases)

IV. Pain without relation to cancer
     (e.g., diabetic neuropathy, rheumatoid arthritis, etc.)

In the present highly unsatisfactory situation concerning our knowledge of cancer pain the following actions are required:
Intensive attempts to improve and standardize the measurement of pain, maybe by setting up an internationally approved and generally employed intensity of pain scale;
Prospective epidemiological studies with large and comparable populations on the type, intensity, and frequency of pain with respect to tumor form, stage, localization, possibly already existing metastases, sex, age, and other factors of interest.
Only by proceeding in such a manner may we hope to decisively deepen our so far fragmentary knowledge of the frequency of pain with cancer. In the United States this has evidently been recognized as an urgent problem in recent times. Within the framework of the Rehabilitation Research Grant Program such studies are to be promoted so that – as the report states: "... as a result of current activities, there will emerge a much clearer understanding of the incidence and magnitude of pain due to cancer" (National Cancer Program 1981).

References

Aitken-Swan J (1959) Nursing the late cancer patient at home. The family's impressions. Practitioner 183:64–69

Andersen R (1959) Carcinoma of the prostate. Clinical observations and treatment. Acta Chir Scand [Suppl] 246

Arvola I, Lilius HG (1972) Malignant testicular tumours presenting with severe pain. Ann Chir Gynaecol 61: 30–32

Bailey L, Rinker M, Stewart C (1979) Pain patterns in patients with advanced cancer. In: Proceedings of the fourth annual congress of the oncology nursing society, New Orleans, La, 17–19 May, p 33 (abstract)

Basset ML, Goulston KJ (1978) Colorectal cancer – a study of 230 patients. Aust NZ J Med 8: 669–670 (abstract)

Bauer KH (1963) Das Krebsproblem, 2nd edn. Springer, Berlin Göttingen Heidelberg

Bladder Tumor Study Group (1977) Report of the bladder tumor study group in Osaka. I. Regional distribution of patients with bladder tumor in Osaka prefecture. Acta Urol Jpn 23: 445–450

Bonica JJ (1979) Importance of the problem. In: Bonica JJ, Ventafridda V (eds) International symposium on pain of advanced cancer. Raven, New York, pp 1–12

Bonica JJ (1981) Cancer pain. Monogra Ser Eur Organ Res Treat Cancer 7: 87–115

Bonica JJ, Bergner M, Moe R (to be published) Pilot study of pain in four selected cancers. (On-going project; cited in Cancerproj Database)

Carpenter RJ, DeSanto LW, Devine KD, Taylor WF (1976) Cancer of the hypopharynx. Analysis of treatment and results in 162 patients. Arch Otolaryngol 102: 716–721

Cornée J, Durbec J-P, Yoro M, Lauret F (1974) Statistiques descriptives de la douleur en pathologie pancréatique. Arch Fr Mal App Dig 63: 375–384

Cukier J, Pascal B, Mangin P (1981) Semiology of the cancer of the kidney in adults: review of 184 cases. Acta Urol Belg 49: 259–262

Descottes B, Cubertafond P, Catanzano G, Caix M (1979) Primary cancer of the gallbladder: report of 55 cases. Sem Hop Paris 55: 1479–1487

Dodd MJ, Livingston CA (1976) Pain and the cancer patient. In: Peterson BH, Kellogg CJ (eds) Current practice in oncologic nursing, vol 1. Mosby, Saint Louis, pp 171–181

Ertl M (1976) Das primäre Gallenblasenkarzinom. Chir Prax 21: 609–612

Fiore D, Zacchi C, Panfilio F, Nitti D, Rossi CR, Favretti F (1978) Analysis of some cases of carcinoma of the esophageal cardia. Acta Chir Ital 34: 557–561

Foley KM (1979) Pain syndromes in patients with cancer. In: Bonica JJ, Ventafridda V (eds) International Symposium on pain of advanced cancer. Raven, New York, pp 59–75

Foley KM, Roger A, Houde RW (1978) Pain in patients with cancer: a quantitative reappraisal. Proc Am Assoc Cancer Res 19: 357

Fuhse J, Schreiber U (1980) Häufigkeit, Symptomatik und Ätiologie maligner Tumoren im Bereich der posthepatischen Gallenwege und des Pankreas. Dtsch Gesundheitsw 35: 71–74

Gullo L, Ventrucci M, Costa PL, Procaccio L, Nestico V, Ripani R (1978) Pancreatic cancer. Etiological and clinical observations of 140 cases. Recent Prog Med (Roma) 64: 90–97

Hamann J, Eckert M, Fux HD (1978) Das Dickdarm-Karzinom. Beobachtungen zu Klinik und Therapie. Fortschr Med 96: 1124–1128

Hernandez Munoz G, Ravelo Celis JA, Martinez LP, Rodriguez Castro C (1978) Five year survival in breast cancer. Bol Organo Soc Med Hosp Munic Emergen 13: 57–63

Herrschaft H (1977) Zur Früherkennung der Gehirntumoren. Fortschr Neurol Psychiatr 45: 383–404

Hirakawa S, Goto H, Takenaka I, Ishida G, Miyagawa I, Rii C (1980) A statistical observation of renal cell carcinoma. Hishinippon Hinyokika 42: 1003–1009

Holland JM (1975) Natural history and staging of renal cell carcinoma. CA 25: 121–133

Inberg MV, Scheinin TM, Voutilainen A, Havia T, Nikkanen TA (1974) Management of oesophageal carcinoma: a report of 267 cases. Scand J Thorac Cardiovasc Surg 8: 220–227

Ito K, Ihara S, Ohara K (1979) Comparison between pancreatic cancer and cholangiocarcinoma. Geka Shinryo 21: 391–399

Kramer A (1960) Das Gallenblasenkarzinom. Münch Med Wochenschr 102: 2082–2087

Lempinen M (1971) Carcinoma of the stomach. I. Diagnostic considerations. Ann Chir Gynaecol 60: 135–140

Lloyd JW, Glynn CJ, Adams CBT, Durrant KR (1978) The pain of cancer. Practitioner 220: 453–457

Minami T, Masuda F, Sasaki T (1975) A clinical study on renal cell carcinoma. Jpn J Urol 66: 474–484

Najem AZ, Hennessey M, Malfitan RC, Cheung NK, Hobson RW (1977) Colon and rectal carcinoma: clinical experience. Am Surg 43: 583–588

National Cancer Program (1981) 1980 Director's report and annual plan f.y. 1982–1986. NIH Publ. No. 81–2290, US Dept. of Health and Human Services, Publ. Health Service, NIH

Olearchyk AS (1978) Gastric carcinoma. A critical review of 243 cases. Am J Gastroenterol 70: 25–45

Oliveux A, Dufour A, Frenkhauser J, Bollack C (1977) Le traitement des formes douloureuses du cancer de la prostate. J Med Strasbourg 8: 67–71

Oster MW, Vizel M, Turgeon LR (1978) Pain of terminal cancer patients. Arch Intern Med 138: 1801–1802

Palacio H, Bedoya MV (1980) Primary carcinoma of the gallbladder: clinical-pathological study of 67 cases. Antioquia Med 29: 8–12

Paterson R, Aitken-Swan J (1954) Public opinion on cancer. A survey among women in the Manchester area. Lancet II: 857–861

Persaud V (1977) Aspects of primary ovarian cancer in Jamaica. West Indian Med J 26: 90–100

Pheils MT, Barnett JE, Newland RC, Macpherson JG (1976) Colorectal carcinoma: a prospective clinopathological study. Med J Aust [Suppl] 1: 17–21

Pillari G, Fulco JD, Lee WJ (1979) Hypernephroma and hypertension: observations. NY State J Med 79: 865–867

Reid DS (1981) Ovarian cancer at Kent General Hospital during the years 1975-1979. Del Med J 53: 399–400, 403–405

Robbie DS, Mennie AT (1974) Analgesics in cancer pain: results of a questionnaire. Postgrad Med J 50: 150–154

Rosomoff HL, Silbret M, Hosek R, Vogel C (1980) Cancer rehabilitation through pain control (project description). Current cancer research, special listing NCI, ICRDB/SL-352

Ross AP, Braasch JW, Warren KW (1974) Carcinoma of the proximal bile ducts. Lahey Clin Found Bull 23: 110–120

Schmid E, Gehl H, Blaich E, Haag S, Lorentz H, Kovarik P, Rettenmayr K, Schwarzkopf H (1981) Early gastric cancer: results in a county hospital. Z Gastroenterol 19: 51–55

Schreml W, Merkle W, Heimpel H (1981) Medikamentöse Schmerztherapie bei Krebspatienten. Med Klin 76: 43–47

Senn HJ, Glaus A (1982) Schmerzen und Schmerzbekämpfung bei Tumorkrankheiten. Schweiz Med Wochenschr 112: 1158–1164

Sung JL, Wang TH, Yu JY (1967) Clinical study on primary carcinoma of the liver in Taiwan. Am J Dig Dis 12: 1036–1049

Tjaden HB, Culp DA, Flocks RH (1965) Clinical adenocarcinoma of the prostate in patients under 50 years of age. J Urol 93: 618–621

Twycross RG (1974) Clinical experience with diamorphine in advanced malignant disease. Int J Clin Pharmacol 7: 184–198

Weingarten LA, Gelb AM, Fischer M (1978) Pancreatic carcinoma: a clinical review and schema for evaluating patients. Gastroenterology 74: 1110 (abstract)

Wilkes E (1974) Some problems in cancer management. Proc R Soc Med 67: 23–27

Wolff J (1911) Die Lehre von der Krebskrankheit von den ältesten Zeiten bis zur Gegenwart. Fischer, Jena

Clinical Pain Syndromes in Cancer Patients and Their Causes

R. Hartenstein and W. Wilmanns

Medizinische Klinik III, Klinikum Grosshadern, Universität München, Marchioninistrasse 15, 8000 München 70, FRG

Introduction

Although reliable data on the frequency of cancer pain do not exist (see Wagner, this volume), it has been estimated that nearly one-third of all nonterminal cancer patients (Foley 1979) and about 60% of all patients with terminal cancer suffer from pain of different degrees of severity (Twycross 1980). These data underline the significance of pain in cancer patients. The predominance of chronic, persistent pain in cancer affects the patient's ability to lead a normal productive life often more than the knowledge of the disease itself and substantially contributes to the physical and psychic decay of the patient.

Corresponding to the concept of pain as a "sensory receptor reaction system" against nociceptive stimuli (Fordyce and Steger 1979), cancer-associated pain can be caused directly by tumorous lesions due to infiltration, expansion, and compression and by their direct consequences, such as spontaneous fracture, myogelosis, ileus, congestion, or ischemia and necrosis.

Indirectly, tumor-related pain can be caused by cancer-accompanying diseases like paraneoplastic syndromes and by cancer-concomitant phenomena like inflammation, infection, or the effect of vasoactive algesic substances produced by the tumor itself. In addition, pain can also be induced indirectly by side effects of the tumor therapy (see Schreml, this volume).

Table 1. Causes of pain associated with cancer

Causes
Directly cancer-related pain due to:
1. Bone involvement
2. Involvement of the nervous system
3. Involvement of a hollow viscus
4. Involvement of a parenchymal viscus
5. Involvement of the head and neck
6. Involvement of blood vessels and lymphatics
Indirectly cancer-related pain due to:
1. Paraneoplastic syndromes
2. Inflammation and infection
3. Vasoactive algesic substances
4. Side effects of tumor therapy
5. Psychological factors

Recent Results in Cancer Research. Vol. 89

Last but not least, psychogenic influences play an important role in the development and intensification of cancer pain.

Of cancer-associated pain syndromes 75% are caused by direct tumor involvement of tissues and organs and by the direct consequences of this involvement. Mostly, the pain originates from damage to pain-sensitive or pain-mediating structures of the skeleton, the nervous system, a hollow viscus, a solid parenchymal viscus, the head and neck, or the blood vessels and lymphatics (Foley 1979; Table 1).

Bone Involvement

The most frequent cause of pain in cancer patients is tumor infiltration of the skeletal system by primary bone tumors, plasmocytomas, or metastases. Breast cancer, prostate carcinoma, bronchogenic carcinoma, renal carcinoma, and thyroid carcinoma are the tumors which most frequently cause bone metastases (Nystrom et al. 1977; Table 2). Vertebrae, ribs, and large joints are often sites on the skeleton where pain is localized. It is assumed that this pain is caused by irritation and damage of the periosteal and endosteal pain receptors (Kottke 1980). As a secondary effect of direct bone involvement, a sensitization of pain receptors in the neighboring muscles, tendons, joints, and nerve elements can result, especially when a spontaneous fracture or a vertebral compression has developed from tumorous bone infiltration.

The clinical pain equivalent varies with the location of the bone lesion and with the secondary manifestations on non-directly tumor-affected tissues. As a consequence of involvement of the spine, dorsalgia, tension headaches, myogelosis and, predominantly, extremely painful root-compression syndromes can appear in addition to pain at the site of the tumorous lesion. Examples of such manifestations are the shoulder-hand syndrome due to involvement of the cervical spine, the so-called intercostal neuralgia or projected pain in the abdomen due to involvement of the upper and lower thoracic spine, and the lumbar vertebral syndromes such as lumbago and ischialgia due to involvement of the lumbar spine and sacrum. Due to incorrect posture, the pain can also be manifested in unaffected parts of the body, distant from the actual lesion, e.g., as coxalgia or as gonalgia.

For differential diagnosis of the tumor-dependent complaints, nonspecific diseases of bone, joint, muscle, tendon, and nervous system, especially of degenerative and inflammatory origin, have to be excluded.

Table 2. Frequency of bone metastases in cancer (Nystrom et al. 1977)

Primary site	Bone metastases (%)
Breast	30–85
Prostate	50–75
Lung	30–50
Kidney	30–50
Thyroid	39
Pancreas	5–10
Colan/Rectum	5–10
Stomach	5–10
Liver	8
Ovary	2– 6

Involvement of the Nervous System

The described indirect tumor-related nerve lesions in primary skeletal tumor invasion can also be initiated by direct tumorous involvement of various structures of the nervous system and can be responsible for a variety of pain syndromes. In this case, the pain arises through the irritation of nociceptive afferent fibres of the spine roots, nerve trunks, plexuses, and the peripheral nerves, or through irritation of pain receptors of the spinal meninges due to tumor compression, tumor-related distention, or tumor infiltration. As a result, painful root-compression syndromes, plexus neuropathy, peripheral neuropathy and – by invasion of the vertebral canal – spinal cordcompression syndromes develop.

In addition to the described tumor manifestations in the area of the spine and the vertebral canal, tumors and metastases with paravertebral localization in the neck, the mediastinum, and the retroperitoneum may create such pain. Here, bronchogenic carcinoma, malignant lymphoma, gastrointestinal, and genito-urinary tract tumors are predominant. Examples of such neurogenic pain syndromes are Pancoast's syndrome, with marked shoulder-hand pain due to an apically located bronchogenic carcinoma, the rootcompression syndrome and the plexus neuropathy in the lumbosacral area due to bulky retroperitoneal metastases of testicular cancer, and the spinal cordcompression syndrome due to tumor metastases in the vertebral canal. Painful neúropathy caused by leukemic infiltration of a nerve should also be mentioned.

Neurogenic lesions can also involve the sympathetic nervous system and can lead to the so-called sympathetic algodystrophy, as in Raynaud's disease, causalgia, and Sudeck's atrophy (Bonica 1979). Disturbances of blood supply due to vasoconstriction and vasodilation as a consequence of a dysregulation of the sympathetic nerves with changes in the environment of the pain receptors are discussed as causes (Zimmermann 1981).

For differential diagnosis, these pain syndromes must be distinguished from rootcompression syndrome, plexus neuropathy, peripheral neuropathy, neuralgia, and algodystrophy of inflammatory, posttraumatic, degenerative, metabolic, or toxic origin. The root pain may also point to visceral sicknesses such as pancreatitis, cholecystitis, and pleurisy.

Headache is not a leading symptom in brain tumors, but when it does occur it is often related to tumors of the posterior cranial fossa (Wolf 1980). Besides primary cerebral tumors like glioblastoma and medulloblastoma and the primarily expansive growing

Table 3. Frequency of brain metastases in cancer (Vieth and Odom 1965)

Primary site	Brain metastases	
	No. of cases	%
Lung	86	(28)
Breast	51	(16)
Melanoma	49	(16)
Unknown	44	(14)
Genito-urinary tract	22	(7)
Colon	16	(5)
Skin and sinuses	14	(4)
Sarcoma	8	(3)
Other	23	(7)

meningioma, hypophyseal tumors, and craniopharyngioma, headache can be caused by brain metastases, in particular from bronchogenic, breast, renal, and testicular cancer, and from malignant melanoma (Vieth and Odom 1965; Table 3). This headache originates from an irritation of pain receptors of the meninges, intracranial sinus veins, and meningeal arteries due to tumorous distension, stretching, compression, or infiltration.

Again, tumor-induced headache has to be differentiated from headache of other causes, like occipital and trigeminal neuralgia, tension headache, vasomotorial headache, neurinomas of the acoustic and trigeminal nerve, inflammatory cerebral and meningeal diseases, and intracranial hemorrhage.

A special form of neurogenic pain syndrome is caused by carcinomatous meningiosis. The tumor infiltration of the leptomeninges of the brain and spinal cord leads to a stretching pain manifesting itself as headache, with or without stiff neck, or as backache (Olson et al. 1974; Foley 1979). Main causes of this type of pain are acute leukemia, malignant lymphoma, breast cancer, and small-cell bronchogenic carcinoma. For differential diagnosis, meningitis must be excluded.

Involvement of a Hollow Viscus

Tumor-caused pain in a hollow viscus occurs when a narrowing of the passage or an obstruction of the hollow organ is present (Fuhse and Schreiber 1980). In any case, this indicates a critical and usually emergency situation due to the risk of organ perforation.

Esophagus, stomach, small and large intestine, gallbladder, and biliary tract, as well as genito-urinary tract including urinary bladder can be affected. The cause of the obstruction is either a primary tumor, a tumor recurrence, or a metastasis, either growing in the organ itself or causing a compression from outside. An example is the obstructing colorectal cancer leading to painful ileus. This pain, poorly localized, diffuse, and often referred to dermatomes supplied by the same spinal cord segments which supply the affected viscus, is caused by distension of the organ and by contraction of the smooth muscle under isometric conditions. It is likely that the ischemia following the organ distension intensifies the pain by lowering the threshold of nociceptors due to the release of pain-mediating substances (Bonica 1979). For differential diagnosis, obstructive diseases caused by benign tumors, postoperative conditions, inflammatory diseases, and lithiasis have to be considered.

Involvement of a Parenchymal Viscus

A pain-causing mechanism similar to that of obstructive disease is assumed to be due to involvement of solid, parenchymal organs, such as liver, spleen, and kidney. The expansion of the tumor due to increased tumor mass leads to intraparenchymal increase of pressure, causing a distension of pain-sensitive structures of the organ capsule. The direct tumor infiltration of the organ can cause pain as well, provided the organ capsule is directly involved. Tumor processes which affect the parenchyma alone do not produce pain. An exception is the involvement of the pancreas. Here, enzymolytic phenomena leading to necrosis and the release of pain-mediating substances are responsible for algogenesis. These tumor-induced pains have to be differentiated from pain due in particular to inflammatory and congestive organ diseases, organ infarctions, or organ cysts.

Involvement of the Head and Neck

In tumors of the head and neck, pain can be found in the oral cavity, pharynx, larynx, nasal cavity, paranasal sinus and, not rarely, in the fossae infratemporales, caused by primary carcinomas, lymphomas, and sarcomas, especially in advanced stages of these diseases (Million et al. 1982; Shapshay et al. 1976).
About 80% of patients with carcinoma of the oral cavity complain of pain (Foley 1979). This pain, due to head and neck malignomas, is either localized at the site of the tumor, manifested as facial pain and headache, or referred to the ear area by sensory cranial nerves (V, IX, X). Frequently the pain is intensified by accompanying ulceration, inflammation, and necrosis.
Trigeminal neuralgia, glossopharyngeal neuralgia, neuritis, herpes zoster, sinusitis, and arthropathy of the temporal mandibular joint must be included in the differential diagnostic considerations.

Involvement of Blood Vessels and Lymphatics

The tumor involvement of blood vessels can be an infiltration of the vessel wall or an occlusion of the vessel lumen, either partial or complete (Bonica 1979). Both of these can produce pain. The infiltration leads to vasoconstriction or vasodilatation, which result in a painful disturbance of blood supply (Zimmermann 1981). The occlusion of blood vessels by infiltration of the vessel lumen or by compression due to an adjacent tumor produces venous engorgement and edema or arterial ischemia. As a consequence of the occlusion, pain is induced by distension and irritation of nociceptive structures of the vessels and of the adjacent tissues. Ischemia, in particular, causes cellular breakdown with production of pain-producing substances which lower the threshold of the nociceptors (Bonica 1979). Corresponding mechanisms of pain induction can be assumed by involvement of the lymph vessels when a painful lymph edema occurs.
An example of pain produced by tumorous vein involvement is the occlusion of the upper vena cava: a vena cava superior syndrome with thoracic and neck vein distension, facial edema, and plethora results, accompanied by chest pain and headache in about 20% of the cases (Carabell and Goodman 1982). Of all vena cava superior syndromes, 97% are caused by tumors, mostly bronchogenic carcinomas, malignant lymphomas, and thymomas.

Pain Caused by Cancer-Concomitant Diseases

Besides the direct tumor invasion causing the venous occlusion, a superior vena-caval syndrome can also develop as a primary thrombotic obstruction due to hypercoagulability associated with the cancer.
The appearance of pain in cancer patients does not necessarily imply that the malignant process is the direct cause of the pain (Twycross 1980). In the course of cancer disease, painful concomitant diseases and accompanying phenomena can occur which are not directly related to malignant tissue lesions but are promoted and supported by the cancerous disease. A large group of disorders secondary to cancer are the so-called paraneoplastic syndromes, which are occasionally found mainly in bronchogenic, gastric, mammary, pancreatic, prostatic, ovarian, and liver-cell carcinoma, in acute leukemias, and malignant lymphomas, and which are accompanied by pain. Examples of such disorders are

Table 4. Indirectly cancer-associated pain caused by paraneoplastic syndromes

Disease	Pain
Nerves	
Neuropathy	Nerve pain, dysesthesias
Muscle	
Dermatomyositis	Muscle pain
Myopathy	
Polymyositis	
Joint	
Rheumatoid arthritis	Joint pain, muscle pain
Polymyalgia rheumatica	
Hypertrophic osteoarthropathy (Marie-Bamberger-Syndrome)	Bone pain
Blood	
Hypercoagulopathy	Pain by embolism (e.g., lung) Pain by thrombosis (e.g., leg) Pain by thrombophlebitis
DIC	Pain by hematoma
Thrombocytopenia (ITP-like syndrome)	

DIC, disseminated intravascular coagulation; *ITP*, idiopathic thrombocytopenia purpura

the dysesthesias causing neuropathy, muscle pain causing dermatomyositis, joint pain causing rheumatoid arthritis, or pain from embolism, thrombosis, or hematoma due to blood coagulation disorders (Minna and Bunn 1982; Table 4).

Painful concomitant symptoms due to inflammation and infection, such as decubitus in bedridden patients, oropharyngeal candidosis and an increased rate of herpes zoster, especially in patients with Hodgkin's and non-Hodgkin's lymphomas, are common indirect forms of cancer pain.

Rare painful reactions caused by vasoactive, algesic substances which are produced by the tumor itself may also be classified here, e.g., the catecholamine-induced headache in pheochromocytoma, the joint pain due to arthropathy induced by serotonin and other metabolites in carcinoid tumors (Brennan 1982), and the tumor pain caused by alcohol as a vasoactive substance in some cases of Hodgkin's disease and occasionally in carcinoma of the uterine cervix, bladder, and lung (Atkinson et al. 1976).

Pain Through Psychogenic Influences

"Pain is an unpleasant sensory and emotional experience . . ." is part of the definition of pain by the International Association for the Study of Pain (1979). This means that pain as a concept essentially comprises more than a simple sensory receptor reaction system to physiopathologic noxae. Emotional and psychic factors play an important role in cancer pain and must be included in the common pain concept. In contrast to patients with acute pain, which is quickly controlled by therapeutical intervention in most cases, in patients suffering from cancer pain, which is mostly chronic and persistent in nature, psychological factors are of striking importance. Anxiety, helplessness, despair, frustration, and depression are able to secondarily increase somatogenic pain (Sternbach 1968). Also, psychological factors are to be considered as a primary cause of chronic pain in cancer patients (Bonica 1979). The poor prognosis in most cancer diseases and the social stigma associated with cancer are able to promote internal and external conflicts initiating pain in patients predisposed to such influences.

References

Atkinson K, Austin DE, McElwain TJ, Peckhorn MJ (1976) Alcohol pain in Hodgkin's disease. Cancer 37: 895–899

Bonica JJ (1979) Introduction to management of pain of advanced cancer. In: Bonica JJ, Ventafridda V (eds) Advances in pain research and therapy, vol 2. Raven, New York, pp 115–130

Brennan MF (1982) Cancer of the endocrine system. In: De Vita VT Jr, Hellman S, Rosenberg SA (eds) Cancer. Principles and practice of oncology. Lippincott, Philadelphia, pp 971–1035

Carabell SC, Goodman RL (1982) Oncologic emergencies: superior vena caval syndrome. In: De Vita VT Jr, Hellman S, Rosenberg SA (eds) Cancer. Principles and practice of oncology. Lippincott, Philadelphia, pp 1582–1594

Foley KM (1979) Pain syndromes in patients with cancer. In: Bonica JJ, Ventafridda V (eds) Advances in pain research and therapy, vol 2. Raven, New York, pp 59–75

Fordyce WE, Steger JC (1979) Chronic pain. In: Pomerlean OV, Brady JJ (eds) Behavioral medicine: theory and practice. Williams and Wilkins, Baltimore, pp 296–349

Fuhse J, Schreiber U (1980) Häufigkeit, Symptomatik und Ätiologie maligner Tumoren im Bereich der posthepatischen Gallenwege und des Pankreas. Dtsch Gesundheitswesen 35: 71–74

IASP Subcommittee on Taxonomy (1979) Pain terms: a list with definitions and notes on usage. Pain 6: 249–252

Kottke FJ (1960) Bone pain from metastases. JAMA 243: 2397

Million RR, Cassisi NJ, Wittes RE (1982) Cancer in the head and neck. In: De Vita VT Jr, Hellman S, Rosenberg SA (eds) Cancer. Principles and practice of oncology. Lippincott, Philadelphia, pp 301–395

Minna JD, Bunn PA Jr (1982) Paraneoplastic syndromes. In: De Vita VT Jr, Hellman S, Rosenberg SA (eds) Cancer. Principles and practice of oncology. Lippincott, Philadelphia, pp 1476–1517

Nystrom JS, Weiner JM, Heffelfinger-Juttner J, Irwin LE, Bateman JR, Meshnik-Wolf R (1977) Metastatic and histologic presentations in unknown primary cancer. Semin Oncol 4: 53–58

Olson ME, Chernik NL, Posner JB (1974) Infiltration of the leptomeninges by systemic cancer: a clinical and pathological study. Arch Neurol 30: 122–127

Shapshay SM, Elber E, Strong MS (1976) Occult tumors of the infratemporal fossa. Arch Otolaryngol 102: 535–538

Sternbach RA (1968) Pain. A psychophysiological analysis. Academic Press, New York

Twycross RG (1980) Incidence and assessment of pain in terminal cancer. In: Twycross RG, Ventafridda V (eds) The continuing care of terminal cancer patients. Pergamon, Oxford, pp 65–74

Vieth R, Odom GL (1965) Intracranial metastases and their neurosurgical treatment. J Neurosurg 23: 375–383

Wolf G (1980) Neurologische Symptome bei Hirntumoren. Fortschr Med 98: 1215–1218

Zimmermann M (1981) Physiological mechanisms of pain and pain therapy. Triangle 20: 7–18

Analysis of Cancer Pain by the Neurologist

M. Berger and F. Gerstenbrand

Neurologische Universitätsklinik, Anichstrasse 35, 6020 Innsbruck, Austria

Introduction

In patients with cancer pain the aim of the neurological diagnosis is the classification of the origin of the pain, with discrimination between structural damage and primary or secondary dysfunction. In cases in which the pain is the first sign of disease, the neurological examination can lead to the detection of the primary lesion. The etiological classification of the pain and its division into individual components allows optimal treatment of the pain and follow-up.

In cancer patients pain can be caused by severe structural damage or, alternatively, it can arise as a combination of several factors. Therefore, it is often not possible to make a diagnosis by the consideration of a single symptom, but only by differential examination of all the body structures in which dysfunction occurs, either from the primary disease or secondarily from the pain syndrome. The cancer pain can be caused by damage of the neuronal structures or can occur as receptor pain.

Pain from Lesions of Neuronal Structures

Lesions of the Peripheral Nerves

Peripheral nerve lesions caused by compression or infiltration of a tumor can lead to an altered afferent pattern, and thus to deafferentation pain through impairment of the integrity of the afferent nerve fibers. Sensory, motor, and vegetative disturbances also occur. The structural lesion can be present in the nerve root, nerve plexus, or peripheral nerve.

Radicular Syndrome

A radicular syndrome arises from primary or secondary blastomatous processes in the region of the vertebrae but can also arise intrathecally from tumors of the nerve roots and their sheaths (Table 1). Paravertebral tumors can also produce root damage. The lesions of the nerve root and the dural sheath lead to violent pain, which usually radiates to the periphery of the relevant dermatome.

Movements which cause stretching or compression of the nerve roots concerned provoke a characteristic radicular pain (Fig. 1). Examination reveals dysfunction of the sensory system in the form of hypoesthesia in the involved dermatome, and in the motor system in

Recent Results in Cancer Research. Vol. 89

Table 1. Radicular syndrome

Pain	*Radiation* usually into the periphery of the dermatome
	Provocation by spinal movement, stretching of nerves, pressure on nerves
	Intensity often toothache-like
Sensibility	*Hypoesthesia* in the dermatome
Motoricity	*Paresis* of the corresponding muscle
	Atrophy – reduced or absent tendon reflex
Associated symptoms	*Dysfunction* and *irritation* in typical parts of the spine

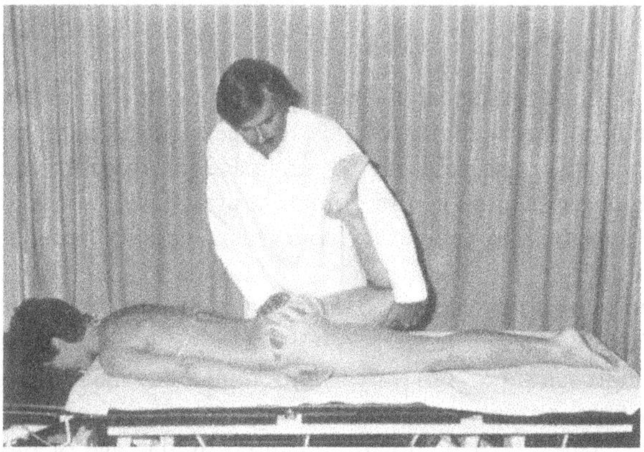

Fig. 1. Femoralis Lasègue: stretch movement of the N. femoralis by bending the knee and stretching the hip

the form of partial paralysis and atrophy of the muscles with reduction or absence of tendon reflexes. Neuro-orthopedic examination usually reveals irritation symptoms of the spinal segments with monosegmental as well as multisegmental dysfunction (e.g., stiff neck, lumbago).

Lesions of the Nerve Plexus

Irritation or lesion of the nerve plexus or peripheral nerves caused by a tumor leads to projection of pain into the areas served by these nerves. Sometimes pain is delayed or may be absent. The sensibility test shows hypalgesia, but also dysesthesia and hyperalgesia in parts of the involved area. Lesions of motor fibres cause partial paralysis and atrophy of the involved muscles, with reduced or absent tendon reflexes. Changes of the autonomic nervous system can lead to alteration of the vasomotor function and cause trophic dysfunction.

Cauda Equina Syndrome

Bilateral paralysis, hypoesthesia, pain in the lower extremities, and bladder and rectal dysfunction are typical symptoms of a cauda equina syndrome, which can be caused by a tumor in the region of the lumbosacral canal.

Paraneoplastic Syndrome

A peripheral neuron lesion does not only occur as a direct result of tumor growth, infiltration, or compression, but also as a consequence of the carcinomatous disease in the form of a paraneoplastic neuropathy, somtimes accompanied by a paraneoplastic myopathy. Because of the poor general condition of the patient, a herpes zoster with severe pain in the affected dermatome may result, usually with involvement of the nerve roots, which exhibit a mechanical lesion from metastases of the spine. This may often be the first sign of a carcinomatous lesion.

Side Effects of Therapy

Peripheral nerve damage can also occur secondarily as a result of cancer therapy. Nerve lesions due to radiation are most frequently found in the region of the plexus brachialis in mammary tumors, in the plexus lumbosacralis, and in the nervus femoralis (Stöhr 1980). Radiogenic vascular damage, in the form of a proliferative radiation vasculopathy or a radiation-induced fibrosis, leads to nerve damage. Moreover, operative therapy, especially radical operations, can lead to lesions of the peripheral nerves. Lymphatic edema can cause lesions of the plexus and peripheral nerves. Phantom stump pain is sometimes experienced following amputation of the limbs. A further iatrogenic impairment of the peripheral nerves is possible following treatment with cytostatic drugs leading to neuropathy with pain, and can be associated also with a myelopathy and encephalopathy. Likewise, polyneuropathy, accompanied by pain, can result from malabsorption and malnutrition.

Spinal Cord Lesions

A carcinomatous process can cause partial paralysis as a result of compression or infiltration of the spine, as well as secondary myelopathy following radiotherapy. At the same time, pain in the affected spastic musculature as well as shooting pains and phantom sensations in the paralyzed limbs can occur (Berger and Gerstenbrand 1981).

Cerebral Lesions

Primary or secondary brain tumors can cause central pain in the form of thalamic pain when the posterior thalamic structures are involved. This can manifest itself as an intolerable pain in one side of the body, accompanied by various dysesthesiae. Headache associated with intracranial tumor can be caused by deposits in the meninges or by increased volume of the brain. According to Weber (1970), headache occurs in 60%–80% of patients with cerebral tumors and in 80%–100% with tumors in the posterior cranial fossa, whereas 40% of brain tumor patients do not complain of headache. Headache and facial pain caused by an intracranial tumor usually start paroxysmally in a projection zone and later become persistent and diffuse.

Pain Caused by Stimulation of Pain Receptors

Whereas it is usually easy to clarify the origin of pain in a carcinomatous lesion of the peripheral or central nervous system, cancer pain as a result of irritation of the pain receptors presents many differential diagnostic problems. Pain receptors, which react to pressure, traction, endogenous or foreign chemicals, temperature, are present in all body structures with the exception of the brain and spinal cord. Provocation of these pain receptors can occur primarily as pressure or traction from the tumors, or secondarily as muscle or joint pain caused by the dysfunction of the motor system. Chemosensitive pain receptors can be stimulated by the liberation of endogenous pain substances, but also by the side effects of chemotherapeutic drugs (Swerdlow 1978). The various causes of receptor pain will not be dealt with in greater detail here.

Lesions of Visceral Structures

Stimulation of pain in the visceral structures can give rise to local pain, as well as referred pain, caused by irritation of larger parts of organs. Moreover, the facilitation and convergence phenomena of the spinal cord can cause a referred visceral pain syndrome, with radiation of organ-specific pain to various parts of the body. As well as this radiating pain, several other objective disturbances in the various body structures can occur, which are not given enough priority in the examination of patients with cancer pain.

The symptoms of the referred visceral pain syndrome (Table 2) are radiation of pain to the organ-specific projection areas of the skin (Head's zone) and the musculature (McKenzie's zone). Pain provocation is partly organ-specific, and complaints of a nocturnal maximum are frequent. Diagnosis of dysesthesic or hyperalgesic zones can help in the etiologic classification of the referred visceral pain syndrome; dysesthesia and hyperalgesia can occur in dermis, epidermis, musculature, or deep structures in a dissociated fashion (Fig. 2).

In the pain region, not only the sensitivity, but also the mechanical quality of the dermis and epidermis is often altered. Impairment can occur in muscles which are functionally or segmentally associated with the diseased organ and can manifest as muscle spasm, tendinopathy, or altered muscle tone. Functional lesions can occur in organ-specific segments of the spine as alteration of active and passive motility and as segmental irritation symptoms.

Lesions of the Locomotor System

Damage to structures of the locomotor system caused by primary or secondary carcinomatous processes can lead to muscular or articular disturbances due to reflex mechanisms, resulting in a pseudoradicular syndrome (Table 3). These symptoms consist of dysesthesia and radiating pain to one or more dermatomes, muscular impairment such as muscle spasm, tendinopathy, or myotendinosis, as well as altered muscle tone in segmentally and functionally associated muscles (Brügger 1980). Disturbances of autonomous nerve function occur in the dermis and epidermis in the form of altered local sweat secretion, skin edema, etc. (Lewit 1977). Involvement of the spinal column or neighboring structures by carcinomatous lesions can lead to a local spinal syndrome or, in severe cases, to a stiff-neck or lumbago syndrome (Brocher and Willert 1980).

Table 2. Referred visceral pain

Pain	*Radiation* in organ-specific projection zones (dermatome, Head's zone; myotome, McKensie's zone) *Provocation* partly organ-specific *Intensity* partly severe, often nocturnal maximum
Sensibility	*Hyperalgesia* and *dysesthesia* in projection zones (dermis, epidermis, musculature)
Motoricity	*Secondary muscle dysfunction* in projection zones (muscle spasm, myogelosis, tendinopathy)
Associated symptoms	Dysfunction of the affected *visceral* organs *Secondary lesions* in typical parts of the spine *Dysfunction* of the autonomous nervous system in the projection zones of the dermis and epidermis (Kibler's zone, etc.)

Table 3. Pseudoradicular syndrome

Pain	*Local pain* in the region of damaged structures *Radiation* often into the dermatome *Provocation* by pressure and movement of the involved joint and muscles *Intensity* usually not severe
Sensibility	*Dysesthesia* and *hyperalgesia* over the damaged structures or in the dermatome
Motoricity	Muscular *hyper-* or *hypotonus,* muscle spasm, myogelosis, tendinopathy
Associated symptoms	*Dysfunction* of the autonomous nervous system in typical zones of the dermis and epidermis (Kibler's zone, etc.)

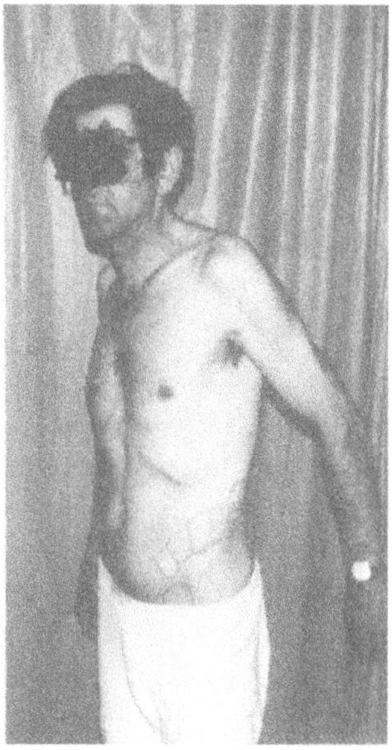

Fig. 2. 53-year-old patient with hypernephroma on left side: referred visceral pain with projection into the dermatome (D.12) and pain caused by pressure on the tip of the 11th rib and on the iliacus muscle

Summary

Pain intensity and the importance of pain for the cancer patient depend on a variety of individual factors and show considerable divergence (Bonica and Ventafridda 1979). They are greatly influenced by the enigma of the cancer disease as well as the consequential psychiatric problems (Frey 1980). An effective neurological analysis of the cancer pain, although demanding for the physician, is important for further specific diagnostic procedures and for the indication of appropriate therapy. Sometimes thorough neurological examination can lead to the first diagnosis of the carcinoma; when there is already evidence of metastases, the unfavorable prognosis can be made at the same time.

References

Berger M, Gerstenbrand F (1981) Phantom illusions in spinal cord lesions. In: Siegfried S, Zimmermann M (eds) Phantom and stump pain. Springer, Berlin Heidelberg New York, pp 66–73

Bonica JJ, Ventafridda V (eds) (1979) Advances in pain research and therapy, vol 2. Raven, New York

Brocher IEW, Willert HG (1980) Differentialdiagnose der Wirbelsäulenerkrankungen. Thieme, Stuttgart

Brügger A (1980) Die Erkrankungen des Bewegungsapparats und seines Nervensystems. Fischer, Stuttgart

Frey M (1980) Diagnose und Therapie des Tumorschmerzes. In: Frey R (ed) Schmerz. Aesopus, Basel, pp 235–242

Lewit K (1977) Manuelle Medizin im Rahmen der medizinischen Rehabilitation. Urban und Schwarzenberg, München

Stöhr M (1980) Iatrogene Nervenläsionen. Thieme, Stuttgart

Swerdlow M (1978) Relief of intractable pain. Excerpta Medica, Amsterdam

Weber G (1970) Kopfschmerzen bei raumfordernden intracraniellen Prozessen. In: Cephalea, Bücherreihe Hommel, Adliswil, pp 185–199

Pain in the Cancer Patient as a Consequence of Therapy (Surgery, Radiotherapy, Chemotherapy)

W. Schreml

Abteilung für Innere Medizin III, Klinikum der Universität, Steinhövelstrasse 9, 7900 Ulm, FRG

Introduction

The problem of pain as a consequence of cancer therapy is of clinical importance in all subspecialities of oncology. A great number of side effects are imposed on the cancer patient by oncological surgery, radiotherapy, and systemic, in particular cytostatic therapy. Frequently, pain is only a secondary, short-lived symptom which accompanies therapy-induced complications. To a certain degree, side effects, including some pain or discomfort, are considered unavoidable by the physician, and the patient feels obliged to cope with them if he wants to qualify as cooperative. Generally, the oncological literature does not pay specific attention to pain as a consequence of cancer therapy, since, in most cases, it is trivial, of short duration, and can be easily managed.

On the other hand, cancer treatment may induce severe and chronic pain syndromes which are of similar impact on the quality of life as the devastating pain of advanced cancer; the true incidence of this type of complication is difficult to estimate from the literature. It should be of major concern for the therapist to avoid or minimize any chronic and severe side effects of therapy – including pain.

Therefore, this contribution is intended to formulate some of the aspects of therapy-induced pain in the cancer patient and to motivate the practising oncologist to devote appropriate attention to this problem in the planning of oncological therapy. Three topics will be considered:

1. The characteristics and range of therapy-induced pain
2. Specific pain syndromes observed in oncological surgery, radiotherapy, and systemic (primarily chemo-)therapy
3. Special (usually recently developed) therapeutic modalities and their impact on the patient in terms of pain

Methodology

Clinical Experience

The oncological therapist is usually well aware of the fact that his therapeutic measures impose a sometimes heavy load of side effects on his patients. Since the amelioration of side effects, such as therapy-induced pain, is a generally accepted task for any physician, relevant data about this problem are frequently omitted from clinical publications; therefore, the author has drawn information from his experience as a clinical oncologist, engaged primarily in systemic therapy, and from the experience of colleagues with whom he has discussed the problem.

Recent Results in Cancer Research. Vol. 89

Literature Search

The usual search in the literature, consulting periodicals, text books, and monographs, was performed, as was a search through DIMDI and CANCERNET[1].

Systematic Search in Cancer

All papers dealing with cancer therapy were screened in Vol. 48 (July–December 1981) and Vol. 49, Issues 1–6 (January–March 1982) of *Cancer*. From more than 4,000 pages all information on toxicity and side effects was checked for its relevance to therapy-induced pain.

This methodology implies that a comprehensive description of the problem could not be accomplished: the data are biased in favor of systemic therapy and of those treatment modalities which happen do have been reported recently in *Cancer*.

Characteristics and Range of Therapy-Induced Pain

Prevalence

It is difficult to estimate from the literature the prevalence of therapy-induced pain in cancer patients; pain is usually not listed as a separate side effect of oncological treatment. Eleven papers in *Cancer* Vol. 48 dealing with systemic or multimodal therapy list side effects in a tabular form (Table 1). Although pain is not listed in any of these tables, the described toxicities are known to be frequently accompanied by pain: infections, e.g., pneumonia, cystitis, cholangitis, and sepsis may be painful complications; gastrointestinal toxicity is accompanied by cramps or colicky pain; mucocutaneous side effects in the form of mouth ulceration constitute a problem of sometimes devastating somatic and psychological distress. Thus, painful episodes are likely symptoms in most of the listed entities. Therefore, although not specified, a high prevalence of therapy-induced pain is documented in these tables.

In a recent issue of *Seminars in Oncology* devoted to the toxicity of chemotherapy, Perry (1982), in addition to the complications shown in Table 1, lists hypersensitivity to cytotoxic drugs and dermatologic, reproductive, neoplastic, and developmental complications. Among these categories of toxicity, hypersensitivity and dermatologic complications may be accompanied by pain.

Although some pain will be experienced by the patient during cancer therapy, most episodes are short-lived and quite acceptable to the patient if he has been well informed about the treatment procedure and has confidence in the skill and care of the therapist. On the other hand, some patients are suffering from such heavy somatic and emotional problems that they are virtually incapable of tolerating any further discomfort. The pain of performing a venipuncture may be unacceptable, limiting further therapeutic measures.

In contrast to acute transient pain, therapy-induced chronic pain syndromes are of great importance to the final outcome of cancer therapy. Their frequency should be an essential

1 The help of Prof. G. Wagner, Institute of Documentation, Information and Statistics, Deutsches Krebsforschungszentrum, Heidelberg, is gratefully acknowledged

Table 1. Toxic effects recorded in tabular form in 11 papers on polychemo- or multimodal therapy studies, published in *Cancer* (Vol. 48, 1981)

Toxic effect	Frequency (total = 11)
Hematologic (infection, sepsis)	11
Gastrointestinal (nausea, vomiting, diarrhea, ileus)	9
Mucocutaneous (stomatitis, dermatitis)	6
Alopecia	6
Cardiopulmonary	5
Renal	3
Cystitis	3
Neurotoxicity	2

factor in designing treatment modalities. Giving a figure for the incidence of therapy-induced pain, if at all possible, would be meaningless without qualification. Of interest are the data from an anesthesiologic pain clinic to which only patients with severe and chronic pain are referred. Inoka et al. (1982) analyzed the etiology of pain in 60 cancer patients treated during 1982, of whom 13% suffered from therapy-induced pain.

Range of the Problem

One of the major difficulties in describing therapy-induced pain in cancer patients lies in the broad range of phenomena related to pain. Four parameters can be used to describe therapy-induced pain syndromes: time scale, pathophysiology, incidence, and impact on the patient (Table 2).

The first parameter ist the *time scale.* A painful event may sometimes acutely accompany a therapeutic measure, e.g., painful irritation of draining veins during injection of DTIC [4(5)-(3.3-dimethy(-1-triazeno)imidazol-5(4)carboxamide] or, quite plainly, the postoperative pain after surgical procedure. Other toxic effects, e.g., neurotoxicity of Vinca alcaloids, develop late during or after completion of therapy, or, with a particularly long delay, the late effects of radiation therapy. Perry (1982) differentiates "immediate", "early", "delayed", and "late" complications of chemotherapy. The time course of possible painful complications may be illustrated by the combined modality approach for Hodgkin's disease (Table 3). Of course, most of these complications are rare and not combined in one individual patient. At the far end of the time scale, the inducing of a secondary neoplasm, which takes about 5–15 years to develop, may be considered. It would be logical to consider any pain experienced from such a secondary tumor as "therapy-induced". This example documents the difficulty in limiting the scope of the problem.

The *pathophysiology* of therapy-induced pain constitutes a second parameter of broad range. Painful toxicity may be a direct consequence of a particular treatment modality; for example, the syndrome including fever, myalgia, bone pain, and chest pain has been observed as a direct effect of the cytostatic drug ara-C, and the term "ara-C syndrome" was

Table 2. Range of parameters of relevance in the description of therapy-induced pain, as illustrated by the examples given

I.	Time scale	
	Acute Irritation of draining veins during injection (e.g., DTIC)	Chronic Peripheral neuropathy (e.g., after vincristine)
II.	Pathophysiology	
	Direct "Ara-C Syndrome"	Indirect Steroid-induced aseptic necrosis of the hip
III.	Incidence	
	Frequent/predictable/unavoidable Mucositis, e.g., after antimetabolites	Infrequent/unpredictable/avoidable necrosis after paravasation (e.g., of adriamycin)
IV.	Impact on patient	
	Light E.g., transient postoperative pain, effectively controlled	Severe E.g., chronic painful neurotoxicity complicated by inability to walk

Table 3. Time course of side effects of treatment of Hodgkin's disease in some cases accompanied by pain

Modality	Immediate	Early	Delayed	Late
Surgical: Staging laparatomy with splenectomy	Postoperative pain	Subphrencial abscess		Intestinal obstruction
Radiotherapy: e.g., involed field (neck)		Parotitis, mucositis	Dry-mouth syndrome	Induration of musculature
Combination chemotherapy (Cyclophosphamide, vincristine, procarbacine, prednisone), repeated monthly courses	Irritation of vein at injection site	Mucositis, cystitis (cyclophosphamide)	Neurotoxicity (vincristine)	Aseptic bone necrosis; induction of secondary neoplasm

used (Castleberry et al. 1981). More often, pain is just one more or less aggravating symptom of a toxic reaction. For each of the toxic reactions listed in Table 1, a sequence of pathophysiological events can be described which leads to tissue damage with pain as a consequence.

Tissues with high proliferating activity are particularly sensitive to radiation and/or cytotoxic drugs, in particular the hemopoietic bone marrow, the mucosa of the gastrointestinal tract, the genitourinary system, and the skin. Damage to the hemopoietic tissue may cause anemia (consequence: e.g., headache), thrombopenia (consequence: e.g., painful muscle hematoma), or granulocytopenia (consequence: e.g., severe cellulitis, abscesses). Damage to the mucous membranes leads to ulceration and infection, which may be extremely painful and poorly healing, particularly when granulocytopenia is present. Inflammatory processes, e.g., radiotherapy-induced enteritis, are a frequent common denominator in the inducing of side effects; they may lead to the formation of scars and indurative changes in the tissue, again causing painful reactions.

Some cytotoxic agents exhibit a specific toxic effect. For instance, the neurotoxicity of Vinca alcaloids is characterized by myelin loss and axonal degeneration in peripheral nerves (Moress et al. 1967). The degradation products of the oxazaphosphorines (e.g., cyclophosphamide) are directly toxic to the mucosa of the urinary bladder. In some instances, rapid destruction of tumor mass with an accumulation of degradation products, hyperemia, changes in tissue pH, and swelling is considered as the mechanism for acute pain syndromes (Castleberry et al. 1981).

Incidence constitutes a clinically important parameter. Some painful toxicities are frequent, predictable, and/or unavoidable. For example, most cytotoxic agents, in particular the antimetabolites, induce mucositis. Aggressive polychemotherapy regimens for inducing remission of acute leukemia cannot be performed unless intensive supportive measures are instituted to reduce the severity and ameliorate the symptoms of mouth ulceration, infection, and bleeding; however, prevention of side effects is only rarely possible if effective therapy is attempted.

Other toxicities are infrequent and their occurrence in an individual patient is unpredictable. For example, pancreatitis as a consequence of asparaginase occurs in less than 15% of patients (Chabner and Myers 1982), but may be very painful and even life-threatening in a few afflicted persons. Sometimes, mistakes in cancer therapy may lead to painful complications, e.g., the paravasation of locally aggressive cytotoxic drugs. Adriamycin or vincristine may lead to necrosis and chronic nonhealing ulceration. Complications of surgery and radiotherapy follow the laws of probability established for the specific type of treatment.

In addition to the above parameters, pain as a subjective experience is greatly influenced in its severity and *impact on the patient* by psychological factors. A hopeful, cooperative state of mind may help a patient to tolerate even severe side effects of therapy without much suffering. On the other hand, a depressive patient with advanced cancer, who is already subject to chronic severe pain from his tumor, may not be able to tolerate any measure which could cause pain, however minimal it may be.

If these parameters of time scale, pathophysiology, incidence, and impact on the patient are considered, the question of therapy-induced pain becomes very broad and quite diffuse at its margins. Therefore, the following sections are directed to those phenomena in which the connection of pain and tumor treatment is characterized by some direct causal or pathophysiological mechanism which justifies the term "specific".

Specific Pain Syndromes

Surgery

There is little specificity connected with the complications of surgical procedures which could be attributed to the neoplastic disease; however, the extent of the surgical procedure which is aimed at removing the entire tumor and its possible regional metastases sometimes exceeds the limits observed for nononcological procedures, and the postoperative pain may, therefore, be more intensive than after other operations. As an example, Fig. 1 describes the case of a young patient with malignant teratoma of the testis in whom retroperitoneal lymphadenectomy was followed by a series of complications which induced long-lasting and severe pain. Considering the patients with osteosarcoma described by Beattie et al. (1975) in whom amputation of an extremity and (several) thoracotomies for

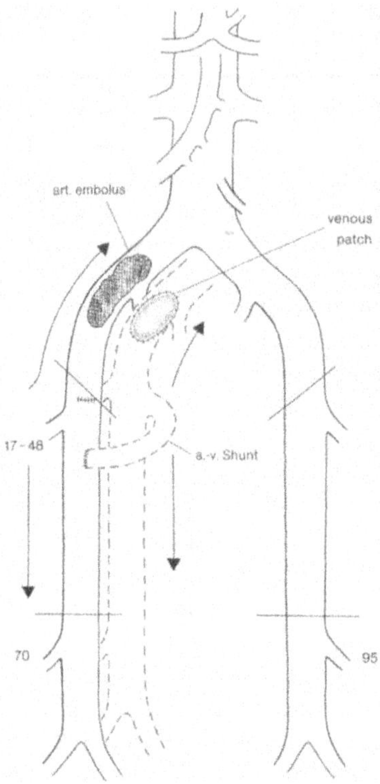

Fig. 1. Drawing of the operative situation after a complicated course of retroperitonal lymphadenectomy for a teratocarcinoma of the testis in a 20-year-old patient; during lymphadenectomy, the right external iliac vein was injured; 1 day later, thrombosis occurred in the iliac vein requiring thrombectomy; an arteriovenous shunt was performed to prevent further thrombus formation; on the following day, complete ischemia of the leg occurred as a consequence of embolization in the iliac artery, which again required embolectomy. As a consequence of ischemia, a painful compartment syndrome with nerve involvement developed in the lower leg. Postoperative complications, although rare, are unavoidable in the extensive surgical procedures for cancer treatment

removal of lung metastases were performed, it becomes evident that the fight for a cure must carry its toll of postoperative discomfort.

Foley (1979) and Bonica (1981) describe some chronic postsurgical pain syndromes. These syndromes follow mastectomy, thoracotomy, and radical neck dissection and are a late consequence of the operation distinct from postoperative pain. Ongoing activity of severed peripheral nerves with formation of small neuromas has been described as the cause of these pain syndromes (Wall and Gutnick 1974). These neurological pain episodes are aggravated by pressure, e.g., from garments and movements; therefore, involved joints are immobilized, leading to atrophy and muscular spasm with additional painful reactions. After amputation of a limb, stump pain and phantom limb pain may develop (Carlen et al. 1978) which are not specific for the cause of surgery, whether oncological or not.

Radiotherapy

Whereas complications of surgery are not specific for tumor therapy, side effects of radiotherapy are: the treatment of neoplastic diseases is the major domain of this therapeutic technique. The acute toxicity of ionizing radiation is directed toward the rapidly proliferating tissues, i.e., hematopoiesis, skin, mucous membranes. In a basic treatise on the principles of radiation therapy, Hellman (1982) lists necrosis, fibrosis, fistula formation, and nonhealing ulcerations among the dose-limiting late effects of radiotherapy.

An episode of acute radiation enteritis or proctocolitis with diarrhea, colicky abdominal pain, and nausea is experienced by the majority of patients following radiation of

Table 4. Radiotherapy studies recently published in *Cancer* with reference to (usually) painful side effects (n = number of patients)

Reference	Diagnosis	Type of treatment	Painful (usually) side effects
Choi and Doucette (1981)	Non-small cell bronchogenic carcinoma	Three modalities escalating to 60–64 Gy large field	Occasional mild to moderate retrosternal discomfort (esophagitis)
Catane et al. (1981)	small cell lung cancer	Seven schedules of combined radio- and chemotherapy	n = 71; severe esophagitis (14%) progressing to stricture (n=3); 24% therapy-related deaths
Borodon (1982)	Vulvo-vaginal cancer	Combined radiotherapy and surgery	n = 33; fistulas (15%); major necrosis (15%)
Hogan et al. (1982)	Carcinoma of the cervix	Radiotherapy after radical hysterectomy	n = 112; complications in 14%: cystitis, proctitis, enteritis, fistula, stricture, bladder perforation
Perez and Camel (1982)	Vaginal cancer	Stage-dependent radiotherapy	n = 134; fistulas, strictures, ulcers, etc. (9%)
Sealy et al. (1982)	Epidermoid lung cancer	Two fractionation schemes	n = 269; esophagitis (19%)

abdominal fields (Kinsella and Bloomer 1980). These authors summarize the experience with dose modifications and supportive measures used in order to minimize acute intestinal toxicity. Late bowel damage occurs in 5%–15% of patients, with 1%–2% showing severe damage (Kinsella and Bloomer 1980). In these patients, the symptoms of diarrhea and intermittent colicky abdominal pain begin from 6 to 18 months after radiotherapy and are progressive and chronic.

Brachial plexus lesions with edema of the arm are sometimes debilitatingly painful after surgery and radiotherapy of breast cancer, although modern operative and radiotherapeutic techniques have greatly reduced this complication by optimizing the relations of time, dose, and irradiated volume. Kori et al. (1981) reported that among 100 cancer patients with brachial plexus lesions, 22 had radiation injury. The severity of the pain induced by irradiation was less marked than that from tumor recurrence. Table 4 summarizes the incidence of radiation-induced complications, which are usually accompanied by pain, from studies recently reported in *Cancer*.

Radiation therapy is frequently used as part of a multimodal treatment strategy. In these situations, complications and pain are a consequence of toxic interactions. Typical examples are prophylactic radio- and chemotherapy of the central nervous system in leukemia and lymphoma and the side effects experienced during bone marrow transplantation. Both methods will be described in the following sections.

Table 5. Pain syndromes which are specific for certain systemic antineoplastic drugs

Reference	Drug	Comment
I. Cytostatic drugs		
Castleberry et al. (1981)	Ara-C	"Ara-C syndrome" = fever, myalgia, bone pain, chest pain, rash, conjunctivitis
O'Regan et al. (1973)	Methotrexate (Mtx)	Bone pain
Sandler et al. (1969)	Vinca alcaloids	Severe jaw pain; in children: myalgias, arthralgias
Campanacci et al. (1981)		Jaw pain in 60% of osteosarcoma patients,
Jackson et al. (1981)	Vincristine	Continuous infusion: 1/3 myalgias
Komp et al. (1980)	Vindesine	Jaw, neck, bone pain "common"
Lucas and Huang (1977)	Vinblastine	Acute pain in tumor area
Haas et al. (1977)	Methyl-CCNU	Sharp, severe pain in or close to the chest
Chabner and Myers (1982)	DTIC, Bleomycin	Flu-like syndrome with headache, malaise, fever
Pottage et al. (1978) Soukop et al. (1978) Von Hoff et al. (1982)	5-Fluorouracil (5-FU)	Angina pectoris-like syndrome
Chabner and Myers (1982)	Mithramycin	Headache, myalgias
Land et al. (1972) Weetman and Baehner (1974) Chabner and Myers (1982)	Asparaginase	Pancreatitis (15%)
Altman et al. (1982)	Ara-C	Pancreatitis (after previous asparaginase)
Griffin and Garnick (1981) Hammersly et al. (1973) Wasserman (1976) Doroshow et al. (1981)	5-FU, BCNU, Highdose Mtx	Eye symptoms: conjunctivitis, burning sensation, pain, itching
II. Hormones		
Rotstein and Good (1957)	Cortison	"Pseudo-rheumatism"
Ihde and DeVita (1975) Sweet et al. (1976) Engel et al. (1981)	Cortison	Aseptic bone necrosis (hip), 1.3%, 3.3% and 1.6% of patients with Hodgkin's disease
Plotkin et al. (1978) Arnold et al. (1979) Veldhuis and Santen (1979) Wallach (1979)	Tamoxifen	"Flare": pain exacerbating in tumor-involved area (breast carcinoma)
Disaia and Morrow (1978)	Megestrol acetate	"Carpal tunnel"-like syndrome
III. Immune–Modulator		
Schreml et al. (1980)	Levamisole	Joint and muscle pain, swelling of hands and feet (adjuvant chemo-immunotherapy of breast cancer)

Systemic Therapy

In recent years, new cytotoxic drugs with high effectiveness and high toxicity have been developed and integrated into treatment schedules frequently comprising more than one drug (polychemotherapy) or additional surgical and radiotherapeutic techniques (multimodal therapy). The primary toxicities and their contribution to pain experienced by the cancer patient have been discussed above (Table 1). In addition, several pain syndromes have been described for individual cytostatic agents, for hormones used in cancer treatment, and for immune modulators. Most of these syndromes are quite infrequent; however, knowledge of them helps to relieve the anxiety of the afflicted patient and to institute appropriate means of treatment. Table 5 summarizes some of the reported pain syndromes.

One important aspect of polychemotherapy is suppression of the immune system; this may lead to the development of infectious disease, e.g, herpes zoster with its sometimes very tiresome and untreatable neurological pain (Reboul et al. 1978). In a recent study, Hyams et al. (1982) reported that lactose malabsorption developed in nine of 27 children during combined chemotherapy; they drew attention to the fact that the use of a high-caloric milk-containing diet may precipitate cramps and diarrhea. This study documents that careful evaluation of toxic effects may help to reduce the incidence of pain during cancer therapy.

Neurotoxicity of cancer therapy requires special consideration, since it is frequently associated with pain; deep, lancinating pain is one of the symptoms of peripheral neuropathy, while neurotoxic manifestations on the gut are frequently accompanied by

Table 6. Therapy-induced neurologic syndroms associated with pain. For review see Weiss et al. (1974) and Kaplan and Wiernik (1982)

Drug	Symptoms
I. Systemic therapy	
Vincaalcaloids, in particular Vincristine	Peripheral neuropathy with deep, lancinating pain (6–8%) Pain in jaw, neck, and shoulder Abdominal colicky cramps with constipation (33–45%)
Vincristine plus VP–16 (Thant et al. 1982)	Increased neurotoxicity (up to 100% at higher doses)
Procarbacine	Myalgias in proximal muscle groups
Misonidazole (Phillips et al. 1981)	Peripheral neuropathy (50%), sometimes with debilitating pain
II. Intrathecal prophylaxis/treatment	
Methotrexate i.t.	Headache, stiff neck, nausea (5–50%)
Mtx/Ara-C, combined with irradiation of CNS (Freeman et al. 1973, Hustu et al. 1973, Wasserstrom et al. 1982) or with i.t.^{198}Au (Metz et al. 1982)	Acute meningoencephalopathy with headache, fever, confusion, apathy syndrome

colicky cramps. Headache is a common problem in prophylactic and therapeutic treatment of the central nervous system by radiotherapy and intrathecal cytotoxic drugs. Several aspects of neurotoxicity are summarized in Table 6 on the basis of the reviews by Weiss et al. (1974) and Kaplan and Wiernik (1982), and more recently published data.

Special Therapeutic Modalities

Recent developments in cancer research have introduced new techniques of therapy, some of which involve a high degree of sophistication. Such recent developments may be induced by the emergence of new concepts, e.g., immunomodulation, hyperthermia, and bone marrow transplantation, or may be a consequence of different ways of application for established modalities, e.g., intra-arterial or local application of cytotoxic drugs. These new modalities are sometimes accompanied by severe pain syndromes. Several examples are briefly described in Table 7.

For eligible patients in remission from acute leukemia, bone marrow transplantation offers a more than 50% chance of cure (Thomas et al. 1979; Blume et al. 1981). This technique pushes physicians to the limits of their skill and involvement and patients to the limits of their tolerance. Major complications are inevitable during the course of bone-marrow transplantation (Fig. 2) and some may cause severe pain. The medical and psychological management of patients with bone marrow transplants represents a great advance also in supportive care and control of therapy-induced pain.

Table 7. Special therapeutic methods which may be connected with painful toxicities

Reference	Type of therapy	Symptoms
Balch et al. (1982)	Immune stimulation (BCG; C. parvum)	C. p.intracutaneously: 41% (n = 260) local pain/abscesses; 4% headache
Hilal et al. (1981)		C. p. IV (n = 38) : 93% "flu-like" syndrome, 71% headache
Watring et al. (1978)	Local chemotherapy	Bleomycin in vulva carcinoma: 7/7 local pain
Wallach (1978) Harbecke (1980)	Intrapleural tetracycline	Induction of painful inflammation aimed at obliteration in malignant effusion; may be ameliorated by local anesthetics
Mavligit et al. (1981)	Intra-arterial chemotherapy	Local pain in infusion area
Manning et al. (1982)	Hyperthermia (plus irradiation)	2nd and 3rd degree burns (4/26)
Kato et al. (1981)	Arterial embolization, arterial chemoembolization	Postembolization pain. Renal chemoembolisation: high fever, severe local pain (4/4). Hypogastric artery: painful necroses in gluteal area (5/9)

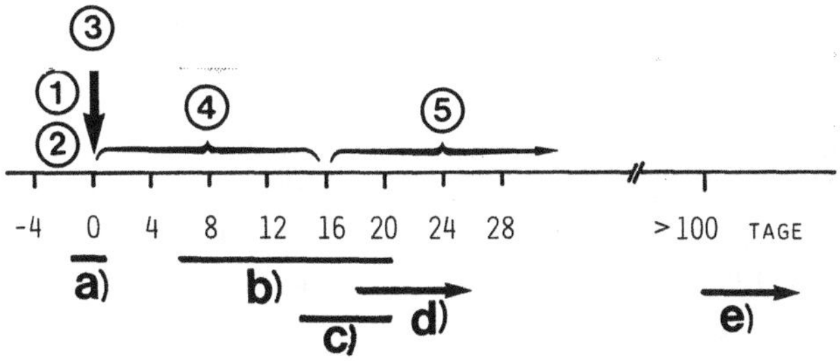

Fig. 2. Schematic course of bone-marrow transplantation used to attempt cure in acute leukemia patients. ① and ② Intensive conditioning with cytostatic drugs (cytoxan) and total-body irradiation to ensure engraftment of transplanted bone marrow and eradication of acute leukemia. ③ Bone-marrow transplantation. ④ Phase of bone-marrow aplasia and take of transplanted marrow; ⑤ regeneration of normal blood cell formation. During the course of therapy, periods of toxic side effects may cause severe pain: a) parotitis beginning 6–18 h after irradiation; usually controllable by symptomatic techniques; cystitis as a consequence of cytoxan is avoidable with adequate support (fluid; mesna); b) mouth ulceration; esophagitis: consequence of chemo- and radiotherapy; agranulocytosis usually prevents healing for approximately 2 weeks; very painful, sometimes requiring regular narcotic medication; c) irradiation dermatitis may develop with painful scaling of the skin; d) acute graft-versus-host disease may occur with severe diarrhea, abdominal cramps and tenesmus; e) chronic graft-versus-host disease may be accompanied by abdominal cramps

Discussion

Some of the pathophysiological and clinical aspects of therapy-induced pain in cancer patients have been reviewed. The importance of these considerations is defined by the psychological consequences and the impact of pain on the cancer patient. Psychological factors play a major role in cancer pain (Chapman 1979). Pain induces anxiety, depression, and anger. If pain is caused by therapeutic measures, the physical and psychological tolerance of a patient may be heavily strained.

In general, the oncologist is always obliged to make his therapeutic decision by weighing the achievable goal against the cost of therapy in terms of toxic side effects. This decision can be made only if the personality of the patient and his physiological and psychological tolerance are carefully taken into account. Most importantly, the therapist must be prepared to give optimal support, both somatic and psychological, during all phases of treatment.

Consideration of the type of therapy-induced pain is important. Acute, short-lived discomfort is usually well tolerated if the patient has been fully informed in advance, if his complaints are taken seriously by the therapist, and if analgesic measures are effectively instituted. Of course, a patient motivated to undergo a therapy with curative potential will cope much more easily with its side effects than would a patient who knows that his disease is in an advanced stage. The examples of testicular tumor (Fig. 1) and of bone marrow transplantation (Fig. 2) show what load of side effects can be imposed on a patient if cure is an achievable goal. When a bone marrow transplantation is considered, the group of experts carefully examine all conditions required for a positive outcome. The psychological situation of the patient, his potential to undergo several weeks of severe side effects, and the support that may be expected from family and friends are major factors in considering bone marrow transplantation.

The individual differences between patients must be considered. Some patients, exhausted by tumor symptoms and the side effects of prior therapy, will not tolerate the discomfort of rather benign treatment. On the other hand, a young patient with a strong will to live may be motivated to withstand the side effects of a much heavier treatment modality. Therefore, no mechanistic rule can be given for the judgement as to how much transient side effects can be accepted for an individual patient; it is a process of weighing arguments in close cooperation with the patient.

The judgement becomes even more difficult when chronic, long-lasting pain syndromes are considered. Usually, these are quite infrequent and not predictable. Every effort has to be made to search for predisposing factors in a patient, to watch carefully for early symptoms, and to institute appropriate measures as soon as possible. Discontinuation of treatment at the beginning of suggestive symptoms frequently prevents the development of serious late effects.

Finally, the possibility of side effects such as pain imposes the obligation on the oncologist to search for improved therapeutic modalities. As a first step, the pathophysiology of the side effects of various treatment modalities should be explored. An example has been given above (Hyams et al. 1982): the development of lactose malabsorption has been observed during combination chemotherapy in children. As a consequence, a diet with lactose restriction may ameliorate the symptoms of abdominal colicky pain. It was the pathophysiological research on intestinal function that led to a clinically relevant treatment modification. Research continues in many fields of oncology with the aim of minimising side effects. For example, newly developed Vinca alcaloids (vindesine) show reduced neurotoxicity, and supportive measures have been improved, e.g., by providing granulocyte substitution in the granulopenic patient. Through this latter measure, severe infections and ulcerations can be ameliorated for a period of time. The goal of avoiding painful side effects should be an incentive for continuing research in clinical oncology.

References

Altman AJ, Dinndorf P, Quinn JJ (1982) Acute pancreatitis in association with cytosine arabinoside therapy. Cancer 49: 1384–1386

Arnold DJ, Markham MJ, Hacker S (1979) Tamoxifen flare. JAMA 241: 2506

Balch CM, Smalley RV, Bartolucci AA, Burns D, Presant CA, Durant JR, and the Southeastern Cancer Study Group (1982) A randomized prospective clinical trial of adjuvant C. parvum immunotherapy in 260 patients with clinically localized melanoma (stage I): prognostic factors, analysis and preliminary results of immunotherapy. Cancer 49: 1079–1084

Beattie EJ, Martini N, Rosen G (1975) The management of pulmonary metastases in children with oesteogenic sarcoma with surgical resection combined with chemotherapy. Cancer 35: 618–621

Blume KG, Spruce WE, Forman SJ, Wolf JL, Farbstein MJ, Scott EB, Fahey JL (1981) Bone marrow transplantation for acute leukemia. N Engl J Med 305: 101–103

Bonica JJ (1981) Cancer pain. In: Klastersky J, Staquet MJ (eds) Medical complications in cancer patients. Raven, New York, pp 87–115

Boronow RC (1982) Combined therapy as an alternative to exenteration for locally advanced vulvo-vaginal cancer: rationale and results. Cancer 49: 1085–1091

Campanacci M, Bacci G, Bertoni F, Picci P, Minutillo A, Franceschi C (1981) The treatment of osteosarcoma of the extremities: twenty year's experience at the Istituto Ortopedico Rizzoli. Cancer 48: 1569–1581

Carlen PL, Wall PD, Nadvorna H, Steinbach T (1978) Phantom limbs and related phenomena in recent traumatic amputations. Neurology 28: 211–217

Castleberry RP, Christ WM, Holbrook T, Malluh A, Gaddy D (1981) The cytosine arabinoside (Ara-C) syndrome. Med Pediatr Oncol 9: 257–264

Catane R, Lichtner A, Lee YJ, Brereton HD, Schwade JG, Glatstein E (1981) Small-cell lung cancer: analysis of treatment factors contributing to prolonged survival. Cancer 48: 1936–1943

Chabner BA, Myers CE (1982) Clinical pharmacology of cancer chemotherapy. In: DeVita VT, Hellman S, Rosenberg SA (eds) Cancer: Principles and practice. Lippincott, Philadelphia, pp 156–197

Chapman CR (1979) Psychologic and behavioral aspects of cancer pain. In: Bonica JJ, Ventafridda V (eds) Advances in pain research, vol 2. Raven, New York, pp 45–56

Choi NCH, Doucette JA (1981) Improved survival of patients with unresectable non-small-cell bronchogenic carcinoma by an innovated high-dose en-bloc radiotherapeutic approach. Cancer 48: 101–109

Disaia PJ, Morrow CP (1978) Unusual side effect of megestrol acetate. Am J Obstet Gynecol 129: 460–461

Doroshow JH, Locker GY, Gaasterland DE, Hubbard SB, Young RC, Myers RC (1981) Ocular irritation from high-dose methotrexate therapy: pharmacokinetics of drug in the tear film. Cancer 48: 2158–2162

Engel IA, Straus DJ, Lacher M, Lane J, Smith J (1981) Osteonecrosis in patients with malignant lymphoma: a review of twenty-five cases. Cancer 48: 1245–1250

Foley KM (1979) Pain syndromes in patients with cancer. In: Bonica JJ, Ventafridda V (eds) Advances in pain research and therapy, vol 2. Raven, New York, pp 59–75

Freeman JE, Johnston PGB, Voke JM (1973) Somnolence after prophylactic cranial irradiation in children with acute lymphoblastic leucemia. Br Med J IV: 523–525

Griffin JD, Garnick MB (1981) Eye toxicity of cancer chemotherapy: a review of the literature. Cancer 48: 1539–1549

Haas CD, Stephens RL, Leite CJ, Goodwin JW, Hoogstraten B (1977) Unexpected pain syndrome during a phase I study of i.v. methyl-CCNU. Cancer Treat Rep 61: 1413–1415

Hammersly J, Luce JK, Florentz TR, Burkholder MM (1973) Excessive lacrimation from fluorouracil treatment. JAMA 225: 747–748

Harbecke RG (1980) Intrapleurally given tetracycline with lindocaine. JAMA 244: 1899–1900

Hellman S (1982) Principles of radiation therapy. In: DeVita VT, Hellman S, Rosenberg SA (eds) Cancer: Principles and practice of oncology. Lippincott, Philadelphia, pp 103–131

Hilal E, Pinsky CM, Hirshaut Y, Wanebo HJ, Hansen JA, Braun DW, Fortner JG, Oettgen HF (1981) Surgical adjuvant therapy of malignant melanoma with corynebacterium parvum. Cancer 48: 245–251

Hogan WM, Littman P, Griner L, Miller CL, Mikuta JJ (1982) Results of radiation therapy given after radical hysterectomy. Cancer 49: 1278–1285

Hustu HO, Aur RJA, Verzosa MS, Simone JV, Pinkel D (1973) Prevention of central nervous system leucemia by irradiation. Cancer 32: 585–597

Hyams JS, Batrus CL, Grand RJ, Sallan SE (1982) Cancer chemotherapy-induced lactose malabsorption in children. Cancer 49: 646–650

Ihde DC, DeVita VT (1975) Osteonecrosis of the femoral heads in patients with lymphoma treated with intermittent combination chemotherapy. Cancer 36: 1585–1588

Inoka PJ, Kossmann B, Dick W, Bowdler I, Schleinzer W (1982) Schmerzursachenanalyse bei Krebspatienten in der Schmerzambulanz. Anaesthesist 31: 651 (abstract)

Jackson DV, Sethi VS, Spurr CL, Willard V, White DR, Richards F, Stuart JJ, Muss HB, Cooper MR, Homesley HD, Jobson VW, Castle MC (1981) Intravenous vincristine infusion: phase I trial. Cancer 48: 2559–5564

Kaplan RS, Wiernik P (1982) Neurotoxicity of antineoplastic drugs. Semin Oncol 9: 103–130

Kato T, Nemoto R, Mori H, Takahashi M, Harada M (1981) Arterial chemoembolization with mitomycin C microcapsules in the treatment of primary or secondary carcinoma of the kidney, liver, bone and intrapelvic organs. Cancer 48: 674–680

Kinsella TJ, Bloomer WD (1981) Tolerance of the intestine to radiation therapy. Surg Gynecol Obstet 151: 273–284

Komp D, Vats T, Shepherd DA, Vietti T, Hoogstraten B, Haas CD (1980) Phase I evaluation of vindesine in children: a Southwest Oncology Group pilot study. Med Pediatr Oncol 8: 243–250

Kori SH, Foley KM, Posner JB (1981) Brachial plexus lesions in patients with cancer: 100 cases. Neurology (Minneap) 31: 45–50

Land VJ, Sutow WW, Fernbach DJ, Lane DM, Williams TE (1972) Toxicity of l-asparaginase in children with advanced leucemia. Cancer 30: 339–347

Lucas VS, Huang AT (1978) Vinblastine – related pain in tumors. Cancer Treat Rep 61: 1735–1736

Manning MR, Cetas TL, Miller RC, Oleson JR, Connor WG, Gerner EW (1982) Clinical hyperthermia: results of a phase I trial employing hyperthermia alone or in combination with external beam or interstitial radiotherapy. Cancer 49: 205–216

Mavligit GM, Benjamin R, Patt YZ, Jaffe N, Chuang V, Wallace S, Murray J, Ayala A, Johnston S, Hersh EM, Calvo DB III (1981) Intra-arterial cis-platinum for patients with inoperable skeletal tumors. Cancer 48: 1–4

Metz O, Stoll W, Plenert W (1982) Meningosis prophylaxis with intrathecal ^{198}Au-colloid and methotrexate in childhood acute lymphocytic leucemia. Cancer 49: 224–228

Moress GR, D'Agostino AN, Jarcho LW (1967) Neuropathy in lymphoblastic leukemia treated with vincristine. Arch Neurol 16: 377–384

O'Regan S, Melhorn DK, Newman AJ (1973) Methotrexate-induced bone pain in childhood leucemia. Am J Dis Child 126: 489–490

Perez CA, Camel HM (1982) Long-term follow-up in radiation therapy of carcinoma of the vagina. Cancer 49: 1308–1315

Perry MC (1982) Chemotherapy, toxicity, and the clinician. Semin Oncol 9: 1–4

Phillips TL, Wasserman TH, Johnson RJ, Levin VA, Van Raalte G (1981) Final report on the United States phase I clinical trial of the hypoxic cell radiosensitizer, misonidazole (Ro-07-0582; NSC No 261037). Cancer 48: 1697–1704

Plotkin D, Lechner JJ, Junge WE, Rosen PJ (1978) Tomaxifen flare in advanced breast cancer. JAMA 240: 2644–2646

Pottage A, Holt S, Lutgade S, Langlands AO (1978) Fluorouracil cardiotoxicity. Br Med J I: 547

Reboul F, Donaldson SS, Kaplan HS (1978) Herpes zoster and varicella infections in children with Hodgkin's disease. Cancer 41: 95–99

Rotstein J, Good RA (1957) Steroid pseudorheumatism. Arch Intern Med 99: 545–555

Sandler SG, Tobin W, Henderson ES (1969) Vincristine-induced neuropathy: a clinical study of fifty leucemic patients. Neurology (Minneap) 19: 367–374

Schreml W, Betzler M, Lang M, Lohrmann HP, Kubitza P, Schlag P, Flad HD, Herfarth C, Heimpel H (1980) Adjuvant intermittent chemo-immunotherapy of breast cancer. A prospective study. In: Mouridsen HT, Palshof T (eds) Breast cancer, experimental and clinical aspects. Pergamon, Oxford, pp 165–168

Sealy R, Lagakos S, Barkley T, Ryall R, Tucker RD, Lee RE, Ehlers G (1982) Radiotherapy of regional epidermoid carcinoma of the lung: a study in fractionation. Cancer 49: 1338–1345

Soukop M, McVie JG, Calman KC (1978) Fluorouracil cardiotoxicity. Br Med J I: 1422

Sweet DL, Roth DG, Desser RK, Miller RB, Ultmann JE (1976) Avascular necrosis of the femoral head with combination therapy. Ann Intern Med 85: 67–68

Thant M, Hawley RJ, Smith MT, Cohen MH, Minna JD, Bunn PA, Ihde DC, West W, Matthews MJ (1982) Possible enhancement of vincristine polyneuropathy by VP-16. Cancer 49: 859–864

Thomas ED, Buckner CD, Clift RA, Fefer A, Johnson FL, Neiman PE, Sale GE, Sanders JE, Singer JW, Shulman H, Storb R, Weiden PL (1979) Marrow transplantation for acute nonlymphoblastic leucemia in first remission. N Engl J Med 301: 597–599

Veldhuis JD, Santen RJ (1979) Tamoxifen flare. JAMA 241: 2506–2507

Von Hoff DD, Rozencweig M, Piccart M (1982) The cardiotoxicity of anticancer agents. Semin Oncol 9: 23–33

Wall PD, Gutnick M (1974) Ongoing activity in peripheral nerves: the physiology and pharmacology of impulses originating from neuroma. Exp Neurol 43: 580–593

Wallach HW (1978) Intrapleural therapy with tetracycline and lindocaine for malignant effusion. Chest 73: 246

Wallach HW (1979) Tamoxifen flare. JAMA 242: 27

Wasserman TH (1976) The nitrosoureas: an outline of clinical schedules and toxic effects. Cancer Treat Rep 60: 709–711

Wasserstrom WR, Glass JP, Posner JB (1982) Diagnosis and treatment of leptomeningeal metastases from solid tumors: experience with 90 patients. Cancer 49: 759–772

Watring WG, Roberts JA, Lagasse LD, Berman ML, Ballon SC, Moore JG, Schlesinger RE (1978) Treatment of recurrent Paget's disease of the vulva with topical bleomycin. Cancer 41: 10–11

Weetman RM, Baehner RL (1974) Latent onset of clinical pancreatitis in children receiving l-asparaginase therapy. Cancer 34: 780–785

Weiss HD, Walker MD, Wiernik PH (1974) Neurotoxicity of commonly used antineoplastic agents. N Engl J Med 291: 75–81, 127–133

Control of Cancer Pain with Analgesics Acting in the Central Nervous System

R. Wörz

Schmerz-Zentrum Mainz, Auf der Steig 14–16, 6500 Mainz, FRG

Introduction

Optimal control of cancer pain requires that the problem of pain be accorded a significance of its own and that it is seen in its complexity. In the context of advanced metastatic malignancies, pain is not only a symptom but also a force with a series of pathophysiologic, psychopathologic, and social consequences (Bonica 1979). Facultatively, we find muscular tension, immobility, disturbances of respiratory and cardiovascular function, inhibition of gastrointestinal motility, disorders of sleep, depressed mood, and misanthropic behavior extending to lamentation, moaning, and crying. These effects of pain may be negatively combined with other manifestations of cancer. For example, lack of appetite due to malignancy can be intensified by pain and thus may contribute to the progress of cachexia by inadequate food intake. In therapy, besides the *pathophysiology* of pain, its *sequelae* as well as its *psychodynamics* and the *behavior* of the patient have thus also to be considered.

Therapy of Cancer Pain with Morphine

Due to its excellent *analgesic action,* morphine has retained its importance in the treatment of carcinoma pain (Houde 1979; Twycross 1980; Vere 1978). Morphine can be applied both orally and parenterally. In chronic persisting cancer pain, the oral route of application has several definite advantages: The nonterminally ill patient is independent of injections from the physician or the nurse. In consequence, his autonomy and dignity are preserved to a better degree and regression is avoided. An effective steady state of plasma and tissue concentration of the analgesic due to continuous absorption involves less toxic risks than peak-and-valley concentrations resulting from injections.

The greatest disadvantages of morphine, which limit its application, are the frequently occurring undesired *side effects* as compiled in Table 1. At a therapeutic dosage, morphine gives rise to *tiredness,* to reduced ability to concentrate and, in some cases, to apathy in persons not used to it. Only a small proportion of the subjects report an improvement of mood or *euphoria* and hallucinations occur in rare cases. If previously intolerable pain is reduced by the analgesic action, then this leads to a reduction of the algogenic psychosyndrome which is characterized by dysphoric-melancholic mood, heightened irritability and restriction of experience capacity and interest exclusively in the constant pain. Moreover, frequent real anxiety plays a role in carcinoma patients. A substantial improvement of the patient's subjective condition thus occurs due to the reduction of pain.

Recent Results in Cancer Research. Vol. 89

Table 1. Main properties of morphine

Analgesic effect
Psychotropic effects
Sedation
Euphoria
Excitation of the vomiting center
Inhibition of the respiratory center
Spastic constipation
Disorder of micturition
Dependence potential
Tolerance development

On the other hand, morphine stimulates the chemoreceptor trigger zone in the area postrema of the medulla oblongata, the center for vomiting. Consequently, *nausea and vomiting* occur in many patients and a deterioration in their subjective condition is associated with this. Following the subcutaneous administration of 15 mg morphine, nausea was observed in 40% of outpatients and vomiting in 15% (Jaffe and Martin 1980).

The reluctance of physicians to administer opiates is partly due to the fact that death from respiratory arrest can occur with overdosage. Most reported cases involve intravenous application of heroin by addicts. The blood-brain barrier is more permeable for heroin than for morphine, so the danger of respiratory arrest is less great with morphine. When it is given *orally,* the risk of *respiratory effect is negligible* at therapeutic doses.

In long-term application of morphine, a *spastic constipation* has to be taken into account from the beginning. This may be due to the action of morphine on the smooth musculature in the gastrointestinal tract, owing to increase in tone in the duodenum, jejunum, and ileum. In addition, the peristaltic waves in the intestine are reduced with simultaneous increase of tone. The tone of the ileocecal valve and the anal sphincter is also raised (Jaffe and Martin 1980).

In some carcinoma patients, morphine leads to *disorders of micturition* via an increase of smooth muscle tone and of the contraction amplitudes in the lower part of the ureter and the detrusor of the urinary bladder. The tone of the sphincter is raised. In pain patients who suffer from disorders of micturition, synthetic opiates should be preferred from the beginning, since their action on the smooth musculature is less pronounced: this is the case with pethidine, tramadol, and also with the partial agonist buprenorphine.

Morphine and its derivatives can lead to psychological and physical *dependence.* In carcinoma patients, above all in those with limited life expectancy, it is inappropriate to apply the unscientific (because it is undefinable) and emotional term "addiction." Dependence obtains significance in carcinoma patients at the point where it can impede the change to another method of therapy. If morphine derivatives are only applied in the advanced stages, this problem plays a minor role.

The *development of tolerance* is of greater clinical interest. It is manifested in carcinoma patients either by the need for higher single doses in the course of time or in a decrease of the duration of action (e.g., from 4 h at the beginning to 3 h). In patients not used to opioids, morphine should be given at 4-h intervals initially. If tolerance develops, a 3 h rhythm is possible without difficulties. At the same time, the dosage can be increased. At the beginning of treatment, single doses of 5–10 mg should be administered orally and then increased to the dose range required for analgesia. In view of the wide spectrum of undesired side effects of morphine, substances have been sought for a long time in which these are present to a smaller extent or not at all.

Novel Substances

Tramadol

This is a pure opiate agonist, but it has some important advantages over morphine. According to information available so far, tramadol has no effects on the cardiovascular system and does not cause a respiratory depression at clinical doses. Constipation and disturbance of micturition are less frequent than with morphine. However, tramadol leads to sedation in the form of fatigue and sleepiness in about two-thirds of the patients at clinical dosage, whereas it does not often result in excitement and mood elevation. Sedation occurs more frequently than euphoria, roughly in the ratio 10:1. Similar to the situation with pentazocine, a euphoric effect is more likely to be expected once more at a higher dosage. Hyperhydrosis is found as the second most frequent undesired effect, and nonspecific weakness takes the third place (Arend et al. 1978). An open trial in 213 terminal malignancy patients did not show any clinically significant tolerance or dependence within a period of 3 weeks (Flohé et al. 1978).

Nefopam

Nefopam is a centrally (but not spinally) acting analgesic (Zimmermann 1979) with a novel activity profile. At clinical dosage, it does not lead to sedation, but rather to a slight stimulation and it brings about neither a respiratory nor a circulatory depression (Schietzl 1979). Further advantages over morphine derivatives are the lack of tolerance development and the absence of danger of dependence. The therapeutic success rate in carcinoma pain has been described as 67.6% (Cronheim and Thiede 1979). In a double-blind study, nefopam at a dose of 60 mg per os proved to have roughly the same analgesic efficacy in carcinoma pain as 50 mg oral pentazocine. There were important differences in the side effects of the two substances: whereas the patients rarely reported fatigue and retching after administration of pentazocine, they complained somewhat more frequently of gastric symptoms after nefopam (De Thibault de Boesinghe 1978).

Opiate Agonist–Antagonists

The opiate agonist–antagonists or partial agonists possess a lower dependence and tolerance potential than morphine. Some also differ from morphine derivatives in other respects. In carcinoma pain, pentazocine and buprenorphine are established as important alternatives to the pure opiate agonists.

Pentazocine

The efficacy of *pentazocine* in carcinoma pain has been verified in several studies (Beaver et al. 1966; Cabanne et al. 1972; Frutschnigg 1973; Kleibel 1972; De Thibault de Boesinghe 1978). An important advantage is that spasmogenic effects occur more rarely than with morphine. It has been shown in animal studies and in clinical application that pentazocine can provoke withdrawal syndromes in opiate dependence (Brauchle 1971; Hoffmeister 1968). The dependence and tolerance potential proved to be clearly lower than with morphine (Eckmann et al. 1975). When applied parenterally, 50 mg pentazocine correspond to about 10 mg morphine in analgesic efficacy (Beaver et al. 1966; Frankendahl and Kjellgren 1971). However, both substances must be given at a roughly three times higher dose orally than parenterally. The most frequent side effects of pentazocine in carcinoma patients are tiredness and sleepiness. Compared with morphine, euphoria occurs more rarely. Pentazocine lowers the hallucination threshold, so that visual or auditory hallucinations can occur at high dosage. Dysphoria occurs more frequently than with pure opiate agonists (Jaffe and Martin 1980). After these psychotropic effects, nausea is the second most frequent side effect. Emesis can also occur at clinical dosage (Beaver et al. 1966; Frutschnigg 1973; Jaffe and Martin 1980).

Tilidine

This is an opiate agonist which is commercially available in a combination with naloxone. This preparation has proved to be a highly effective analgesic in the treatment of carcinoma pain (Groh et al. 1971). Tilidine leads to constipation, disorders of micturition, and tiredness more rarely than morphine. It was previously discredited because of abuse by opiate addicts. In 1978, when the manufacturer mixed tilidine with naloxone (Valoron N) in the ratio 50 : 4 mg, the abuse of tilidine disappeared. A clinical comparison of tilidine and tilidine-naloxone did not reveal any significant difference in the relief of cancer pain (Krell and Hanke 1979).

Buprenorphine

This drug proved to be a potent analgesic in cancer pain. An important advantage over morphine is that it rarely leads to constipation and disorders of micturition. The most prominent undesired effects are tiredness and sleepiness, dryness of the mouth, and nausea. Vomiting occurs not rarely (Robbie 1979). Since carcinoma patients frequently suffer from nausea and emesis of other origin, it is a clinically important advantage that buprenorphine can also be administered sublingually.

Guidelines for the Application of Centrally Acting Analgesics

Control of cancer pain is not possible without taking into account the *dimension of time*. Some empirical evidence to document these observations is compiled in Table 2. The table shows the diagnoses in 50 malignancy patients who were referred to us for pain therapy. Without exception, they had incurable diseases at an advanced stage. None of these patients had lymphoma or leukemia. The diagnosis had been obtained from 2 weeks up to a maximum of 125 months (median: 40 months) previously. Patients were aged from 21 to 81 years (median: 60 years). In two cases, violent attacks of pain occurred. In 48 patients, there was continuous pain with a duration of from 1 to 36 months (median: 9 months). The intensity of pain was estimated by the patients on the visual analog scale[1] 24–98 (mean:

1 The visual analog scale is a horizontal line 100 mm long with the boundary values 0 = free of pain and 100 = worst conceivable pain, which would lead to suicide within minutes. The patient himself assesses the intensity of his pain by a vertical line on this scale

Table 2. Cancer pain and the kind of tumor

Diagnosis	Male	Female	Total
Bronchial carcinoma	5	–	5
Mammary carcinoma	–	5	5
Colorectal carcinoma	8	6	14
Bladder carcinoma	2	2	4
Prostate carcinoma	5	–	5
Collum carcinoma	–	5	5
Vulvar carcinoma	–	3	3
Bone metastases in unknown primary tumor	2	2	4
Other malignancies	3	2	5
Total	25	25	50

The kind of tumor in 50 patients who were referred to the Pain Center in Mainz for therapy of pain

Table 3. Cancer pain and analgesics used

Kind of analgesic	Patients
Peripherally acting	11
Centrally acting	26
Application of both kinds	13
Total	50

The kind of analgesics employed so far in 50 cancer pain patients admitted to the Pain Center at Mainz

Table 4. Regimen of application of analgesics

Administration	No. of patients	Intervals too long
On request	19	
Regular time schedule	31	17
Total	50	

Principle of analgesic application employed so far in 50 patients with incurable malignancies admitted to the Pain Center at Mainz

62). At the time of referral to the Pain Center in Mainz, all 50 patients were being treated with analgesics (Table 3). For various reasons, in all cases the treatment results were unsatisfactory, so that admission to our Pain Center was indicated. The unsuccesful treatment methods are compiled in Table 4. These figures reflect the tendency to treat states of pain resulting from advanced malignancies with centrally active analgesics. In some cases, a peripherally acting analgesic was indeed unnecessarily replaced by a centrally acting analgesic when the pain syndrome was recognized to be due to cancer. The correct application (especially of centrally acting analgesic drugs) unfortunately is not part of general medical knowledge: although 48 patients suffered from continuous pain, only 31 patients received analgesics according to a regular time schedule. Four patients came into difficulties due to early parenteral administration of opiates: due to development of tolerance, 6 to 12 injections were necessary per day at the time of admission. For this reason, too, oral medication should be preferred, especially in outpatients (Houde 1979; Vere 1978).

In seven patients, the analgesics were underdosed. In 17 out of 31 patients who took the analgesics in accordance with a fixed scheme, the intervals were appreciably longer than the duration of action of the drug used. The majority of patients who took analgesics on request, i.e., when pain recurred, also allowed the intervals to become too long, so that they suffered violent pain for prolonged periods. The duration of action of morphine as the prototype of a centrally acting analgesic is about 4 h. The pharmacokinetics of levorphanol and methadone provide these drugs with a 1 to 2 h longer effectiveness (Jaffe and Martin 1980). The weakly acting opiate dextropropoxyphene has a duration of action of about 8 h in a special galenic preparation (Brauchle 1971).

In conclusion, we should like to emphasize that in the use of analgesic drugs in continuous carcinoma pain it is very important that the substances be administered at regular intervals depending on their duration of action and at a sufficient dosage. There is much evidence that oral administration has several definite advantages over parenteral application in the conscious patient.

Summary

Systemic administration of opioids is one of the traditional, but by no means optimized therapeutic procedures in cancer pain. Besides the underlying pathophysiology, appropriate treatment has to take into account the psychodynamics and behavior of the patient as well as his life expectancy. In view of this, therapy with centrally acting analgesics can be considered after administration of analgesics with peripheral action first and then of psychoactive agents. Nefopam is a centrally (but not spinally) acting analgesic with a novel activity profile. Its advantages and disadvantages in the treatment of carcinoma pain are outlined. The opiate agonist–antagonist principle has the advantage of a lower dependence and tolerance potential. In addition, the preparations pentazocine, tilidine plus naloxone, and buprenorphine deviate from the morphine derivatives in various constituent effects. Their actions and side effects are outlined.

The optimization of control of cancer pain is not possible without taking into account the time dimension. In 50 pain patients with advanced cancer, the following main errors were observed in previous treatment of pain syndromes: (1) too early parenteral administration in the course of the disease; (2) underdosage; (3) application intervals that were too long; and (4) use of analgesics as needed by the patient or on request and not according to a time schedule.

References

Arend J, von Arnim B, Nijssen J, Scheele J, Flohé L (1978) Tramadol und Pentazocin im klinischen Doppelblind-Crossover-Vergleich. Arzneim Forsch Drug Res 28: 199–208

Beaver WT, Wallenstein SL, Houde RW, Rogers A (1966) A comparison of the analgesic effects of pentazocine and morphine in patients with cancer. Clin Pharmacol Ther 7: 740–751

Bonica JJ (1979) Importance of the problem. In: Bonica JJ, Ventafridda V (eds) Advances in pain research and therapy, vol 2. Raven, New York, pp 1–12

Brauchle W (1971) Erfahrungen mit einem neuen Depot-Analgetikum (Develin retard). Z Allgemeinmed 47: 1465–1467

Cabanne F, Guerrin J, Wilkening M (1972) Die Behandlung von Tumorschmerzen mit Pentazocin. In: Janzen R, Keidel WD, Herz A, Steichele C (eds) Pain. Thieme, Stuttgart, pp 444–446

Cronheim G, Thiede W (1979) Ergebnisse einer Feldstudie mit Nefopam. In: Gerbershagen HU, Cronheim G (eds) Nefopam. Ein neuartiges Analgetikum. Fischer, Stuttgart, pp 142–147

De Thibault de Boesinghe L (1978) Double blind study of the analgesic effect of nefopam hydrochloride (Acupan) and pentazocine (Fortral) in cancer patients with pain. Curr Ther Res 24: 646–655

Eckmann F, Kubicki SK, Mazaheri P (1975) Zur Frage einer Pentazocin-Abhängigkeit. In: Neuhaus GA, Kubicki SK (eds) Pentazocin, ein neuer Weg. Thieme, Stuttgart, pp 61–64

Flohé L, Arend J, Cogal A, Richter W, Simon W (1978) Klinische Prüfungen der Langzeitapplikation von Tramadol. Arzneim Forsch Drug Res 28: 213–217

Foley KM (1976) Pain syndromes in patients with cancer. In: Bonica JJ, Ventafridda V (eds) Advances in pain research and therapy, vol 2. Raven, New York, pp 59–78

Frankendahl B, Kjellgren O (1971) Severe pain in gynecologic cancer. Cancer 27: 842–847

Frutschnigg E (1973) Schmerzbehandlung bei Karzinomen. Aerztl Praxis 25: 4429–4432

Groh R, Schindera A, Werringloer M (1971) Klinische Erfahrungen mit dem neuen Analgetikum Tilidin-HCL. Med Klinik 66: 1241–1245

Hoffmeister F (1968) Untersuchungen über die analgetischen, morphinantagonistischen und morphinartigen Wirkungen von Morphinantagonisten an normalen und morphinabhängigen Tieren. Pharmakopsychiatrie 1: 239–260

Houde RW (1979) Systemic analgesics and related drugs: Narcotic analgesics. In: Bonica JJ, Ventafridda V (eds) Advances in pain research and therapy, vol 2. Raven, New York, pp 263–273

Jaffe JH, Martin WR (1980) Opoid analgesics and antagonists. In: Goodman LS, Gilman A (eds) The pharmacological basis of therapeutics. MacMillan, New York, pp 494–534

Kleibel F (1972) Erfahrungen mit Pentazocin in der klinischen Onkologie. In: Janzen R, Keidel WD, Herz A, Steichele C (eds) Pain. Thieme, Stuttgart, pp 446–448

Krell R, Hanke M (1979) Klinische Prüfung der analgetischen Wirksamkeit von Valoron N im Vergleich zu Valoron bei Tumorschmerzen. Krankenhausarzt 52: 760–764

Robbie DS (1979) A trial of sublingual buprenorphine in cancer pain. Br J Clin Pharmacol 7: 3155–3175

Schietzl M (1979) Nefopamhydrochlorid, ein neuartiges Analgetikum mit geringen Nebenwirkungen. In: Gerbershagen HU, Cronheim G (eds) Nefopam. Ein neuartiges Analgetikum. Fischer, Stuttgart, pp 129–131

Twycross RG (1980) Overview of analgesia. In: Bonica JJ, Ventafridda V (eds) Advances in pain research and therapy, vol 2. Raven, New York, pp 617–633

Vere DW (1978) Pharmacology of morphine drugs in terminal care. In: Vere DW (ed) Topics in therapeutics 4. Pitman, London, pp 75–83

Zimmermann M (1979) Neurophysiologische Untersuchungen über einen spinalen Wirkungsort von Nefopam. In: Gerbershagen HU, Cronheim G (eds) Nefopam. Ein neuartiges Analgetikum. Fischer, Stuttgart New York, pp 18–26

Epidural Opiates for the Treatment of Cancer Pain

M. Zenz

Abteilung IV, Krankenhaus Oststadt, Zentrum für Anästhesiologie,
Medizinische Hochschule Hannover, Podbielskistrasse 380, 3000 Hannover 51, FRG

Epidural Opiates in Cancer Pain

Epidural opiate analgesia represent an alternative to the systemic application of opiates in the treatment of chronic pain. The efficacy of this new method – particularly in the therapy of cancer pain – has been demonstrated by a great number of clinicians (Poletti et al. 1981; Christensen 1982; Howard et al. 1981; Zenz et al. 1981a; Magora et al. 1980; Chayen et al. 1980). Even in cases of unsuccessful treatment with high doses of opiates parenterally given, analgesia can be achieved with significantly lower doses of opiates by epidural administration (Coombs et al. 1981; Howard et al. 1981; Poletti et al. 1981). Nevertheless, epidural opiates are not ideal in every case of cancer pain treatment. A catheter must be inserted and checked regularly and, moreover, the epidurally injected opiate can induce severe side effects, among which are life-threatening side effects such as respiratory depression (Gustafsson et al. 1982). Epidural opiates do not help in every case of pain and they cannot be used in every localization of pain. Therefore, guidelines are required for the safe use of epidural opiates in patients suffering from cancer pain.

Basic Research on Spinal Opiates

Specific opiate receptors were identified in the brain and the substantia gelatinosa of the spinal cord (Pert and Snyder 1973; Pert et al. 1976). Yaksh and Rudy (1976) reported that morphine administered directly into the spinal subarachnoid space in animals produces a dose-dependent elevation in the nociceptive threshold. These experiments were soon followed by the demonstration that the intrathecal injection of morphine gives profound pain relief in man (Wang 1977). The epidural administration of morphine also produced long-lasting analgesia (Bahar et al. 1979). Subsequent clinical work demonstrated the effectiveness of spinal opiates in relieving postoperative, posttraumatic, ischemic, and cancer pain (Magora et al. 1980). The main advantages of the new method are long duration of analgesia with minimal doses, no interference with other neurologic functions, no effect on the gut, and no autonomic changes, but a serious risk is respiratory depression (Scott and McClure 1979; Gustafsson et al. 1982). However, the total incidence of side effects from epidural opiates is low compared to parenteral administration, although some side effects of this method are potentially dangerous enough to raise the question of whether this promising analgesic method can be recommended for general use in the treatment of cancer pain.

Recent Results in Cancer Research. Vol. 89

Methods

Our results and observations were obtained from 92 patients suffering from severe cancer pain. The diffuse pain was induced by multiple bone metastases in most instances or by primary invasion of the carcinoma. The treatment in our pain clinic was preceded by oncologic and neurologic examinations. Only those patients were referred to us to whom simpler methods did not give sufficient pain relief.

When blood coagulation was within the normal range, an epidural catheter was inserted via a Tuohy needle as near as possible to the spinal segment where the pain projected. Thoracic epidurals were performed only when treatment via a lumbar catheter was unsuccessful. The epidural catheter was sutured and the puncture site was covered with povidone iodine (Zenz et al. 1981b). To exclude an intrathecal catheter position, 20 mg bupivacaine was injected. The first dose of opiates was given – either 2–5 mg morphine hydrochloride or 0.15–0.3 mg buprenorphine in 10–20 mg saline solution. The analgesic effect of this initial dose was recorded and subsequent injections were given according to the degree and time of action of the first dose at 6-h to 24-h intervals. These injections were given at the hospital by nurses or at home by family physicians, home nurses, or relatives who received training from us. The patients were instructed to take a bath in povidone-iodine-containing water every second day and to change the cover and the bacterial filter of the catheter. Once a week, the patients came to our clinic to have the catheter and puncture site, the degree of pain relief, and the dosage of opiates checked. The catheters were left in situ as long as the therapy was necessary. In cases of infection at the puncture site, the catheter was removed, and on the same day a new one was placed in a cranially or caudally adjacent segment.

Results

The mean age (± SD) of the 92 patients (25 men and 67 women) was 58 ± 13 years. Fifty were treated as inpatients, 42 as outpatients. We inserted a total number of 163 *epidural catheters,* 150 at lumbar segments, 11 at thoracic segments, and two via the sacral route. The catheters were in place for 36 ± 39 days (mean ± SD; range 1–190 days), 14 catheters were in place for more than 100 days, six catheters for more than 150 days, and three for up to 190 days (Fig. 1). The *complications* arising from the epidural catheters are listed in Table 1: Seven catheters were obstructed due to intervals of more than 50 h between the injections, and 11 catheters were broken. At the very beginning of this pain therapy, 11 catheters were accidentally removed, but after that we fixed the catheter, as described above, with a suture. In two instances there was subcutaneous kinking of the catheter, making injections impossible. These catheters had to be withdrawn by about 1 cm until a free injection could be performed. In ten patients there was local infection at the puncture site. In two cases a spinal infection developed which was confirmed by dural puncture; we removed the catheter and performed antibiotic therapy. Both patients became free of symptoms. One of them received a new catheter at his own request, the other died of his cancer before a new course of therapy could be instituted.

The mean *duration of therapy* was 63 ± 65 days. Twenty patients were treated for more than 100 days, nine patients for more than 150 days, and two patients for more than 300 days (Table 2). The *mean daily dosage* of morphine was 10 ± 8 mg (range 2–80 mg), the mean single dose being 5 ± 3 mg (range 1–20 mg). The analgesic effect of each dose lasted for 14 ± 7 h (range 1–93 h). The mean daily dose of morphine had to be increased slightly

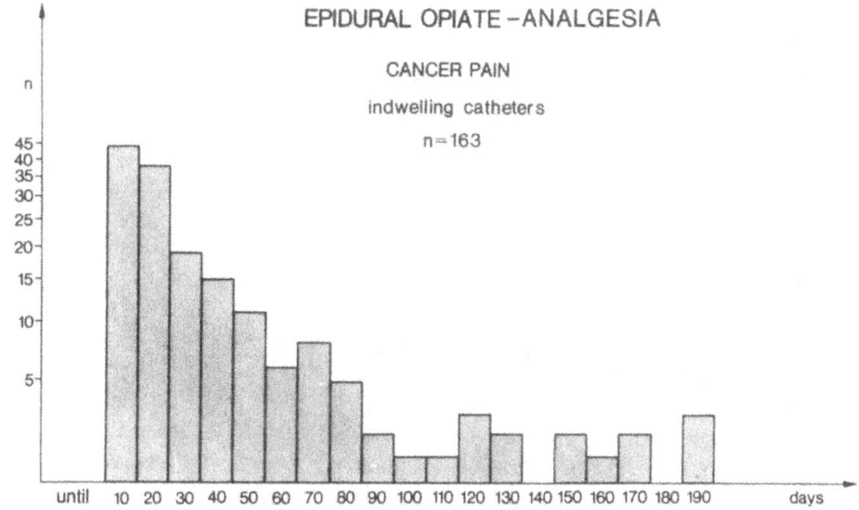

Fig. 1. Distribution of insertion time of epidural catheters

Table 1. Complications arising from epidural catheters. Epidural opiate analgesia in cancer pain in 92 patients

Epidural catheters	(total 163)
Obstructed	7
Broken	11
Accidentally removed	11
Subcutaneous kinking	2
Accidentally cut	2
Local infection	10
Spinal infection	2

Table 2. Duration of therapy with epidural opiates in cancer pain in 92 patients

1– 50 days	n = 51
51–100 days	n = 21
101–150 days	n = 11
151–200 days	n = 6
218 days	n = 1
339 days	n = 1
348 days	n = 1

within the first 20 days of treatment from 6 mg on the 1st day to 9 mg on the 20th day (Fig. 2). This increase in dose was probably necessitated by increasing pain stimulus through the continuing infiltration of cancer in the terminal stage. In the last 20 days of treatment periods lasting longer than 45 days, i.e., mostly the 20 days before death, the mean daily dose was 15 mg.

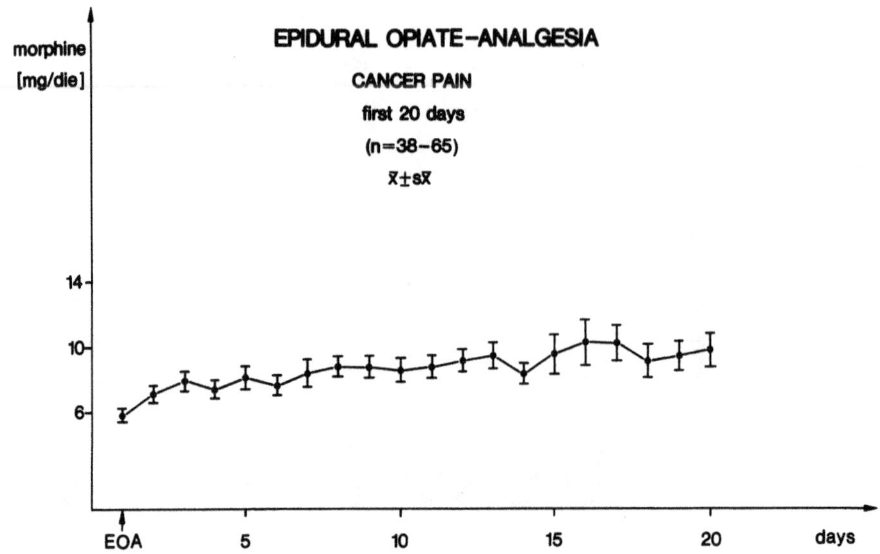

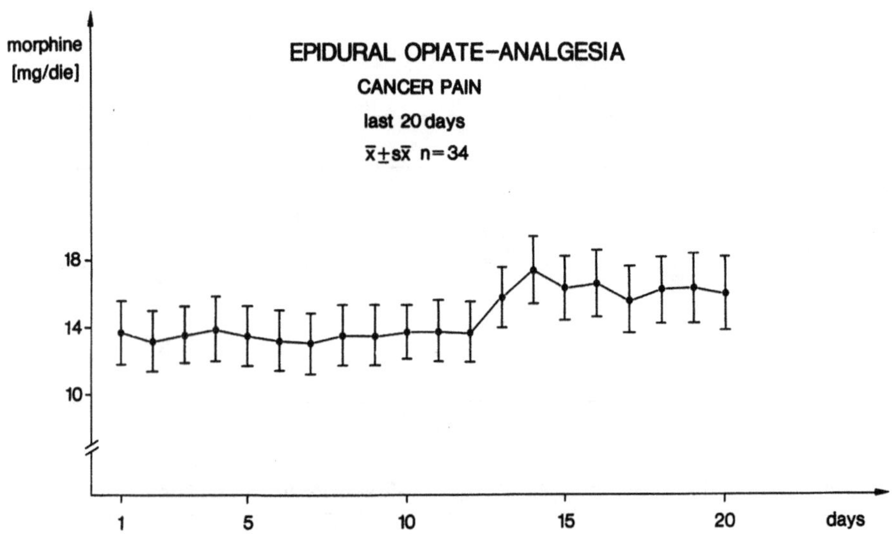

Fig. 2. Dosage of morphine given during the first 20 days and during the last 20 days of treatment ($\bar{x}$ *mean;* $s\bar{x}$, SD)

Satisfactory *analgesia* was obtained in 90% of patients with epidural opiates alone. Some patients received in addition nonnarcotic analgesics (aspirin, paracetamol) or sedatives at night. In some patients, a mixture of local anesthetics (5 ml bupivacaine 0.25%) and opiates was administered epidurally. This was only performed in cases where we wanted to achieve a greater degree of pain relief by the additional sympathetic block. Normally we do not combine opiates with local anesthetics in outpatients to avoid the side effects of sympathetic blockade and loss of sensation in the lower extremities.

Side effects were registered in 15% of our patients. Four patients had nausea and three vomiting. With three daily doses of 1–2 ml domperidon this side effect was successfully treated. One patient complained of severe diffuse itching. Six patients had urinary retention which disappeared after some days without treatment. Respiratory depression was never observed. The total incidence of side effects was lower during treatment with buprenorphine than with morphine. In six patients we changed from morphine to buprenorphine because of the side effects of epidural morphine. One patient had obstipation, three nausea, one vomiting, and two urinary retention. With epidural buprenorphine there was only one patient with a minor degree of vomiting.

Discussion

Epidural administration of opiates proved to be a valuable new technique in the treatment of cancer pain. The degree of pain relief is higher than with oral or intravenous narcotics, as is known from objective investigations during the postoperative period (Welchew and Thornton 1982; Jörgensen et al. 1982). A major proportion of our patients had been treated with systemic opiates without success, but the change from the systemic to the epidural route resulted in a marked increase in pain relief. The same was demonstrated by Glynn et al. (1981) and Woods and Cohen (1982). This might be due to the fact that the blood–brain barrier is bypassed by epidural application. In consequence, the concentration of the narcotic in the CSF might be rather high and the CSF: blood ratio of concentration is much higher than can be achieved by parenteral administration (Weddel and Ritter 1981; Glynn et al. 1981). This might explain the very intense and long-lasting analgesic effect. One of our patients had analgesia lasting 93 h after one administration. Glynn et al. (1981) were able to increase the intervals between administrations significantly by changing from oral to epidural narcotics. The average duration of analgesia of 14 h in our patients clearly exceeds that known for enteral or parenteral administration. The analgesia initially has a segmental topography, relieving the blunt pain by modulation of input via small afferents of C- and A-delta nociceptors. In contrast, all other functions, e.g., motor, sympathetic, and somatosensory, remain unaffected (Yaksh 1981).

The central effects of epidural opiates on the brain are minimal, indicating that the epidural narcotics predominantly effect the spinal cord. Analgesia is spinal not central (Yaksh 1981). Nevertheless, some side effects of epidural narcotics are potentially dangerous enough that this technique should be reserved for severe pain states only (Bromage 1981). The only patients we have treated were those to whom other simpler approaches did not give sufficient pain relief. Only less severe side effects occurred, such as vomiting, itching, and urinary retention. In no case did we observe a potentially life-threatening side effect such as respiratory depression. To keep the risk of central side effects down to a minimum, the catheter has to be inserted as far away from the brain as possible. This means that, even in case of thoracic pain, the catheter should be positioned at a lumbar segment (Gustafsson et al. 1982). Our results confirm that this technique provides successful pain relief. Only 11 out of 163 catheters were inserted at the thoracic level because a lumbar catheter did not relieve the thoracic pain sufficiently. All other patients, even with pain from high thoracic dermatoma, were free of pain by lumbar epidural opiates alone. In all patients with multiple rib fractures also the pain could be relieved by lumbar epidural narcotics (Hüsch and Zenz 1981).

The risk of respiratory depression in cancer patients following epidural opiate administration seems to be very low (Gustafsson et al. 1982). Respiratory depression in cancer pain treatment was only reported when systemic opiates were given concomitantly (Gustafsson et al. 1982). This is in apparent contrast to measurements of the CO_2 sensitivity after administration of epidural opiates (Knill et al. 1981; Nielsen et al. 1981), where even after 6 h a marked depression of the CO_2-response curve was detectable. But all these experiments were carried out on painfree patients and they are not comparable with cancer patients. It can be concluded that pain is a potent stimulator of the respiratory center in patients who are receiving narcotic drugs (Hanks et al. 1981). Woods et al. (1982) have reported that in a cancer patient up to 240 mg morphine were given epidurally each day without any sign of respiratory depression.

Perhaps the use of lipophilic narcotics would further decrease the side-effect rate. We have seen this in a small number of cancer patients successively treated with morphine (hydrophilic) and buprenorphine (lipophilic), as well as in a study on postoperative pain (Zenz et al. 1981a). Buprenorphine produced a similar analgesia but had a lower incidence of side effects. This might be explained by the different pharmacokinetics in accordance with the physicochemical properties (de Castro and Lecron 1981; Bromage 1981). The lipophilic drug has a rapid blood reabsorption after entering the CSF. Consequently, the portion of the drug which is not bound to spinal opiate receptors and can, therefore, be carried rostrally within the CSF is minimal. The drugs most used for epidural administration in cancer pain were morphine, pethidine, fentanyl, and buprenorphine. Glynn et al. (1981) used pethidine with good results but with shorter duration of analgesia than we found using morphine and buprenorphine. Fentanyl was only used as a continuous infusion (Bowen-Wright and Goroszeniuk 1980), which is not possible in home care. Thus, there remain morphine and buprenorphine, with buprenorphine seeming to have some advantages.

With regard to the dose of opiates, we only had to inject small amounts: 6 mg morphine on the first day and 15 mg on the very last day of treatment are low doses compared with those given in systemic application (Selz and Bürgi 1979). The increase of dose is, in our opinion, a consequence of increasing pain due to the rapid growth of the cancer and is not a result of tolerance to the drug (Coombs et al. 1981). In any case, the slightly increasing need for opiates in not a practical problem (Twycross 1979).

Contrary to simpler techniques of pain relief, in epidural opiate analgesia a catheter has to be inserted and checked regularly over a rather long period of time. Therefore, whenever oral medication is possible, it should be preferred. Epidural opiates are a very valuable and effective second-choice method. When oral opiates are no longer effective or result in sedation and somnolence, the epidural route may provide regional analgesia without these side effects. However, great care has to be taken with the catheter to protect the patients from spinal or general infections. We prefer percutaneous cannulation to a surgically implanted system. With our method, we can change the catheter and remove it very easily when the localization or character of pain changes. The risk of spinal infection in our experience is low in comparison with immunosuppressed patients. An alternative technique of systems with an implanted reservoir of opiates was only used in a small number of patients (Poletti et al. 1981; Coombs et al. 1981). Thus, the infection rate in these anecdotal cases is difficult to compare with our results.

Our patients accepted this method of pain therapy very well, although the catheter was combined with some discomfort. They preferred epidural opiates to oral or intramuscular narcotics because they gave greater pain relief. Above all, those patients previously treated with other methods of pain relief were very content with epidural opiates.

Conclusion

The administration of epidural opiates is a valuable technique in the treatment of cancer pain. It should be reserved for terminal care and for those patients in whom other methods are not sufficiently effective. If possible, oral narcotics, neurolytic blockade, or chordotomy should be given preference. Epidural narcotics are a reasonable method in patients with pain diffusely distributed over wide areas, whereas in patients with radiculitis epidural opiates fail to provide analgesia. The catheter should be inserted as near as possible to the site of spinal projection of the pain and as far as possible from the brain to minimize the risk of central side effects such as respiratory depression. Under close supervision and care, the epidural catheter can be held in place for periods of up to 6 months. The opiate doses needed are low in comparison with systemical application. The increase in dosage is rather slow and tolerance is no practical problem, even in cases of long periods of treatment. The differential action of epidural opiates on pain favors this method for selected cancer patients in a terminal stage of illness. It frees the patients of pain, leaves them clearminded, and enables them to spend their last weeks or months at home with their families instead of in the hospital.

References

Bahar M, Magora F, Olshwang D, Davidson JT (1979) Epidural morphine in treatment of pain. Lancet 1:527

Bowen-Wright RM, Goroszeniuk T (1980) Epidural fentanyl for pain of multiple fractures. Lancet 2:1033

Bromage PR (1981) The price of intraspinal narcotic analgesia: basic constraints. Anesth Analg 60:461

Chayen MS, Rudick V, Borvine A (1980) Pain control with epidural injection of morphine. Anesthesiology 53:338

Christensen FR (1982) Epidural morphine at home in terminal patients. Lancet 1:47

Coombs DW, Saunders RL, Gaylor MS, Pageau MG, Leith MG, Schaiberger C (1981) Continuous epidural analgesia via implanted morphine reservoir. Lancet 1:425

De Castro J, Lecron L (1981) Peridurale Opiat-Analgesie. Verschiedene Opiate. Komplikationen und Nebenwirkungen. In: Zenz M (ed) Peridurale Opiat-Analgesie. Fischer, Stuttgart, p 103

Glynn CJ, Mather LE, Cousins MJ, Graham JR, Wilson PR (1981) Peridural meperidine in humans: analgetic response, pharmacokinetics, and transmission into C.S.F. Anesthesiology 55:520

Gustafsson LL, Schildt B, Jacobsen K (1982) Adverse effects of extradural and intrathecal opiates: report of a nationwide survey in Sweden. Br J Anaesth 54:479

Hanks GW, Twycross RG, Lloyd JW (1981) Unexpected complication of successful nerve block: Morphine induced respiratory depression precipitated by removal of severe pain. Anaesthesia 36:37

Howard RP, Milne LA, Williams NE (1981) Epidural morphine in terminal care. Anaesthesia 36:51

Hüsch M, Zenz M (1981) Peridurale Morphin-Analgesie bei Rippenserienfrakturen. In: Zenz M (ed) Peridurale Opiat-Analgesie. Fischer, Stuttgart, p 69

Jörgensen BC, Andersen HB, Engquist A (1982) Influence of epidural morphine on postoperative pain, endocrinemetabolic, and renal responses to surgery. A controlled study. Acta Anaesth Scand 26:63

Knill RL, Clement JL, Thompson WR (1981) Epidural morphine causes delayed and prolonged ventilatory depression. Can Anaesth Soc J 28:537

Magora F, Olshwang D, Eimerl D, Shorr J, Katzenelson R, Cotev S, Davidson JT (1980) Observations on extradural morphine analgesia in various pain conditions. Br J Anaesth 52:247

Nielsen CH, Camporesi EM, Bromage PR, Bukowski EM, Durant PAC (1981) CO_2 sensitivity after epidural and i.v. morphine. Anesthesiology 55:372

Pert CB, Snyder SH (1973) Opiate receptor: demonstration in nervous tissue. Science 179:1011

Pert CB, Kuhar MJ, Snyder SH (1976) Opiate receptor: autoradiographic localisation in rat brain. Proc Natl Acad Sci USA 73: 3729

Poletti CE, Cohen AM, Todd DP, Ojemann RG, Sweet W, Zervas NT (1981) Cancer pain relieved by long-term epidural morphine with permanent indwelling systems for self-administration. J Neurosurg 55: 581

Scott DB, McClure J (1979) Selective epidural analgesia. Lancet 2: 1410

Selz B, Bürgi H (1979) Erfahrung mit einer oralen Cocain-Morphin-Lösung ("Brompton-Mixture") in der Behandlung schwerer Schmerzzustände bei Krebspatienten. Schweiz Med Wochenschr 109: 1161

Twycross RG (1979) Overview of analgesia. In: Bonica JJ, Ventafridda V (eds.) Advances in pain research and therapy, vol 2. Raven, New York, p 617

Wang JK (1977) Analgesic effect of intrathecally administered morphine. Regional Anesth 2: 8

Weddel SJ, Ritter RR (1981) Serum levels following epidural administration of morphine and correlation with relief of postsurgical pain. Anesthesiology 54: 210

Welchew EA, Thornton JA (1982) Continuous thoracic epidural fentanyl. Anaesthesia 37: 309

Woods WA, Cohen SE (1982) High-dose epidural morphine in a terminally ill patient. Anesthesiology 56: 311

Yaksh TL (1981) Spinal opiate analgesia: characteristics and principles of action. Pain 11: 293

Yaksh TL, Rudy TA (1976) Analgesia mediated by a direct spinal action of narcotics. Science 192: 1357

Zenz M, Schappler-Scheele B, Neuhaus R, Piepenbrock S, Hilfrich J (1981a) Long-term peridural morphine analgesia in cancer pain. Lancet 1: 91

Zenz M, Piepenbrock S, Hüsch M, Schappler-Scheele B, Neuhaus R (1981b) Experience with long-term peridural catheters-peridural morphine analgesia in cancer pain. Regional Anaesthesie 4: 26

Zenz M, Piepenbrock S, Hübner B, Glocke M (1981c) A double-blind comparison of epidural buprenorphine and epidural morphine in postoperative pain. Anaesth Intensivther Notfallmed 16: 333

*Opiates and Respiratory Function in Advanced Cancer**

T. D. Walsh

Department of Clinical Pharmacology, Guy's Hospital, St. Thomas Street, London SE1 9RT, United Kingdom

Introduction

Oral administration of opiates is the preferred method of relieving chronic pain in advanced cancer. Morphine, methadone and diamorphine (heroin) are the main drugs used for severe pain. Saunders (1979, personal communication) and Mount (1980) reported that respiratory depression in such patients is uncommon when oral morphine (in aqueous solution) is given 4-hourly in individually determined doses, titrated against the patient's level of pain. These reports were surprising in view of the known effect of opiates on respiratory function (Bellville et al. 1968) and the clinical condition of the patient population in question. Oral morphine is known to provide effective pain relief in up to 95% of cancer patients (Mount 1980) despite low relative bioavailability (Brunk and Delle 1974) compared with parenteral administration. It is likely too that oral administration is associated with lower peaks and less rapid change in morphine plasma levels. Examination of the literature on the effects of opiates on respiratory function (Murray and Grant 1966) reveals that studies have been largely conducted on surgically treated patients following parenteral administration (Rigg 1978) of opiates. The methodology employed has not always had direct clinical relevance, nor have the impairments in respiratory function demonstrated clinical significance (Betcher and Barber 1966).

Because of its pharmacokinetic characteristics (Kitahata and Collins 1982), repeated oral administration of morphine might allow effective pain relief without compromising respiratory function. It was decided to conduct a prospective study amongst advanced cancer patients using conventional clinical measures of respiratory function: all patients examined were receiving in excess of 100 mg morphine sulphate/24 h.

Material, Methods and Results

Twenty pain-free patients (median age 59 years; range 45–79 years) were examined at rest by means of respiratory rate (counted clinically), peak-flow rate ("mini" Wright peak-flow meter), arterial blood gases and plasma morphine levels (radioimmunoassay). Each was examined on one occasion only in the 30-min period preceding a regular 4-h dose of morphine. All patients had been receiving regular morphine for more than 7 days and had been on a steady dose for more than 48 h. Patients with an acute condition likely to cause impaired respiratory function were excluded. Twelve patients had a history of chronic bronchitis and eight were dying from carcinoma of the bronchus. Respiratory rates were all

* Supported by DHSS grant number OCS (3) A

Recent Results in Cancer Research. Vol. 89

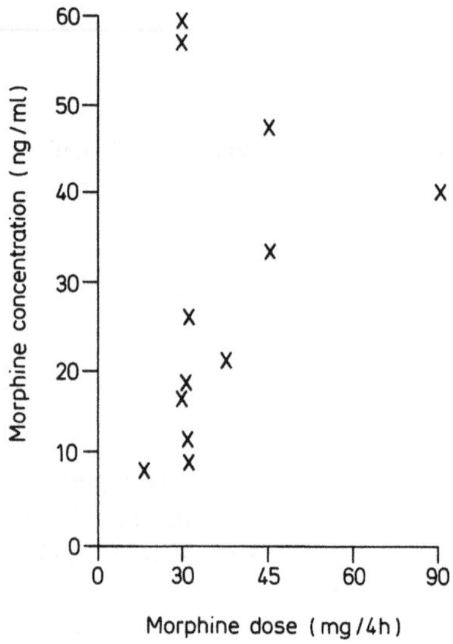

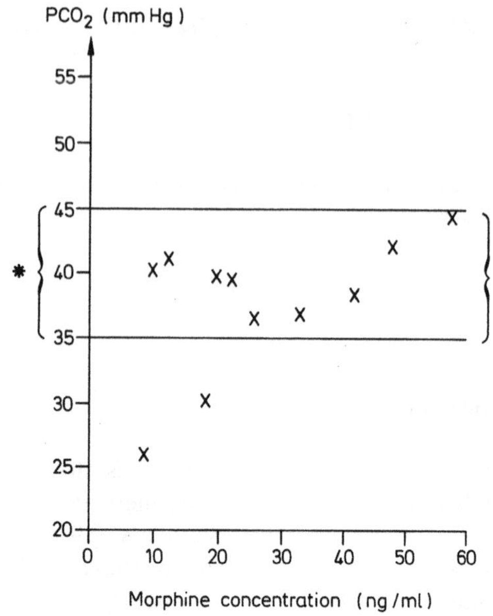

Fig. 1. (*left*) Scatter diagram of 4-h morphine dosage and morphine plasma levels (expressed as morphine equivalents) after measurement by a radioimmunoassay employing an extraction procedure (Grabinski et al. 1982); *ng per ml = nanogrammes per millilitre; plasma morphine concentration (post extraction) measured as morphine equivalents

Fig. 2. (*right*) Scatter diagram of arterial PCO_2 (mm Hg) and morphine plasma levels (expressed as morphine equivalents) after measurement by a radioimmunoassay employing an extraction procedure (Grabinski et al. 1982); *ng per ml,* nanogrammes per millilitre; plasma morphine concentration (post extraction) measured as morphine equivalents. *Reference range of arterial PCO_2 35–45 mm Hg (Cotes 1979)

12/min, mean peak-flow rates were all 350 l/min. All had significant amounts of morphine present in their plasma (Grabinski et al. 1982; Fig 1). Correlation coefficient of log morphine dose and extracted plasma morphine level (ng/ml) was $r = 0.438$ ($P < 0.05$). One patient had an elevated PCO_2 level (Fig. 2), 12 were hypoxic but only one severely so (PO_2 = 48 mm Hg).

Discussion and Conclusions

Given the advanced condition of the patients, the prevalence of chronic respiratory disease and the fact that all were receiving substantial amounts of oral morphine, the results are surprising. Arterial PCO_2 is a sensitive index of ventilatory failure; chronic ventilatory failure appears to be neither common nor severe when oral morphine is used to treat chronic severe pain in advanced cancer – even in the presence of pre-existing respiratory tract disease. Some degree of hypoxia would be expected in this population given the frequency of respiratory tract disease. Respiratory depression via ventilatory failure from opiates may be dependent on the rate of change (or on the peak levels) of morphine in the plasma. Titration of the dose (rather than employing standard doses) and oral administration with dosage increments (if required) at 48–72 h intervals may thus allow tolerance to the respiratory depressant effect of morphine to develop whilst continuing to provide pain relief.

References

Bellville JW, Escanaza LA, Wallenstein SL, Houde RW (1968) The respiratory effects of codeine and morphine in man. Clin Pharmacol Ther 9: 435–441

Betcher G, Barber JL (1966) Lung mechanics and physiologic shunt during spontaneous breathing in normal subjects. Anaesthesiology 27: 638–647

Brunk SF, Delle M (1974) Morphine metabolism in man. Clin Pharmacol Ther 16: 51–57

Cotes JE (1979) Lung function, 4th edn. Blackwell, London

Grabinski PY, Kaiko RF, Walsh TD, Foley KM, Houde RW (1983) Morphine radioimmunoassay specificity before and after extraction of plasma and cerebrospinal fluid. J Pharm Sci 72: 27–30

Kitahata LM, Collins JG (1982) Narcotic analgesics in anesthesiology. Williams and Wilkins, Baltimore

Mount BM (1980) Narcotic analgesics. In: Twycross RG, Ventafridda V (eds) The continuing care of terminal cancer patients. Pergamon, Oxford, pp 79–116

Murray WD, Grant IW (1966) Effects of opiates in chronic bronchitis. Thorax 21: 57–64

Rigg JRA (1978) Ventilatory effects and plasma concentration of morphine in man. Br J Anaesth 50: 759–764

The Use of Psychotropic Drugs in the Treatment of Cancer Pain

R. Kocher

Psychiatrische Universitätsklinik, Wilhelm-Klein-Strasse 27, 4025 Basel, Switzerland

Introduction

Psychotropic drugs – especially antidepressants and neuroleptics – have become an important element in the treatment of cancer pain. Soon after the introduction of neuroleptics in 1951/52 and antidepressants in 1957 in psychiatry, the first publications appeared reporting their beneficial analgesic effect. Later publications emphasized that psychotropic drugs may potentiate the effects of analgesics and help to reduce their use.

Survey of Psychotropic Drugs Used for Cancer Pain

Antidepressants and neuroleptics are particularly efficacious in the treatment of cancer pain. Tranquilizers alone or in combination with antidepressants are not recommended for treatment of pain because of the risk of dependence in long-term use. As yet we do not have enough experience of the efficacy of carbamazepine alone or in combination with antidepressants and/or neuroleptics in the treatment of carcinomatous pain. Furthermore, there are no proven beneficial results of the treatment of cancer pain with valproate sodium.

Antidepressants

These drugs block the re-uptake of serotonin and noradrenaline into the nerve cell near the synapse and thus cause increased noradrenergic and serotoninergic activity in the central nervous system. Successfully used antidepressants are, in particular, those that both improve mood and relieve depression. These effects are primarily found with clomipramine, imipramine, maprotiline, amitriptyline, and trimipramine.

Neuroleptics

Of this group, levomepromazine has been reported to be analgesically efficacious. However, even in low doses levomepromazine causes some side reactions (somnolence, orthostasic problems).
Therefore, haloperidol, a butyrophenone derivate that has a high neuroleptic efficacy but does not cause the side effects mentioned for levomepromazine, is more widely used today.

Recent Results in Cancer Research. Vol. 89

Neuroleptics block the receptors for dopamine at the synapses. Recently, four papers have been published claiming good effects in the treatment of cancer pain with tiapride, a derivative of benzamide, a kind of orthopramide (Dilhuydy et al. 1979; Lepille and Bastit 1979; Pressey and Lacomme 1980; Gennari et al. 1981). On the basis of the first publications reporting the beneficial analgesic effect of neuroleptics and antidepressants in the treatment of all chronic pains caused by different diseases, we decided on a combination therapy. Our good results (Kocher 1969) were confirmed by others (Merskey and Hester 1972; Taub and Collins 1974) and the reports about the beneficial analgesic effect of psychotropic drugs began to spread throughout the world. The reasons why combination therapy is to be recommended will be mentioned later. Combination therapy is today well established for all chronic pain.

Modes of Action

General

The high rate of success attained in treatment with antidepressants or neuroleptics has been explained by the hypothesis that these agents cause a change in pain perception. This has been called "depersonalisation of pain" and "pain removing effect" (Linke 1963). Having their major site of action in the limbic system, the psychotropic drugs are particularly suited to reducing the averse effects of pain perception. According to neuropsychology, these changed attitudes are associated with functions of the frontal cortex as part of the limbic system. In cancer pain, there is often a vicious circle of pain → anxiety → depression → pain (Kocher 1976). Combined treatment with an antidepressant and a neuroleptic can break this vicious circle more effectively than the use of either an antidepressant or a neuroleptic alone. One of the effects is either lacking or insufficient if only one drug is used.

According to Linke (1963) psychotropic drugs, especially neuroleptics, can also break the fatal vicious circle: pain → vegetative excitability → psychological reaction → pain. The more the pain is influenced by a disorder of the emotional, psychological, and vegetative balance, the more impressive the beneficial effect of these drugs. They have an effect on the medial structures of the thalamus and hypothalamus, areas that are thought to be of crucial importance for the afferent pain system. Thus the patients' attitude to their chronic pain is changed: they are less aware of it, it can be overcome more easily and can also be removed from subjective perception. There is no excruciating perception of pain (Linke 1963).

Worldwide research in the area of pain has made important progress during the past 10 years. In particular, the discovery of opiate receptors in the central nervous system in 1973 and soon afterward the discovery of enkephalins and endorphins offered new perspectives for the understanding of pain. It has been speculated that the analgesic action of antidepressants and neuroleptics might be due to an interference in the endogenous opioid system, for example by way of their well-known pharmacologic effects on the central metabolism of the neurotransmitters (Spencer 1976; Spencer et al. 1979).

Neuroleptics

Clay and Brougham (1975) showed that haloperidol binds to opiate receptors. This binding is strongly reduced when sodium ions are present, as in the case of opiate agonists. It has

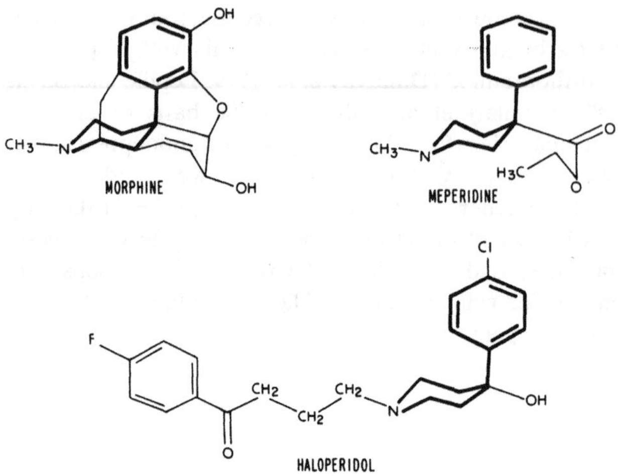

Fig. 1. Similarity in the chemical structures of morphine, meperidine, and haloperidol (according to Karkalas and Lal 1973)

been concluded, therefore, that haloperidol might have a small opiate-agonistic effect which, however, is different from that of morphine. Simon (1976) confirmed this contention. Based on his research in animals, he supposed haloperidol had a slight but definite analgesic effect. Creese et al. (1976) examined some butyrophenones and other neuroleptics with respect to their influence on opiate receptors. They discovered that haloperidol acts in a similar way as agonists-antagonists on sodium ions located at the opiate receptors. Furthermore, they found that two other butyrophenones, pimozide and benperidol, have a stronger analgesic effect than propoxyphene and meperidine. Their pharmacologic effect is similar to that of opiate agonists. Maltbie et al. (1979) pointed out that there are similarities in the structures of morphine, haloperidol, and meperidine. According to Creese et al. (1976), the piperidine ring of the butyrophenones is important for their opiate activity (see Fig. 1).

Antidepressants

Apart from its analgesic effect, morphine causes an improvement in the psychological condition. Spencer (1976) believed this to be the result of an interaction with certain neurotransmitters, such as acetylcholine, dopamine, noradrenaline, and serotonin. The effect of morphine is bound to cholinergic, dopaminergic, noradrenergic, and serotoninergic pathways, and the nature of interaction between morphine and these substances differs according to location. Disorders in the central metabolism of serotonin cause a change in pain perception and in the analgesic effect of morphine. In general, a reduction of serotonin leads to more pain and vice versa. Acetylcholine and dopamine also play a role in the action of analgesics. Cholinomimetics have an antinociceptive effect. Cholinesterase inhibitors intensify the analgesic effect of morphine in man. Dopamine is necessary for normal morphine analgesia, which is diminished by a depletion of the dopaminergic reservoir. Mayer and Price (1976) found that serotonin plays an important role in morphine analgesia. A reduction of serotonin caused by the destruction of the afferent or descending pathways in animals completely blocks the analgesic effect of morphine. The analgesia

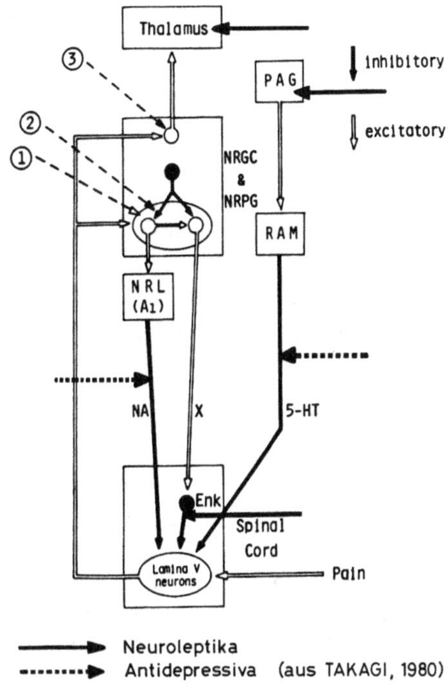

Fig. 2. Possible mechanisms of action of morphine and enkephalin in the nucleus reticularis gigantocellularis (NRGC) and the nucleus reticularis paragigantocellularis (NRPG; according to Takagi 1980). *1*, direct activation of two descending pain inhibitory systems originating from the nucleus reticularis paragigantocellularis (NRPG): noradrenergic system (NA) and enkephalinergic system (Enk). *2*, suppression of inhibitory interneurons in the nucleus reticularis gigantocellularis (NRGC) which, in turn, causes activation of two descending inhibitory systems. *3*, suppression of a pain afferent neuron in the nucelus reticularis gigantocellularis (NRGC). *PAG-RAM*, periaqueductal gray – Raphe magnus, a descending inhibitory system providing another possible site of action of morphine; *NRL*, nucleus reticularis lateralis; *5-HT*, serotoninergic nerve; *X*, unknown transmitter

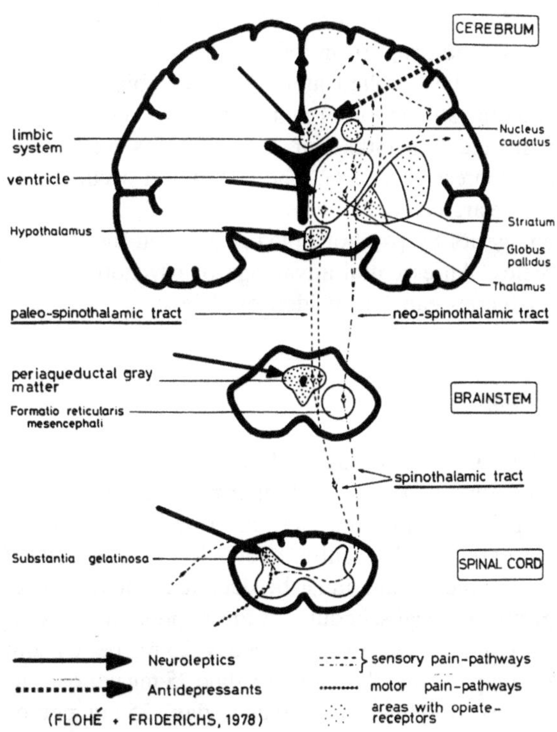

Fig. 3. Sites of action of neuroleptics and antidepressants in the central nervous system in chronic pain (according to Flohé and Friderichs 1978)

produced by β-endorphine is also linked to the activation of serotoninergic pathways. Beaumont (1976) showed that clomipramine, a specific serotonin re-uptake inhibitor, increases enkephalin analgesia. Spencer et al. (1979) found a better analgesic effect of morphine, pentazocine, and cyclazocine in mice that had been pretreated with clomipramine. In their opinion, the increase in the central serotonin activity is a common characteristic of the analgesic effect of narcotic analgesics and might also mediate the analgesic effect of antidepressants.

In 1980, Takagi reported that noradrenaline might also be a neurotransmitter in descending inhibitory pathways in the spinal cord (Fig. 2). According to this view, a noradrenergic descending pathway originates in the bulbar reticular formation. Figures 2 and 3 show the supposed action of neuroleptics and antidepressants at different levels of the central nervous system in chronic pain.

Results of Clinical Studies

Analgesic Effect in Cancer Patients

Table 1 is a compilation of the most important publications stating the drugs used, the number of patients treated, and the proportion of cases where an alleviation of cancer pain could be achieved. All reviews of Table 1 produce agreement on the following definition of improvement: results either good (less pain, reduction of intake of analgesics) or very good (no more pain at all, no analgesics used). The compilation in Table 1 shows that psychotropic drugs caused a marked decrease of cancer pain in 50% to 90% of the patients. Unfortunately, we do not know of any controlled long-term studies. Usually the treatment of cancer pain is started with non-narcotic analgesics and when their analgesic effect is insufficient, in general, psychotropic drugs are added as a next step. In the above mentioned proportion (50% to 90%), psychotropic drugs, especially antidepressants and neuroleptics applied alone or in combination with non-narcotic analgesics, produce an essential alleviation of pain. The general condition of the patients is better physically (less pain and less intake of analgesics) as well as psychically (through the anxiolytic and antidepressive effect). The alleviation occurs in general in the 1st week (Kocher 1969). There are no controlled studies on the percentage of reduction of non-narcotic or narcotic analgesics by psychotropic drugs or on the general condition by means of specific rating scales. An essential advantage of psychotropic drugs is the fact that the use of narcotic analgesics can be avoided or delayed.

Dosage

The following dosage schedules, which in our experience proved successful, give a guideline; however, each pharmacologic treatment requires adaptation to the individual. In principle, the treatment must be started with a low dosage, which should be carefully increased until essential alleviation is achieved. If severe and/or disturbing side effects occur, the dosage must be decreased or the drug replaced by another one of the same group. Dosage schedule for antidepressants: Clomipramine: three times a day, 25 mg per os; imipramine: three times a day, 25 mg per os; amitriptyline: three times a day, 25 mg per os; maprotiline: three times a day, 25 mg per os; trimipramine: three times a day, 25 mg per os; nortriptyline: two times a day, 25 mg per os (in the morning and at noon). For

Table 1. The analgesic effect of psychotropic drugs in cancer pain

Author	Drug	Number of patients	Indication	Percentage of patients reporting alleviation of pain
Antidepressants:				
Daxelmüller (1966)	Imipramine	40	Neurologic patients, including cancer pain	80
Gebhardt et al. (1969)	Clomipramine	52	Cancer pain	67
Mönkemeier and Steffen (1970)	Imipramine	20	Cancer pain	75
Adjan (1970)	Imipramine	31	Cancer pain	80
Adjan (1970)	Clomipramine	50	Cancer pain	90
Barjou (1971)	Imipramine	30	Surgical patients, including cancer pain	70–80
Deutschmann (1971)	Imipramine	44	Cancer pain	80
Neuroleptics:				
Bloomfield et al. (1964)	Levomepromazine	18	Cancer pain and arthritis	> 50
Combinations of neuroleptics and antidepressants:				
Bernard and Scheurer (1972)	Clomipramine and levo-mepromazine or haloperidol	83	Cancer pain (inoperable)	87
Put (1974)	Fluphenazine and melitracene	17	Cancer pain (visceral)	67

long-term treatment, a single evening dose of an antidepressant without analeptic side effects is sufficient, e.g., amitriptyline, imipramine, maprotiline, trimipramine, 50–75 mg a day per os.

Dosage schedule for neuroleptics: Haloperidol: three times a day, 0.5–1 mg per os; levomepromazine: three times a day, 12.5–25 mg or 25–75 mg in the evening per os; chlorpromazine: three times a day, 25 mg or 50–75 mg in the evening; thioridazine: three times a day, 25 mg or 50–100 mg in the evening.

Dosage schedule for combined treatment with neuroleptics and antidepressants, as recommended by us: a) Inpatients. Clomipramine: continuous drop infusion (25–50 mg in 250 ml 5% glucose solution for 3–4 h once per day, after 1 week three times, 25 mg a day per os) in addition to haloperidol: three times a day 0.5–1 mg per os. b) Outpatients. Clomipramine: three times a day 25 mg per os, in addition to haloperidol: three times a day, 0.5–1 mg per os. The advantages of a combined treatment of neuroleptics and antidepressants, as recommended by us, are as follows: first, a combined treatment generally requires a lower dosage than with either drug alone; therefore, severe and/or disturbing effects can be avoided. The patients may also receive ambulatory treatment. Gram (1974) was able to demonstrate that in combined antidepressant-neuroleptic therapy the plasma level of the antidepressant is increased, so that lower dosages of antidepressants are sufficient. Furthermore, the analgesic effect is more rapid and more intensive. Second, a combined treatment has both antidepressive and neuroleptic effects often required to interrupt the vicious circle of pain → anxiety → depression → pain (Kocher 1976). Third, in a combined treatment, the positive effect of the antidepressants on serotoninergic and noradrenergic (pain) inhibitory pathways is increased by the action of neuroleptics, in particular, haloperidol, which might be due to its slight but definite opiate-agonistic activity.

Side Effects

Neuroleptics

Extrapyramidal motor disorders very seldom appear when the low dosages mentioned are used, but include dyskinesia at the start of therapy (acute dystonic reaction), akathisia (restlessness), and a slight Parkinson syndrome. More than 200 patients (Kocher 1979) were treated with low doses of neuroleptics and in no case could important side effects of this kind be found. In early dyskinesia (acute dystonic reaction), the neuroleptic has to be withdrawn immediately and an intravenous injection of biperidine must be given. If akathisia or a slight Parkinson syndrome appear, an antiparkinsonian drug must be given in addition. Other side effects caused by neuroleptics are dryness of the mouth, fall in blood pressure, sweating, hypocyclosis (accommodation disorders), and obstipation.

Antidepressants

Antidepressants can cause the following side effects in particular: dryness of the mouth, sweating, hypocyclosis (accommodation disorders), obstipation, orthostatic disorders, dysuria (particularly retention of urine), tachycardia, and tremor. In low doses as recommended by us, side effects can be minimized. It is important and vital that the possible side effects are explained to the patient before the medication is started. When low doses are given, the side effects caused by psychotropic drugs are a minor problem compared with the relief of pain experienced by the patient.

Summary

Treatment of cancer pain with psychotropic drugs offers the following advantages:
- It helps patients who do not normally respond to the usual analgesics.
- The effect of analgesics is enhanced.
- There is reduction in the use of analgesics.
- The antidepressive and anxiolytic effects improve the psychological condition.
- The use of opiate analgesics may be avoided or delayed.

References

Adjan M (1970) Zur therapeutischen Beeinflussung des Schmerzsymptoms bei unheilbaren Tumorkranken. Ther Ggw 109: 1620–1627

Barjou B (1971) Etude du Tofranil sur les douleurs en chirurgie. Revue Med Tours 6: 473–482

Beaumont G (1976) The use of psychotropic drugs in other painful conditions. J Int Med Res [Suppl 2] 4: 56–57

Bernard PhA, Scheurer H (1972) Action de la clorimipramine (Anafranil) sur da douleur des cancers en pathologie cervico-faciale. J Fr Otorhinolaryngol 21: 723–729

Bloomfield S, Simard-Savoie S, Bernier J, Tretault L (1964) Comparative analgesic activity of levopromazine and morphine in patients with chronic pain. Can Med Assoc J 90: 1156–1159

Clay GS, Brougham LR (1975) Haloperidol binding to an opiate receptor site. Biochem Pharmacol 42: 1363–1367

Creese J, Feinberg AP, Snyder SH (1976) Butyrophenone influences on opiate receptor. Eur J Pharmacol 36: 231–235

Daxelmüller L (1966) Zur Therapie schwerer Schmerzzustände mit Tofranil. Med Welt 43: 2339–2340

Deutschmann W (1971) Tofranil in der Schmerzbehandlung der Krebskranken. Med Welt 22: 1346–1347

Dilhuydy JM, Miguel Y, Oyon J (1979) Etude en double insu du tiapride dans les algies en carcinologie. Sem Hop Paris 55: 2020–2021

Flohé L, Friderichs E (1978) Alte Probleme und neue Aspekte in der Analgesieforschung. Drug Res 28: 99–106

Gebhart KH, Beller J, Nischk R (1969) Behandlung des Karzinomschmerzes mit Chlorimipramin (Anafranil). Med Klin 64: 751–756

Gennari C, Nami R, Pizzuti M, D'Ascenzo G, Bianchini C (1981) Effects du tiapride en perfusion sur le taux plasmatique de betaendorphine, prolactine et dopamine chez des patients souffrant d'algies cancereuses. Sem Hop Paris 57: 795–800

Gram LF (1974) Influence of neuroleptics and benzodiazepines on metabolism of tricyclic antidepressants in man. Am J Psychiatry 131: 863

Karkalas Y, Lal H (1973) A comparison of haloperidol with methadone in blocking heroin withdrawal symptoms. Int Pharmacopsychiatry 8: 248–251

Kocher R (1969) Zur Behandlung schwerer Schmerzzustände mit einer Kombination von Tofranil (Imipramin) und Nozinan (Laevopromazin). Praxis 57: 1459–1464

Kocher R (1976) The use of psychotropic drugs in the treatment of chronic, severe pains. In: Bonica JJ, Albe-Fessard D. (eds) Advances in pain research and therapy, vol 1. Raven, New York, pp 285–289

Kocher R (1979) The use of psychotropic drugs in the treatment of cancer pain. In: Bonica JJ, Ventafridda V (eds) Advances in pain research and therapy, vol 2. Raven, New York, pp 579–582

Lepille D, Bastit Ph (1979) Essai thérapeutique dans les algies néoplasiques. Sem Hop Paris 55: 791–795

Linke H (1963) Die Entpersönlichung des Schmerzes durch Phenothiazinderivate. Ther Berichte 35: 94–99

Maltbie AA, Cavenar O, Sullivan JL, Hammet EB (1979) Analgesia and haloperidol: a hypothesis. J Clin Psychiatry 40: 323–326

Mayer DJ, Price DP (1976) Central nervous system mechanism of analgesia. Pain 2: 379–404

Merskey H, Hester RA (1972) The treatment of chronic pain with psychotropic drugs. Postgrad Med J 48: 494–598

Mönkemeier D, Steffen U (1970) Zur Behandlung mit Imipramin bei Krebserkrankungen. Med Klin 65: 213–215

Pessey JJ, Lacomme Y (1980) Tiapride use in neoplasic algia. Sem Hop Paris 56: 351–353

Put TR (1974) Traitement des douleurs rebelles à l'aide du flupenthixol et du mélitracène. Ars Medici 29: 1401–1413

Simon EJ (1976) The opiate receptors. Neurochem Res 1: 3–28

Spencer PSJ (1976) Some aspects of pharmacology of analgesia. J Int Med Res 4: 1–14

Spencer PSJ, Lee RL, Sewell RDE (1979) Centrally-acting analgesics. A brief review of opiates and psychotropic drugs. Pharmaceut Med 1: 6–20

Takagi H (1980) The nucleus reticularis paragiganto-cellularis as a site of analgesic-action of morphine and enkephalin. Trends Pharmacol Sci 1: 182–184

Taub A, Collins WF (1974) Observations on the treatment on denervation dysaesthesia with psychotropic drugs: postherpetic neuralgia, anaesthesia, dolorosa, peripheral neuropathy. Adv Neurol 4: 309–315

Local Anesthetics in the Treatment of Cancer Pain

P. Porges

Klinik für Anästhesie und Intensivmedizin, Universität Wien, Spitalgasse 23, 1090 Wien, Austria

Local anesthetics play only a minor role in the treatment of cancer pain, but they are still important in three different ways.

Diagnostic and Prognostic Blocks

Diagnostic blocks are a useful tool in determining the path of pain transmission along neighboring sensory nerve routes as well as in differentiating between somatic and visceral pain (Bonica 1953, 1959). They may also help to localize the lesion in cases of projected pain (Fig. 1). Ahlgren et al. (1966) described graduated spinal block technique, which is a refined differential block. At 10-min intervals they injected 1. 5 ml isotonic saline, 2. 10 ml 0.2% procaine for sympathetic block, 3. 10 ml 0.5% procaine for sensory block, and 4. 10 ml 1% procaine for motor block. Wherever possible, we prefer to block anatomically distant structures in separate sessions, e.g., for differentiation of somatic pain of the abdominal wall from visceral pain in the upper abdomen we used, first, intercostal blocks and, second, celiac plexus blocks (Fig. 2). Before a diagnostic block is carried out, the patient should abstain from taking analgesics and hypnotics or, if this is impossible, at least should be on a clear-cut course of medication and should not receive premedication. Sedated patients who are taking a variety of drugs will make it impossible to interpret the outcome of the block. For quantification of their pain, patients may be asked to mark one of the verbal, numerical, or visual analogue pain scales (Rosen 1977; Fig. 3).

Drugs

Any local anesthetic may be used, but we prefer to use the long-acting drug bupivacaine so the patient has plenty of time to assess the effect of the block. In practice, one must be

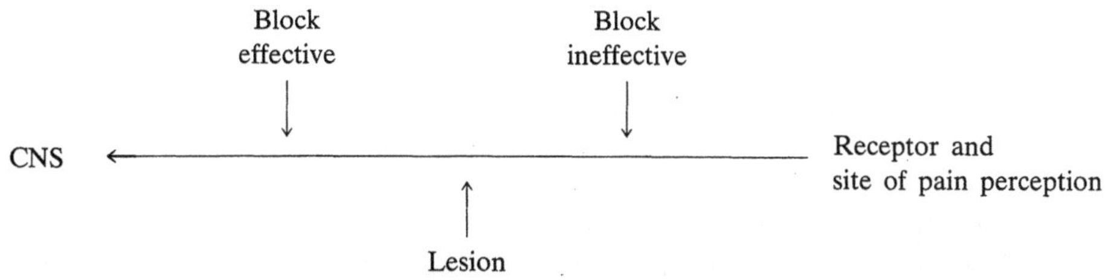

Fig. 1. Diagnostic block to locate the site of the noxious lesion. A lesion in an afferent nervous pathway produces projected (or referred somatic) pain in the area of the pysiological receptor. A local block will only work when performed proximal to the lesion

Recent Results in Cancer Research. Vol. 89

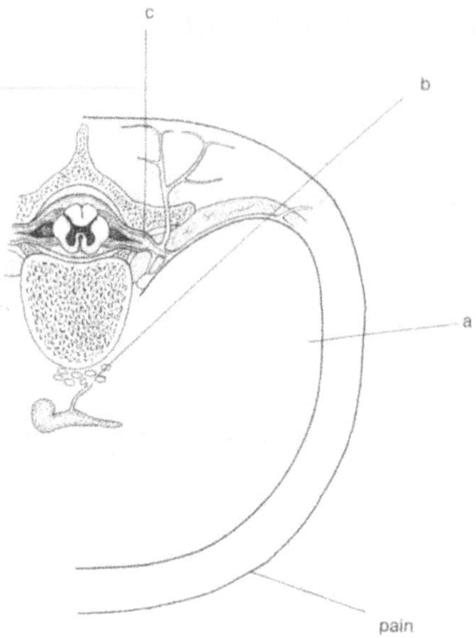

Fig. 2. Diagnostic blocks. *a,* Intercostal blocks will work in case of local pain. *b,* Celiac plexus block will work in case of visceral referred pain. *c,* Paravertebral blocks or epidural block will work in *a* and *b* and in spondylogenic projected pain

— none
— mild
— moderate
— severe

— no improvement
— slight improvement
— great improvement
— pain free

1 no pain
2
3
4
5
6
7
8
9
10 as much as you can imagine

no pain ——————————————— as bad as it could possibly be

Fig. 3. Scoring scales for assessment of pain. Verbal scale, verbal pain relief scale, numerical scale, and visual analogue scale

aware of the fact that placebo effects of blocks (Papper 1967) can confuse a diagnostic blocking program. It is also important to repeat diagnostic nerve blocks and, if there is any doubt about the result, a placebo block with saline might help to clarify the situation. If the patient does not get relief from the block, then either the messages on the noxious stimuli are traveling via another neural pathway or the pain complaint has other causes than noxious stimulation in the periphery. A prognostic block performed before neurolysis with alcohol or phenol enables the patient to familiarize himself with the postneurolytic situation and may help him to decide whether he will accept neurolysis.

Temporary Blocks

This is the use of local anesthetics in the sense of their definition as drugs for the local and reversible block of pain receptors and/or their afferent nerve fibers. In this field, the epidural catheter is of practical importance. By the continuous epidural application of local anesthetics, a patient can be freed from his pain for a limited period of time, e.g., before or after an operation or during the last few days of his life. An epidural block gives instant relief and provides the time to try a longer-lasting method of pain relief, e.g., radiotherapy, cytostatic therapy, or neurosurgery.

Choice of Drugs

Tetracaine, bupivacaine, and etidocaine are the long-acting local anesthetics in clinical use. Etidocaine, which has excellent motor blocking but weak sympathetic blocking properties (Foldes and Porges 1976), is least qualified for chronic pain therapy. For surgical purposes, tetracaine seems to be the more popular drug in America, whereas bupivacaine is more widely used in Europe. For pain therapy, bupivacaine is the drug of choice. Its longer onset time is not a disadvantage in this field. Bromage (1975) compared etidocaine, tetracaine, lignocaine, and bupivacaine and found that bupivacaine in dilute solutions gave the least motor block for any given degree of sensory block. Clinical doses have no sedative effect (Niederlehner et al. 1981). The addition of a vasoconstrictor to a long-acting local anesthetic for pain therapy is not indicated, as no apparent prolongation of the block can be achieved with it. Adrenaline has only a minor influence on the absorption of bupivacaine (Boyes 1981). Doses used for pain relief are always well below the recommended maximum doses; approximately one-third of the dose needed for surgery in the same region is sufficient. The effective dose depends on a variety of factors (Table 1), but the usual dose is 5–10 ml 0.25% bupivacaine at 4- or 6-h intervals. The dose of the epidural local anesthetic must be carefully chosen and adapted and readjusted to the needs of the individual patient.

Tachyphylaxis plays a minor role where long-acting local anesthetics are used. A constant drip infusion is no more effective than intermittent administration (Renck 1980). When relieved from their principal pain by the block, most patients with malignant disease will complain of pain in other areas. In spite of an effective epidural blockade, they will not be able to come off their sedative and analgesic medications completely. The caudal epidural catheter introduced via the sacral hiatus has no advantages over the lumbar route. For reasons of hygiene, we have used it only occasionally in patients with colostomy. Epidural catheters may be introduced at any level, but, for anatomical reasons, the introduction is more difficult in the midthoracic level (D_4–D_7). Thoracic catheters are rarely used. As a rule, paravertebral test blocks followed by intrathecal alcohol neurolysis are preferred. We can keep epidural catheters in situ for up to 14 days, but longer periods have been reported, especially since the injection of opiates into the epidural space has become a clinical method (Farcot et al. 1982).

In our opinion, a visible inflammatory reaction with a thin necrotic seam around the catheter should be a reason to remove it. If necessary, a catheter can be replaced at another vertebral level. Pilon and Baker (1976) reported a case of pain control by means of an epidural catheter that remained in situ for $4^1/_2$ months. However, in this case the catheter was connected to a subcutaneously situated shunt reservoir. The aim of the temporary block should be to use the time to institute a longer-lasting method of pain relief by other

Table 1. Factors influencing the dose of local anesthetic required for epidural block

Dose	Influencing factors
More	Somatic pain Great extension of area to be blocked Lumbar area
Less	Thoracic area Old age Increased intraabdominal pressure (tumor, ascites, obesity) Burning pain Visceral pain

means. The epidural opiate application in cancer pain (see Zenz, this volume p. 107 ff.) has reduced the use of local anesthetics in this field today. The combined epidural application of opiates and local anesthetics has been advocated (Müller et al. 1980, 1982). The development of extremely long-acting local anesthetics (Scurlock and Curtis 1981) might result in new applications in the future.

Therapeutic Blocks

The crucial question is: It is possible that a local anesthetic agent exerts a permanent or at least a long-lasting effect? Can the analgesic effect persist when there is no longer an effective concentration of the agent at the site of injection? Empirically we must admit that there are lasting analgesic effects. This can be partially explained by the interruption of skeletomotor and vasomotor efferents, producing pathophysiologic reflex responses resulting in vasoconstriction, ischemia, and local acidosis that may be new sources of noxious stimulation (Bonica 1974). The assumption that there are ongoing depolarizing stimuli to the nociceptive afferents, which, once blocked off, do not reappear, is also plausible. In fact, cardiologists use local anesthetics for ectopic excitation and extrasystoles and they have lasting therapeutic effects (Kuschinsky and Lüllmann 1978). In this respect, the heart is a model for the nervous system. Not only local anesthetics, but several other drugs have analogous effects on the nervous system and the heart. For instance, barbiturates depress excitability in both structures, and cardioactive pressor agents are also central-nervous-system stimulators.

Local blocks are not a suitable form of treatment for severe states of pain as common in patients with bone metastases or with nerve compression syndromes due to expanding tumors. However, some symptoms of pain indicate their possible use: painful muscle spasms due to a malignant affection of the vertebral column, trigger points, and the tumor-induced sympathetic reflex dystrophy (Dargent 1948; Challenger 1978; Gerbershagen 1979) are indications of when therapeutic local anesthetic blocks can be used. An X-ray or scintigram that shows vertebral metastases should never be the end of our diagnostic efforts. The painful condition of the patient must be investigated and the region examined visually and manually. Pain mediated by trigger points can be treated successfully with small volumes of dilute solutions (e.g., 3–5 ml 0.25% bupivacaine). If a trigger point cannot be found, spastic muscles should be infiltrated directly. The addition of hyaluronidase for better spreading of the solution is advisable (5–10 ml 0.25% bupivacaine + 100 U hyaluronidase).

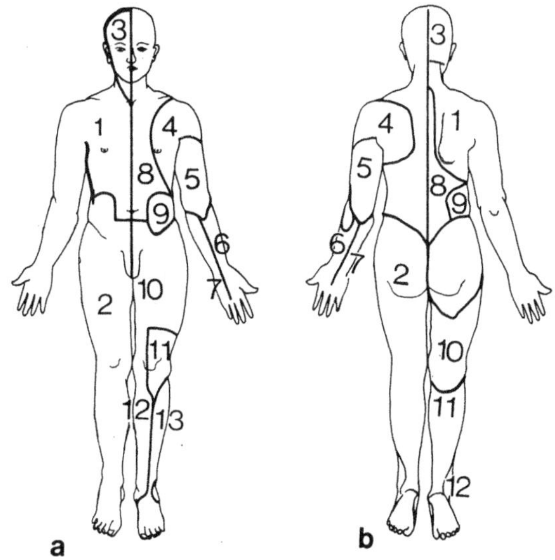

Fig. 4a, b. Distribution of vascular-zone disturbances as described by Gross (1972) in one or more arterial supply zones of the skin. *1,* Subclavian artery (upper quadrant of the body); *2,* iliac arteries (lower quadrant of the body) and subdivisions of these major trunks; *3,* common carotid artery; *4,* axillary artery; *5,* brachial artery; *6,* radial artery; *7,* ulnar artery; *8,* thoracic aorta; *9,* abdominal aorta; *10,* femoral artery; *11,* popliteal artery; *12,* posterior tibial artery; *13,* anterior tibial artery (Gerbershagen 1979)

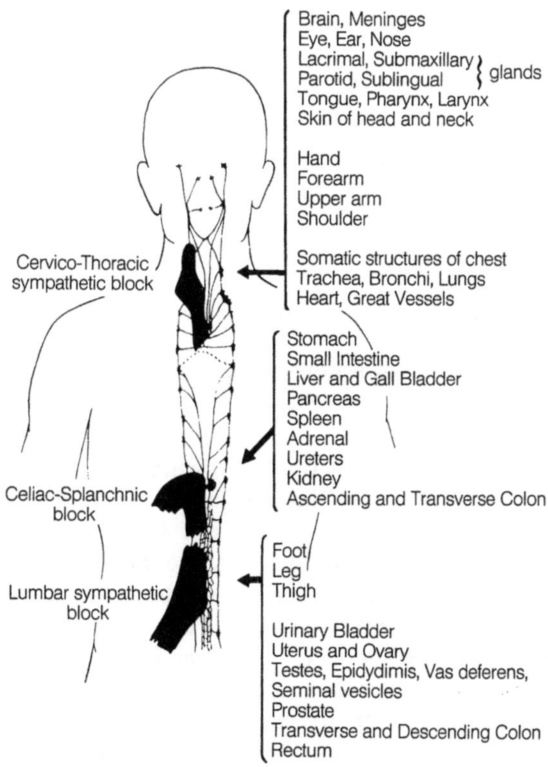

Fig. 5. The three principal sites to interrupt the regional sympathetic nervous supply. On the left is the pattern of diffusion of local anesthetic solutions injected into the fascial planes of the stellate ganglion, the celiac plexus, and the lumbar sympathetic ganglia. On the right are the names of the structures affected with each block. After F. A. D. Alexander (Bonica 1959)

Sympathetic nerve blocks are a valuable tool in treating the type of pain that is associated with carcinomatous neuritis. The symptoms are the same as for sympathetic reflex dystrophy: pain (often burning), hyperpathia, sudomotor disturbances, skin cyanotic or pale, and edema followed by dystrophic alterations of skin, osteoporosis. Characteristically, these pains are burning and dull. Their spatial distribution does not correspond to segmental or peripheral nerve distribution but involves one or more vascular zones (Gross 1972; Fig. 4a, b). The regional sympathetic nervous supply can be blocked at three sites (Fig. 5).

Stellate Ganglion Block

More than 30 methods of stellate ganglion block have been described (Jenkner 1980). The anterior paratracheal technique is simple and most widely used (Fig. 6). The patient lies in the dorsal recumbent position with a pillow under the shoulder and the neck slightly hyperextended. A thin 3–4 cm needle with the syringe attached is inserted horizontally at the level of the cricoid cartilage, while the sternocleidomastoid muscle and the carotid artery are pressed laterally with the index and middle fingers of the left hand. The needle impinges on the transverse process of C_6 at a depth of about 2 cm and is then withdrawn by 0.3 cm. The tip of the needle is now in the prevertebral fascia, which is the plane of the stellate ganglion. After injection of 8–10 ml 0.5% bupivacaine, the patient is sat up to induce a downward spread of the solution.

The celiac plexus is far from any somatic nervous pathway that could be damaged, so alcohol may be employed for the relief of upper-abdominal cancer pain.

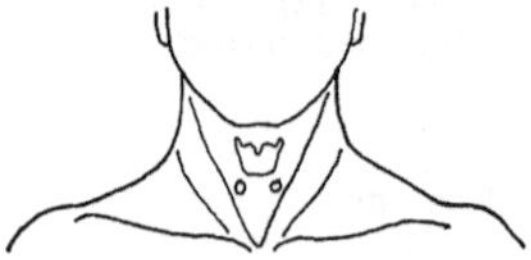

Fig. 6. Stellate ganglion block. Site of puncture for the anterior paratracheal technique

Lumbar Sympathetic Block (Moore 1978)

The lumbar sympathetic ganglia lie along the anterolateral surface of the vertebrae, medial to the psoas muscle. The patient lies in a prone position with a pillow placed under the abdomen. The spines of the lumbar vertebrae are identified and marked (Fig. 7a, b) and horizontal lines are drawn through the middle of the spines L_2, L_3, and L_4. The intersections of these lines with a vertical line 4.5–5 cm from the midline mark the points of insertion of the needles. On one level, a 10-cm needle is now passed cephalad at a 45-degree angle to the skin until the transverse process of the vertebrae is contacted. The distance (3.8–5 cm) is marked on the needle, the needle retracted, and redirected into a transverse plane with the tip pointing slightly medially. In this new direction, the needle is readvanced to a level 4.5 cm deeper than before. There will be a minimal resistance if the needle is well placed in the loose areolar tissue around the lumbar sympathetic ganglia. If the needle is within the psoas muscle, a definite resistance to injection will be felt. A test injection of 2 ml air may be given to discern better the area of high resistance. The distance from the plane of the transverse processes to the lumbar sympathetic ganglia is fairly constant, whereas the distance from the skin to the transverse processes is more variable. It is sufficient to determine it at one level only. Ten milliliters of 0.25% bupivacaine injected at each level will give an efficient sympathetic block of one lower extremity. For bilateral sympathetic blockade of the legs, a caudal or lumbar epidural block with 20 ml 0.25% bupivacaine is an alternative method that yields good results.

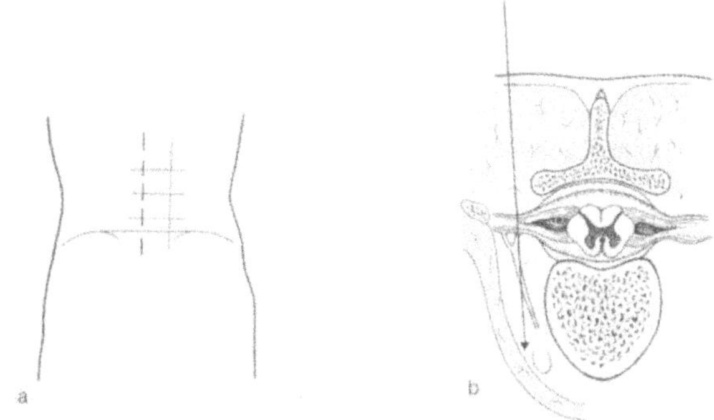

Fig. 7a, b. Landmarks for lumbar sympathetic block. Sagittal section showing the path of the needle

Complications

All those who perform major blocks with local anesthetics must be aware of the possible complications and must know the relevant precautions and therapies. Although the doses employed for pain therapy are only about one-third of those used for surgery and are always well below the recommended maximum dose, this is no guarantee against toxic reactions. Whereas surgical blocks are, as a rule, performed in or near an operating theater, it is tempting to carry out therapeutic blocks in the ward or in an insufficiently equipped outpatients department.

Systemic Toxicity

The majority of toxic reactions are caused by high blood levels of the local anesthetic due to intravascular injection, overdose, or to rapid absorption from highly vascular regions or inflamed tissue. The speed of absorption is also increased when hyaluronidase has been added. Preventive measures are as follows: Avoid overdoses; inject slowly with frequent aspiration tests; and before all major blocks, give 5 mg diazepam i.v. or 10 mg i.m.

Central-Nervous-System Complications

Unconsciousness. The unconscious patient who is pink and breathing spontaneously should be placed on his side and respiration and circulation should be closely observed. Administration of oxygen is recommended. Instruments for intubation and ventilation must be available.

Seizures. Therapy should begin as early as possible so prodromes, such as anxiety, drowsiness, muscle twitching, numbness of lips and tongue, and flickering of the eyelids must not be overlooked. Most seizures are short and will end even before therapy has begun.
The first therapeutic step is to give oxygen as, during convulsions, the patients' respiration is disturbed and oxygen consumption is high. Thus a dangerous hypoxic state ensues; 5 mg diazepam are given then. Sustained convulsions (Moore 1978) are very rare and need

Table 2. Equipment and drugs to counteract complications of regional block

Oxygen supply masks
Suction apparatus
Laryngoscope, tubes, airways
ECG monitor
Cardiac defribrillator
Drugs: diazepam, atropine, vasoconstrictor drugs, relaxants, methylprednisone, calcium cloride, sodium bicarbonate
i.v. sets
i.v. fluids

further treatment: the patient should be relaxed, intubated, ventilated with oxygen, and anesthetized with normal doses of barbiturates (e.g., 5 mg/kg thiopental). Subsequent doses of barbiturates and relaxants should keep the patient in anesthesia for 30 min before being brought round to ascertain that convulsions are no longer present.

Cardiovascular Complications

These must be treated according to the symptoms present. Atropine, ephedrine or another alpha- plus beta-adrenergic vasoconstrictor, and all means of cardiovascular resuscitation must be available (Table 2). Albright (1979) reports several cases of seizures induced by bupivacaine followed by cardiac arrests. The common features of these arrests were their long duration and resistance to therapy.

Allergy

Allergies to local anesthetics are occasionally claimed by patients who have experienced unpleasant systemic effects from an added vasoconstrictor while in the dentist's chair. True allergies accompanied by, e.g., itching, wheezing, and dermal reactions, are rare and occur rather with the ether type of local anesthetic than with the amide type (Fisher and Pennington 1982). Allergy to methylparaben, a preservative in many preparations, is also possible (Moore 1978; our own experience). Treatment is as for any allergic reaction: administration of fluids, vasoconstrictors, methylprednisone, calcium, oxygen, and cardiovascular support as required.

Complications of Epidural Blocks

Bradycardia and/or hypotension are common sequelae of thoracic epidural blocks, especially in elderly patients. Epidural administration of local anesthetics is contraindicated in hypovolemic situations. Local anesthetics in the upper thoracic epidural space will also block parts of the thoracic sympathetic system and the Nn. accelerantes of the heart. These cardiovascular changes may sometimes require therapy. Bradycardia responds readily to 0.5 mg atropine and hypotension responds to administration of fluid and/or vasoconstrictors (e.g., 10 mg ephedrine i.v.).

Pneumothorax

This is a complication of a paravertebral block. It may also occur when stellate ganglion, brachial plexus, or intercostal nerve blocks are performed. Coughing and subscapular pain are the indications and a chest X-ray will confirm the diagnosis. In most cases, admission to hospital, observation, and bed rest for 24 h will be sufficient.

General Effects

Independent of any local anesthetic effect, a series of parenteral local anesthetic injections has proven to be advantageous for the general condition of the cachectic and restless patient, a finding gerontologists make use of (Aslan 1951). This is probably a major factor for the success of many neural therapeutic procedures (Dosch 1981; Göbel 1979–1982) that include regular procaine injections (Schlitter 1979; Böcker 1974).

Summary

Local anesthetics are in general not suitable for the treatment of patients with severe cancer pain. Local blocks are useful for diagnostic and prognostic purposes. As their action is instantaneous and reliable, they can be used to relieve pain for a limited period of time. The use of local anesthetics may yield long-lasting relief in some specific pain syndromes, such as tumor-related reflex dystrophies, in painful muscle spasms, and trigger points due to tumor-affected vertebrae. In addition, local anesthetics may have a generally beneficial effect in the restless, cachectic, and aged patient.

References

Ahlgren EW, Stephen CR, Lloyd AC, McCollum DE (1966) Diagnosis of pain with a graduated spinal block technique. JAMA 195: 813–816

Albright GA (1979) Cardiac arrest following regional anesthesia with etidocaine or bupyvacaine, Anesthesiology 51: 285–287

Althoff H (1973) Therapie mit Novocain. In: Killian H (ed) Lokalanästhesie und Lokalanästhetika. 2nd edn. Thieme, Stuttgart

Aslan A (1951) Neue Erfahrungen über die verjüngende Wirkung des Novocains nebst experimentellen, klinischen und statistischen Hinweisen. Therapiewoche 8: 10

Böcker R (1974) Procainhydrochlorid per os hat Schutzeffekt bei Tumorbildung. Med Trib 22: 28

Bonica JJ (1953) The managment of pain. Lea and Febiger, Philadelphia

Bonica JJ (1959) Clinical applications of diagnostic and therapeutic nerve blocks. Thomas, Springfield

Bonica JJ (1974) General clinical considerations (including organization and function of a pain clinic). In: Bonica JJ, Procacci P, Pagni CA (eds) Recent advances on pain. Thomas, Springfield, pp 274–298

Boyes RN (1981) Some aspects of the systemic absorption and toxicity of local anaesthetic agents. In: Rugheimer E, Zindler M (eds) Anaesthesiology, int cong ser 538. Exerpta Medica, Amsterdam, pp 907–909

Bromage PR (1975) Mechanism of action of extradural analgesia. Br J Anaesth 47: 199–211

Challenger JH (1978) Sympathetic nervous system blocking in pain relief. In: Swerdlow M (ed) Relief of intractable pain, 2nd edn. Biomedical, Amsterdam, pp 157–182

Dargent M (1948) Role of sympathetic nerve in cancerous pain, inquiry into 300 cases. Br Med J 1:440

Dosch P (1981) Lehrbuch der Neuraltherapie nach Huneke, 10th edn. Haug, Heidelberg

Farcot JM, Laugner B, Muller A (1982) Therapeutic and diagnostic uses of morphine epidurals in the management of pain: In: Yaksh TL, Müller H (eds) Spinal opiate analgesia. Springer, Berlin Heidelberg New York, pp 40–46 (Anaesthesiology and intensive care medicine, vol 144)

Fisher M McD, Pennington JC (1982) Allergy to local anaesthesia. Br J Anaesth 54:893–894

Foldes FF, Porges P (1976) Cerebrospinal fluid and plasma levels of etidocaine after peridural administration. In: Anaesthesia and pharmacology. Boerhave series for postgraduate medical education Nr 12. Leiden University Press, Leiden, pp 78–85

Gerbershagen HU (1979) Blocks with local anesthetics in the treatment of cancer pain. In: Bonica JJ, Ventafridda V (eds) Advances in pain research and therapy, vol 2. Raven, New York, pp 311–323

Göbel J (1979–1982) Die Neuraltherapie nach Huneke. Phys Med u Rehab 12/79; 7/80; 12/80; 8/82

Gross D (1972) Therapeutische Lokalanästhesie. Hippokrates, Stuttgart

Jenkner FL (1980) Nervenblockaden auf pharmakologischem und auf elektrischem Weg, 3rd edn. Springer, Wien New York

Kuschinsky G, Lüllmann H (1978) Kurzes Lehrbuch der Pharmakologie und Toxikologie, 8th edn. Thieme, Stuttgart, p 122

Moore DC (1978) Regional block. A handbook for use in the clinical practice of medicine and surgery, 4th edn. Thomas, Springfield, pp 211–218

Müller H, Börner U, Hempelmann G (1980) Tissue and cerebrospinal fluid tolerance of epidural opiate application. In: Cools AR, Nijhus GMM (eds) Analgesia by peridural and spinal opiates, Proceedings of Nijmegen Congress, pp 171–187

Müller H, Stoyanov M, Börner U, Hempelmann G (1982) Epidural opiates for relief of cancer pain. In: Yaksh TL, Müller H (eds) Spinal opiate analgesia. Springer, Berlin Heidelberg New York, pp 125–137 (Anaesthesiology and intensive care medicine, vol 144)

Niederlehner JR, Cosma A, DiFazio A (1981) Comparison of bupivacaine and lidocaine: general anesthetic potency and therapeutic index. Reg Anesth 6:95–98

Papper EM (1967) Regional anesthesia. A critical assessment of its place in therapeutics. Anesthesiology 28:1074–1084

Pilon RN, Baker AR (1976) Chronic pain control by means of an epidural catheter. Cancer 37:903–905

Renck H (1980) Tachyphylaxis during postoperative peridural analgesia of long action. In: Wüst HJ, Zindler M (eds) Neue Aspekte in der Regionalanaesthesie 1. Springer, Berlin Heidelberg New York, pp 188–191 (Anaesthesiology and intensive care medicine, vol 124)

Rosen M (1977) The measurement of pain. In: Harcus AW, Smith R, Whittle B (eds) Pain, new perspectives in measurment and management. Churchill Livingstone, Edinburgh, pp 13–19

Schlitter HE (1979) Erfahrungen mit der Neuraltherapie bei fortgeschrittenen Krebserkrankungen. Krebsgeschehen 1:2–13

Scurlock JE, Curtis BM (1981) Tetraethylammonium derivates: ultralong-acting local anesthetics. Anesthesiology 54:265–269

Treatment of Cancer Pain with Neurolytic Agents

U. Drechsel

Deutsche Klinik für Diagnostik, Aukammallee 33, 6200 Wiesbaden, FRG

Introduction

Whenever we are dealing with cancer pain we are also – owing to Bonica's indefatigable efforts (Bonica 1953, 1954, 1978, 1979) – dealing with neurolytic blocks. Injection of neurolytic agents – substances that destroy the nerve tissue – is a special type of regional anesthesia.

Ethyl alcohol and phenol are the neurolytics used almost exclusively today. Despite an abundance of published data in favor of it, this method is only rarely practiced, although it has advantages such as technical simplicity, applicability to patients in poor physical condition, a fair success rate, a low complication rate, and economy (Gerbershagen 1981). But it demands knowledge of the benefits and risks and its limitation to pain in special areas. In principle, it could be carried out by a physician versed in regional anesthesia, but mostly it is performed by experienced anesthesiologists. In the treatment of pain neurolytic agents are used for subarachnoid blocks, sympathetic blocks, and injections into the sella turcica. Among the less important peripheral nerve blocks, the subdural, and epidural blocks, only the latter are again receiving increasing attention (Colpitts 1978; Maher and Mehta 1977; Swerdlow 1978). This paper gives an outline of substances used as neurolytic agents and their indications, methods of administration, complications, and results involved.

Pitres and Vaillard (1888) were the first to inject alcohol for the treatment of trigeminal neuralgia. Dogliotti (1931) reported on the intrathecal application of alcohol in order to relieve pain. Then Maher used the already known neurolytic agent phenol in 1955 also for intrathecal pain therapy. Other neurolytic agents, however, such as chlorocresol, ammonium sulfate, and hypertonic saline solution, did not gain lasting recognition (Katz 1974; Maher 1963; Swerdlow 1973). Up to the beginning of the 1970s, there was intensive publication of results (Bonica 1953, 1954; Gerbershagen et al. 1972; Lifshitz et al. 1976; Papo and Visca 1974, 1976; Stovner and Endresen 1972), but later no essentially new aspects were presented, although very little evidence has been produced so far. Furthermore, it has not been established which neurolytic agent can be used in what concentration or where to inject it; moreover, there have been no controlled studies comparing the use of neurolytics with other methods. In the following, a survey is given of the present state of research on neurolytic blocks based on the literature and personal experiences.

Mechanisms of Action

For a long time it was believed that neurolytics predominantly affect the thin pain-conducting C fibers, the A-delta and A-gamma fibers (Mahler 1957), hardly involving

Recent Results in Cancer Research. Vol. 89

the thicker ones (Iggo and Walsh 1960; Nathan and Sears 1960) and thus having a selective effect. This could not be confirmed, however, in animal experiments (Nathan et al. 1965; Stewart and Lourie 1963). Protein denaturation is not selective for fibers of different diameters but severe damage to the perineural vascular elements is noted (Burkel and McPhee 1970), depending only on the quantity and concentration of the neurolytic agent and its possible range of distribution in the tissue. The results of histopathologic analyses following alcohol or phenol treatment are practically identical (Møller et al. 1969): Phenol results in a more transient and alcohol in a more permanent interruption of impulse conduction (Moore et al. 1957). The latter also accounts for the dreaded secondary neuritis occurring in about 15% of the cases, above all when alcohol is applied at the peripheral nerves (White and Sweet 1955). Phenol diffuses more easily and thus does not cause such circumscribed lesions (Feldmann 1974). Therefore, if chemical neurolysis of a peripheral nerve is necessary, phenol should be preferred. In the subarachnoidal space, however, only the posterior roots are exposed; so the destructive effect rarely causes significant neurological deficits (Iggo and Walsh 1960; Maher 1957, Nathan and Sears 1960), depending, of course, on the number rather than on the type of fibers affected, whereas the motor fibers of the anterior roots should not be involved. Degeneration of the ascending pathways is a sequel secondary to the histologic changes in the dorsal root. The spinal ganglion is rarely found to be affected.

Substances Used for and Technique of Subarachnoid Block

As ethanol (98%) is highly hypobaric with a specific weight of from 0.79 to 0.81 compared to cerebrospinal fluid (CSF) with its specific weight of 1.007, gradually injected alcohol accumulates in the upmost portion of the vertebral canal. The posterior roots to be blocked must be located at this maximal point (Fig. 1); therefore, the patient has to be placed in the so-called anterolateral position (a forward tilt of 45° from the lateral position) for unilateral dorsal-root block with the painful side facing upward. In addition, pillows are placed under the patient until maximal curvature of the vertebral spine is achieved in the area of the pain-conducting dorsal roots. This position – uncomfortable at times – is maintained by straps or tape to prevent involuntary movement of the patient causing the neurolytic agent to spread (Gerbershagen 1981).

The choice of the site of puncture depends on the segments to be blocked. Of course, the neurolytic agent must be introduced at the origin of the dorsal roots from the cord, not at its point of passage through the foramen intervertebrale, because, at its origin, the root still consists of eight to ten fila radicularia which provide a larger area for the neurolytic agent to work on. A short beveled cannula is used for puncture (gauge 25 for alcohol, gauge 22 for phenol) with the opening pointing upward. After free passage of the cerebrospinal fluid, 98% alcohol is injected by a tuberculine syringe in a volume of 0.2 to 1 ml per segment and at a speed not faster than 0.1 ml per min. Cutaneous hypalgesia is tested by needle stimulation after each partial injection. The total volume depends on the degree of hypalgesia and on the degree of pain reduction. For a period of up to 15 min post injection, the patient often has a sensation of heat as well as segmental paresthesias. These sensations, which start after 30 s, indicate whether the injection is acting in the precise area of pain aimed at, thereby allowing adjustment of needle placement (Swerdlow 1978). We do not block more than two segments per session.

If bilateral neurolysis is required, it can be carried out with the patient in the prone position. Adjustment of the operation table will bend the patient's spine in such a way that

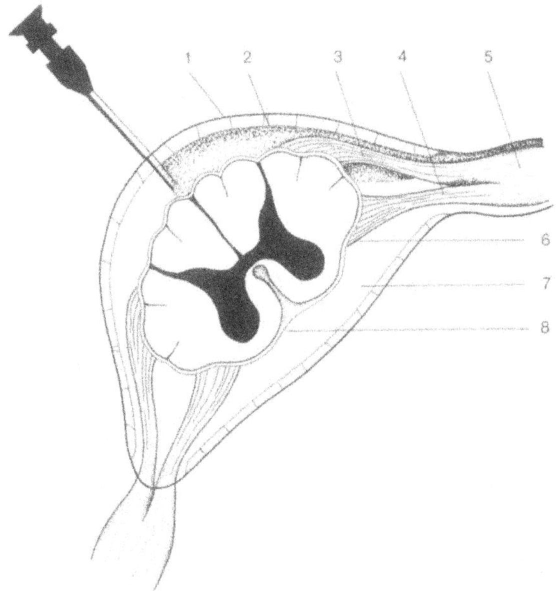

Fig. 1. Subarachnoid alcohol block. With the patient in the anterolateral position, hypobaric alcohol forms a layer on the CSF reaching the dorsal roots only. *1,* dura mater; *2,* arachnoidea; *3,* dorsal root; *4,* ventral root; *5,* ganglion spinale; *6,* fila radicularia; *7,* cavum subarachnoidale; *8,* pia mater (Gerbershagen et al. 1972)

the roots to be blocked will be located at the highest point of the vertebral canal. Here 1 to 1.5 ml ethyl alcohol per segment is needed. Two unilateral injections, one on each side given with the patient in the lateral position treating the side with severest pain first and the other in a subsequent session, will, however, be more efficient. The distal sacral fibers can also be blocked in cases of pain in the small pelvis and in the perineum related to tumors in that area. The patient is placed in a prone position, his sacral region being as elevated as possible, and lumbar puncture through intervertebral space L5/S1 is carried out with aspiration of CSF and slow injection of 1 to 1.5 ml alcohol.

Phenol is soluble in water at concentrations up to 6.7% and at higher concentrations in glycerine. Phenol-glycerine (5% to 10%) is used for intrathecal neurolysis. With its specific weight of 1.027 it is hyperbaric to CSF and therefore accumulates at the lowest point. The patient must lie on the painful side with the segment to be blocked at the bottom, then follows dorsal tilting through 45° and attachment of straps to maintain this position (see Fig. 1, turned through exactly 180°). A cannula of at least gauge 22 is needed as the solution is viscous. With the opening pointing downward, 0.1 ml/min is injected with a tuberculine syringe giving up to 0.2–0.5 ml per segment. To block several segments several cannulas should be used because of more precise positioning of the neurolytic agent in relation to the dorsal roots. For the sacral fibers, in the case of pain in the pelvis-perineum area, 0.3–0.7 ml 6% phenol-glycerine is injected with the patient sitting. After injection, the patient is tilted by a dorsal flexion of 45°. This is preferred in patients who already have colostomy with a permanent bladder catheter, since a so-called saddle block frequently leads to paralysis of the sphincter ani and the detrusor vesicae. Motor disorders in the lower extremities need not occur with the appropriate procedure. Of course, continuous checking of hypalgesia is mandatory when injecting these neurolytic agents and this calls for a cooperative, nonsedated patient.

One of the reasons why we prefer to use alcohol instead of phenol is that the patient does not have to remain lying motionless on the side suffering pain for at least 20 min. This is necessary when using hyperbaric phenol as this neurolytic agent takes so long for fixation at the roots and for diffusion in the remaining CSF without risk (Brodauf 1974; Pietsch 1974). After termination of the alcohol or phenol injection, the mandrin of the cannula is reintroduced, although the cannula itself still remains in situ, to avoid CSF turbulence. Now the patient may be sedated as necessary. After 20 min, the cannula is slowly rinsed with 0.1 ml normal saline solution to avoid irritation of the tissue by the neurolytic agent on removal of the cannula.

Diagnostic Local-Anesthetic Block

A preceding diagnostic spinal anesthesia with a local anesthetic is of particular importance (0.05 ml hyperbaric local-anesthetic solution per segment if a phenol block is planned; Gerbershagen 1981). Only in complete pain relief do we consider injection of a neurolytic agent. The patient will then know what to expect and the therapist can collect the relevant data on pain conduction and pain response.

Indications for Performing Subarachnoid Blocks with Neurolytic Agents

These are as follows:
- Advanced stage of neoplastic disease
- Severely debilitated patient
- Life expectancy less than 6 months
- Contraindication of neurosurgical procedures or their refusal by the patient
- Inefficacy of peripherally acting analgesics
- Inefficacy of transcutaneous nerve stimulation
- No pain relief after a series of blocks with local anesthetics
- Localization of cancer pain: segmentally limited pain of the trunk wall between T3 and T10 and pain of the pelvic wall and of the retroperitoneum between S2 and S5
- Types of pain: of nonvisceral and of nonparenchymatous origin.

This list may read like a negative catalog, but it is important that the site, type, and extent of pain are the main criteria in the proper selection of patient for this treatment.

Contraindications

These are:
- Inefficiency of diagnostic nerve block with local anesthetic
- Extended and mainly nonlocalized pain areas
- Tumor within the spinal cord or the spinal column at the level of injection
- Pain of the limbs due to major nerve compression with edema (on account of the accompanying sympathetic reflex dystrophic component)
- Patients unable to lie still (because of increased complication rate from CSF turbulence)
- Addiction to narcotics (depending on the individual case: if narcotics are used merely on account of pain, their administration will be reduced by other pain-relieving measures).

Results of Subarachnoid Neurolytic Blocks

The reported results are difficult to compare since there are a number of factors involved, such as the assessment of pain relief and also the nature of the malignant disease itself, i.e., the site and growth of the tumor, the tissues involved, and the sequelae of the accompanying cancer therapy. The utilizable cases of subarachnoid alcohol blocks with categories of assessment in the literature found by Papke (1974) and those treated with phenol reported by Swerdlow (1979a) are summarized in Table 1, in which "good" means either complete pain relief for more than 1 month or being free from pain till death; "fair" means complete pain relief for less than 1 month or reduction of pain for more than 1 month; and "poor" means relief for several days only or no analgetic effect at all. These almost identical results are difficult to evaluate since they are not subdivided into groups according to site and type of tumor and the associated complications. The results concerning the duration of pain relief, are also not beyond doubt, as shown by some more recent reports (see Table 2).

Whereas Ventafridda and Martino (1976) achieved a mean duration of pain relief of 15.5 days only, Swerdlow (1979a) reported better results. However, approximately 30% of the patients needed a second injection before a stable painfree period was reached. This proportion was also confirmed by a review of 789 patients from the literature (Papke 1974). More than two injections does not increase the success rate further. The proper selection of patients with respect to the site of the tumor is obviously of utmost importance. Detailed data on this subject obtained in recent years are given by only some authors who are, however, true experts in this technique. Swerdlow (1979a) quotes particularly good and/or longer-lasting results of pain relief in tumors of the rectum, cervix, breast, and colon (see Table 3). According to the data reported in Table 3, we only use subarachnoid neurolytic blocks in circumscribed – preferably unilateral – somatic pain of the trunk or in bilateral saddle pain in patients with colostomy and permanent bladder catheter. We never use it in visceral, parenchymatous, nerve compression, or limb pain.

Table 1. Results of subarachnoid neurolytic blocks without subdivision

	Efficacy of therapy (% of patients)			
	No. of patients	Good relief	Fair relief	Poor relief
Review of alcohol blocks (Papke 1974)	1,908	60	21.3	18.7
Review of phenol blocks (Swerdlow 1979a)	1,387	61	15	24

Table 2. Results of subarachnoid neurolytic blocks with subdivision

Author	No. of patients	No. of blocks	Good results (% of patients)	Mean duration of pain relief
Ventafridda and Martino (1976)	227	319	56	15.5 days
Swerdlow (1979a)	130	200	64	2–3 months

Table 3. Results of subarachnoid neurolytic block depending on the localization of pain

Region		Authors		
		Ventafridda et al. (1976)	Papo and Visca (1976)	Gerbershagen (1981)
C7–Th5	Chest wall	+	±	+
	Chest and lung	–	–	–
	Lung and brachial plexus	±	–	0
	Vertebral	–	0	0
Th6–Th12	Splanchnic	–	–	–
	Kidney	–	–	–
	Abdominal wall	+	+	+
	Vertebral	±	0	0
L1–S5	Visceral	–	–	–
	Visceral and bone	–	0	–
	Pelvic wall	+	+	+
	Sciatic pain	0	–	0
	Perineum	+	+	+
	Sacral wall	+	+	0
	Lower limbs	+	–	0
Other	Bone pain	0	+	0
	Radicular pain	0	–	–

+, Good results
±, Fair results
–, Poor results
0, No information

As the authors' criteria for "good, fair, poor" are not identical, only unambigious information from single reports supporting the same tendencies has been selected

Complications

Two aspects should be observed: the complication rate related to the site of the subarachnoid injection and the duration of the complication. Motor pareses occur when a ventral root is hit unintentionally: paresis of the extremities in the case of intrathecal injections on a level with the roots of the plexus brachialis (C4 to Th1) or the plexus lumbosacralis (L1 to S2). Respiration may be affected by complete blocking of dorsal and ventral roots of several thoracic segments. Patients with severe ventilatory obstruction or borderline insufficiency should not be given thoracic blocks, two segments already may become dangerous even if the ventral roots are only transiently blocked. Bladder dysfunction is seen after intrathecal blocks of the sacral segments in 50% of cases, lasting from some days to 4 weeks and, in a few cases, even longer (Ventafridda 1979). Deficits in cutaneous sensibility occur transiently and are often similar to those experienced by the patient during the preceding diagnostic block (see Table 4).

Table 4. Complications with > 2,125 alcohol subarachnoid blocks in 1,478 patients (Gerbershagen 1981)

Complications	Duration of complication		Total (%)
	Transient	Permanent	
Paresis/paralysis	92	18	5
Bladder dysfunction	137	14	7
Bowel disorder	8	3	0.5
Others	19	10	1.5
Total	256 (12%)	45 (2%)	14

The duration of 232 complications has been stated exactly: 28% disappeared within 3 days, 23% passed within 1 week, 21% within 1 month, 9% within 4 months, and only 18% lasted longer than 4 months (Gerbershagen 1981). In contrast to these favorable data, taking the overall complication rate of different injection sites together, there are reports showing an elevated risk with special localization of injection. Ventafridda and Martino (1976) found bladder and/or lower-limb disorders in up to 67% of patients when injecting the neurolytic agent between L1 and S5. Generally, however, it can be stated that the complication must be related to the intensity of pain, on the one hand, and the side effects of narcotics used or neurosurgical procedures on the other hand (Gerbershagen 1981).

Sympathetic Blocks with Neurolytic Agents

The rationale for producing a sympathetic block for pain relief is twofold: (1) some pain is enhanced by the pathophysiologic influence of the sympathetic (efferent) nervous system to the region where the pain originates (algodystrophies, sympathetic reflex dystrophies) and (2) nociceptive afferent fibers, particularly those with nociceptors in the viscera and blood vessels, course through the sympathetic ganglia before they enter the spinal cord. Thus, indications for neurolysis of the sympathetic nervous system are pain from visceral tumors and pain showing signs of sympathetic dysfunction, whereby the latter may be successfully treated with a series of local anesthetic blocks. There are three targets of sympathetic blocks: The cervicothoracic sympathetic trunk for pain arising in the head, upper extremity, lung, and pleura; the ganglion celiacum for pain from the viscera between stomach and colon transversum; and the lumbar sympathetic trunk for pain from the pelvic viscera, the descending colon, and the lower extremity.

A diagnostic block with a local anesthetic is mandatory in testing the susceptibility to pain before carrying out a neurolytic injection. For this correct placement of the needle has to be monitored using X rays or computer tomography, after a contrast medium has been injected into the compartment confined by the fasciae around the sympathetic ganglia (Boas et al. 1976; Ferrer-Brechner and Brechner 1976; Moore et al. 1981).

The concentrations and volumes of neurolytics needed for sympathetic blocks are as follows. Plexus solaris, n. splanchnicus: 30 ml 50% ethanol, 6% phenol in water, or 7.5% in X-ray contrast medium lumbar sympathetic block: 5 ml 50% ethanol, 6% phenol in water, or 7.5% in X-ray contrast medium (with two cannulas in adjacent ganglia, the amount is to be doubled).

Absolute alcohol may be diluted with normal saline or local anesthetic to a concentration of 50%. The patient will feel an intense burning pain with the injection. Considering the technique and radiologic monitoring in two positions, there is practically no risk of injuring lung, kidney, or any other organ. If blood has been aspirated from the vena cava or aorta, one should not inject a neurolytic agent at the same session because it might be too diluted. The injection should be carried out slowly and should be discontinued at once if the cutaneous sensibility test, which is performed continuously, indicates hypesthesia.

Indications for neurolytic blocks of the cervicothoracal chain, in particular of the ganglion stellatum, are rarely present since tumor pain from the upper thoracic region and upper extremities is additionally transmitted via somatic nerves (Batzdorf and Brechner 1979). More important and more successful is the block of the celiac ganglion (Itoh et al. 1979; Thompson et al. 1977). The lumbar sympathetic block – also carried out in the case of impaired circulation (Boas et al. 1976) – may be helpful with visceral pelvic pain (Moore 1979b). As tumors in the pelviperitoneal area rarely grow viscerally only, but infiltrate their environment, a lumbar sympathetic block will help for a limited time only, although it should still be tried because of its low risk of complications (Moore 1979b; Ventafridda and Martino 1976). Results of sympathetic blocks with neurolytics agents against cancer pain have been less frequently reported than blocks against vascular disorders or reflex dystrophies. Since Bonica (1953) injected neurolytics at all levels of the sympathetic chain, the method has been widely used, but even the report of Reid et al. (1970), which involved 1,666 blocks in 1,028 patients, for different reasons left the number of satisfactory results open. Moore's data (1979a) showed the effect of a celiac plexus block with alcohol on upper intra-abdominal visceral cancer pain. In his study, 168 patients (75% with pancreas tumors) received 186 blocks; 94% had good to excellent pain relief ranging from 5 days to 1 year, but no data are given on the ratio of number of patients/duration of pain relief. Growth of the tumor and its infiltration beyond the organs innervated by the celiac plexus are the reasons for failure. Results of a lumbar sympathetic block with neurolytic agents only reveal temporary relief for 1 to 4 weeks with bladder and prostate pain (Moore 1979b), but complications are less frequent than with intrathecal administration of neurolytics. Reid et al. (1970) found in 9% of patients neuritis related to adjacent nerves of the lumbosacral plexus, subsiding after some weeks. Other complications, such as pneumothorax or renal injury with hematuria, occur in 0.5% of the cases. Impotence accompanying a bilateral lumbar sympathetic block is frequent and must be discussed with male patients in advance (Challanger 1978). Hypotension subsequent to a plexus solaris block may occur by severe dilatation of the splanchnic vessels, which lasts for several days, and should be treated – particularly in the beginning – by increasing the circulating volume and by administering vasoconstrictors (Itoh et al. 1979). Intravasal injections of phenol must be avoided as this may lead to convulsions (Benzon 1979).

The neurolysis of peripheral somatic nerves is carried out rather less often now compared with the past. Alcohol leads to secondary neuritis in 15% of the cases (White and Sweet 1955) and phenol acts too inefficiently and, besides, for too short a time. This method is still carried out only by some groups very experienced in pain treatment, such as the groups of Swerdlow (1979b), Churcher (1978), Ventafridda et al. (1980), and Bonica and Madrid (1979), the latter two using it in cases of facial pain. One approach, the interscalenus block of the brachial plexus, performed with phenol, especially against the almost unmanageable shoulder-arm pain with Pancoast's tumor is still noteworthy (Bonica 1953; Swerdlow 1979b). The plexus is situated between fascial layers, including the perivascular sympathetic supply. Mullin uses 10 ml 3% phenol in water, an otherwise weak neurolytic concentration (Mullin 1980).

Finally let us come to the question of which neurolytic agent should be used for the different blocks – alcohol or phenol? Since the histopathology of the nerves is the same after both of these treatments, it is a matter of what one has been used to (Swerdlow 1978). However, the literature deals predominantly with phenol for subarachnoid blocks, apparently because anesthesiologists are more familiar with the use of hyperbaric solutions, a preference regarded as a prejudice (Katz 1974). Like Gerbershagen (1981), we prefer alcohol because the patient is usually unable to lie down on the side where the pain originates. There is one other procedure using neurolytic agents for pain relief in cancer patients, namely the injection of alcohol into the sella turcica. This is discussed in the chapter by Siegfried et al. in this volume (p. 148 ff.).

Conclusions

The use of neurolytic agents is recommended for intrathecal injection between segments T3 and T10 for pain of the thoracic wall, but not for pain of parenchymatous origin; between S2 and S5 for pain of the retroperitoneum and the pelvic wall (patients with colostomy and permanent bladder catheter); and in the sympathetic system, in the ganglion celiacum for visceral pain of the upper abdomen and in the lumbar sympathetic chain for reflex dystrophies associated with tumors. Neurolytics are not advisable for the cervical segments (paresis of the brachial plexus), for the thoracic segments in the case of severe bronchial obstruction, for intraspinal tumors, or for pain in the extremities due to nerve lesions. Only localized cancer-related pain is subject to neurolytic treatment. If this is found to be advisable it should be carried out in due time, as long as the patient can be expected to resume his normal activities which had been hampered by pain. In the advanced cachectic and final stage, this therapy is an additional burden to the patient and one should then resort to other methods.

References

Batzdorf U, Brechner VL (1979) Management of pain associated with the Pancoast syndrom. Am J Surg 137: 638–646

Benzon HT (1979) Convulsions secondary to intravascular phenol: a hazard of celiac plexus block. Anesth Analg (Cleve) 58: 150–151

Boas RA, Hatangdi VS, Richards EG (1976) Lumbar sympathectomy – a percutaneous chemical technique. In: Bonica JJ, Albe-Fessard D (eds) Advances in pain research and therapy, vol 1. Raven, New York, pp 685–689

Bonica JJ (1953) The management of pain. Lea and Febiger, Philadelphia

Bonica JJ (1954) The management of pain of malignant disease with nerve blocks. Anesthesiology 15: 280–301

Bonica JJ (1978) Cancer pain. A major national health problem. Cancer Nurs J 4: 313–316

Bonica JJ (1979) Cancer pain, introduction. In: Bonica JJ, Ventafridda V (eds) Advances in pain research and therapy, vol 2. Raven, New York, pp 1–12, 115–130

Bonica JJ, Madrid JC (1979) Therapy of cancer pain in the head and neck. Role of nerve blocks. In: Bonica JJ, Ventafridda V (eds) Advances in pain research and therapy, vol 2. Raven, New York, pp 537–542

Brodauf H (1974) Äthanolkonzentrationsbestimmung an benachbarten Segmenten nach intraspinaler Injektion bei der Katze. MD Thesis, University of Mainz, Germany

Burkel WE, McPhee M (1970) Effect of phenol injection into peripheral nerve of rat: electron microscope studies. Arch Phys Med Rehabil 51: 391–398

Challanger JH (1978) Sympathetic nervous system blocking and pain relief. In: Swerdlow M (ed) Relief of intractable pain, 2nd edn. Elsevier, Amsterdam, pp 157–182

Churcher M (1978) Peripheral nerve blocks in relief of intractable pain. In: Swerdlow M (ed) Relief of intractable pain, 2nd edn. Elsevier, Amsterdam, pp 99–120

Colpitts MR, Levy BA, Lawrence M (1978) Treatment of cancer-related pain with phenol epidural block. In: Abstracts of the Second World Congress on Pain, vol 1. International Association for the Study of Pain, Seattle, p 147

Dogliotti AM (1931a) Traitement des douleurs de la périphérie par alcoolisation subarachnoidienne des racines posterieures à leur émergence de la moelle épinière. Presse Med 39: 1248

Dogliotti AM (1931b) Nouvelle méthode thérapeutique pour les algies périphériques. Injection d'alcool dans l'espace sous-arachnoidienne. Rev Neurol (Paris) 2: 485

Feldmann SA (1974) Chemical neurolysis in the treatment of chronic pain. In: Hart DF (ed) The treatment of chronic pain. MTP, Lancaster, p 163

Ferrer-Brechner T, Brechner VL (1976) Accuracy of needle placement during diagnostic and therapeutic nerve blocks. In: Bonica JJ, Albe-Fessard D (eds) Advances in pain research and therapy, vol 1. Raven, New York, pp 679–683

Gerbershagen HU, Baar HA, Kreuscher H (1972) Langzeitnervenblockaden zur Behandlung schwerer Schmerzzustände. I. Die intrathecale Injektion von Neurolytika. Anaesthesist 21: 112–121

Gerbershagen HU (1973) Behandlung chronischer Schmerzzustände mit Nervenblockaden. In: Killian H (ed) Lokalanästhesie und Lokalanästhetika. Thieme, Stuttgart, pp 760–792

Gerbershagen HU (1981) Neurolysis. Subarachnoid neurolytic blockade. Acta Anaesthesiol Belg 32: 45–57

Iggo A, Walsh EG (1960) Selective block of small fibers in the spinal roots by phenol. Brain 83: 701–708

Itoh T, Fujimo Y, Yamada S (1979) The management of the intra-abdominal celiac plexus block for the intractable abdominal pain. Jpn J Anesth 28: 197–204

Katz J (1974) Current role of neurolytic agents. Adv Neurol 4: 471–476

Lifshitz S, Debacker LJ, Buchsbaum HJ (1976) Subarachnoid phenol block for pain relief in gynecologic malignancy. Obstet Gynecol 48: 316–320

Maher RM (1955) Relief of pain in incurable cancer. Lancet I: 18–20

Maher RM (1957) Neuronal selection in relief of pain, further experience with intrathecal injections. Lancet I: 16–19

Maher RM (1963) Intrathecal chlorocresol in the treatment of pain in cancer. Lancet I: 965–967

Maher RM, Mehta M (1977) Spinal (intrathecal) and extradural analgesia. In: Lipton S (ed) Persistent pain. Academic Press, London; Grune and Stratton, New York, pp 61–99

Mehta M (1973) Intractable pain, Saunders, London

Møller JE, Helweg-Larson J, Jacobsen E (1969) Histopathological lesions in the sciatic nerve of the rat following perineural application of phenol and alcohol solutions. Dan Med Bull 16: 116–119

Moore DC, Bridenbaugh LD, Baker JW, Stone CS (1957) The postoperative mastectomy syndrome. Arch Surg 75: 946–951

Moore DC (1979a) Celiac (splanchnic) plexus block with alcohol for cancer pain of the upper intra-abdominal viscera. In: Bonica JJ, Ventafridda V (eds) Advances in pain research and therapy, vol 2. Raven, New York, pp 357–371

Moore DC (1979b) Role of nerve block with neurolytic solutions for pelvic visceral cancer pain. In: Bonica JJ, Ventafridda V (eds) Advances in pain research and therapy, vol 2. Raven, New York, pp 593–596

Moore DC, Bush WH, Burnett LL (1981) Celiac plexus block: a roentgenographic, anatomic study of technique and spread of solution in patients and corpses. Anesth Analg (Cleve) 60: 369–379

Mullin V (1980) Brachial plexus block with phenol for painful arm associated with Pancoast's syndrome. Anesthesiology 53: 431–433

Nathan PW, Sears TA (1960) Effects of phenol on nervous conduction. J Physiol (Lond) 150: 565–580

Nathan PW, Sears TA, Smith MC (1965) Effects of phenol solutions on the nerve roots of the cat: An electrophysiological and histological study. J Neurol Sci 2: 7–29

Papke H (1974) Indikationen, Möglichkeiten und Grenzen der subarachnoidalen Alkoholinjektionen. MD Thesis, University of Mainz, Germany

Papo J, Visca A (1974) Phenol rhizotomy in the treatment of cancer pain. Anesth Analg (Cleve) 53: 993–997

Papo J, Visca A (1976) Intrathecal phenol in the treatment of pain and spasticity. Prog Neurol Surg 7: 56–130

Pietsch A (1974) Konzentrationsbestimmungen von Phenol nach intraspinaler Applikation bei der Katze. MD Thesis, University of Mainz, Germany

Pitres A, Vaillard L (1888) Des névrites provoquées par le contact de l'alcool pur ou diloué avec les nerfs vivants. C R Soc Biol (Paris) 5: 550

Reid W, Watt JK, Gray TG (1970) Phenol injection of the sympathetic chain. Br J Surg 57: 45–50

Stewart WA, Lourie H (1963) An experimental evaluation of the effects of subarachnoid injection of phenol-pantopaque in cats. J Neurosurg 20: 64–72

Stovner J, Endresen R (1972) Intrathecal phenol for cancer pain. Acta Anaesthesiol Scand 16: 17–21

Swerdlow M (1973) Intrathecal chlorocresol, a comparison with phenol in the treatment of intractable pain. Anaesthesia 28: 297–301

Swerdlow M (1978) Intrathecal and extradural block in pain relief. In: Swerdlow M (ed) Relief of intractable pain. Elsevier, Amsterdam, pp 121–156

Swerdlow M (1979a) Subarachnoid and extradural neurolytic blocks. In: Bonica JJ, Ventafridda V (eds) Advances in pain research and therapy, vol 2. Raven, New York, pp 325–337

Swerdlow M (1979b) Role of nerve blocks in pain involving the chest and brachial plexus. In: Bonica JJ, Ventafridda V (eds) Advances in pain research and therapy, vol 2. Raven, New York, pp 567–576

Thompson GE, Moore DC, Bridenbaugh LD (1977) Abdominal pain and alcohol celiac plexus nerve block. Anesth Analg (Cleve) 56: 1–5

Ventafridda V, Martino G (1976) Clinical evaluation of subarachnoid neurolytic blocks in intractable cancer pain. In: Bonica JJ, Albe-Fessard D (eds) Advances in pain research and therapy, vol 1. Raven, New York, pp 699–703

Ventafridda V, Fochi C, Sganzerla EP, Tamburini M (1979) Neurolytic blocks in perineal pain. In: Bonica JJ, Ventafridda V (eds) Advances in pain research and therapy, vol 2. Raven, New York, pp 597–605

Ventafridda V, Fochi C, de Como F (1980) Nerve blocks. In: Twycross RG, Ventafridda V (eds) The continuing care of terminal cancer patients. Pergamon, Oxford, pp 135–145

White JC, Sweet WH (1955) Pain, its mechanisms and neurosurgical control. Thomas, Springfield

Wood KM (1978) The use of phenol as a neurolytic agent: a review. Pain 5: 205–229

Neurosurgical Treatment of Cancer Pain

J. Siegfried[1], A. Kühner[2], and V. Sturm[2]

[1] Abteilung für Neurochirurgie, Rämistrasse 100, 8049 Zürich, Switzerland
[2] Abteilung für Neurochirurgie, Im Neuenheimer Feld 110, 6900 Heidelberg 1, FRG

Introduction

Neurosurgery for cancer pain should always be considered when, in an advanced stage of the disease, the pain no longer responds to conservative treatment methods or only at the cost of undesired side effects. Appreciable progress has recently been achieved in this field. Almost all the operations that can be considered for the cancer patient can be performed percutaneously, without general anesthesia, without loss of blood, and with a short hospital stay. Parallel to the advances in the field of pain physiology, the neurosurgical therapeutic spectrum has also extended. In the choice of operation, it is of decisive importance to distinguish between deafferentation pain and somatic pain. Deafferentation pain is taken to mean pain in an area of disturbed sensitivity, as can be observed, e.g., after radiation damage to the brachial plexus. Somatic pain occurs because of irritation of pain receptors, for instance, bone pain in bone metastases. In accordance with this clinical pain classification, there are in principle two methods available for neurosurgery: (1) Interruption of the tracts conducting pain between the periphery and the cerebral integration centers. These are the destructive methods that are primarily considered in cases of somatic pain. (2) Intermittent electric stimulation of a tract or of a center aimed at producing inhibition of the pain information. These techniques are designated as neuroaugmentative, since here relief from pain is attained by stimulation of pain-inhibiting systems. These techniques are mainly used for treatment of deafferentation pain. A third (nondestructive) technique using a percutaneous approach consists of administration of opiates to the spinal cord via a catheter which can also be connected to a subcutaneously implanted reservoir.

On the basis of the experience of two neurosurgery departments in which all presently possible operations are performed, the most important treatment methods are described and analyzed critically.

Destructive Techniques

Interruption of the pain-conducting pathways can take place on various levels, from the periphery to the cerebral centers. Depending on the level of the operation and the technical procedure, almost selective destruction is possible: thus, pain conduction is suppressed and analgesia is produced with maintenance of the epicritic sensitivity, i.e., avoiding anesthesia. The interruption of afferent pain pathways is a very attractive approach in the treatment of somatic pain in the advanced stage of cancer.

Recent Results in Cancer Research. Vol. 89

Interruption of Peripheral Nerves

Neurolytics. Chemical neurolysis with alcohol or phenol is treated in detail by Drechsel. A few critical comments might be useful. A chemical blockade of peripheral nerves not only leads to anesthesia, but also to motor deficits. Unfortunately, the relief from pain attained is mostly only temporary. The situation is similar for chemical blockades of the sympathetic plexus.

Neurotomies. Transection of a peripheral nerve leads to analgesia, anesthesia, and motor deficits in the area supplied by this nerve. In about 10% of the cases, dysesthesias or anesthesia dolorosa occur as a sequel of the transection. Because of this severe side effect, in our opinion neurotomy should not be used even for localized facial pain. There is no doubt that retroganglionic operations (rhizotomies) afford better results. Finally, it must be pointed out that, outside the face area, pain syndromes concerning the area innervated by a single peripheral nerve are extremely rare.

Sympathectomies. Sympathectomies are not usually performed by the neurosurgeon, but fall within the field of general surgery. They may be useful in the treatment of visceral or causalgiform pain. The often poor results are due above all to the fact that it is almost impossible to eliminate all afferents from a visceral organ coursing through the sympathetic ganglia.

Rhizotomies

Surgical Rhizotomy. A rhizotomy or radicotomy is the interruption of the dorsal root between the spinal cord and the spinal ganglion. This interruption leads to a complete and definitive loss of somatic sensation, i.e., anesthesia and analgesia without motor deficits. Recently, a certain selectivity has been claimed, i.e., a predominant elimination of the pain-conducting A delta and C fibers (Sindou et al. 1976), resulting in analgesia without complete anesthesia. However, this technique requires open surgery under complete general anesthesia (laminectomy). Percutaneous controlled thermocoagulation of the dorsal roots is less burdensome. This likewise enables more or less selective elimination of the pain fibers, which only have a small degree of myelination since they react more sensitively to heat than the more highly myelinated fibers that conduct epicritic sensation. Because of overlapping of the innervation areas, it is necessary to eliminate more roots than the number of dermatomes into which the pain projects. Since carcinoma pain in only one dermatome is extremely rare, a relatively large number of dorsal roots would have to be eliminated in most cases. For this reason, rhizotomy is only very rarely indicated in carcinoma pain. It has been applied above all in cases of Pancoast tumors and carcinomas in the throat and neck region. Recently, rhizotomies have been largely replaced by percutaneous chordotomy with the exception of those cases of cancer pain localized in the region supplied by the trigeminal or glossopharyngeal nerves. Here, controlled thermocoagulation of the trigeminal ganglion via the foramen ovale or of the glossopharyngeal nerve via the foramen jugulare can produce adequate analgesia in many cases (Broggi and Siegfried 1979; Tew 1977).

Intrathecal Neurolytics. A detailed description is given by Drechsel. We should like to restrict ourselves to a few critical comments. This is a chemical rhizotomy to which the same limitations apply as to surgical rhizotomy. In addition, the limitation already mentioned with regard to neurolytic treatment of peripheral nerves also applies: a complete and definitive block of conduction is frequently not attained, so that pain relief is mostly of limited duration. In addition, the spatial distribution of the neurolytics is difficult to control, so that a distinct elimination of a dermatome is often difficult to attain. In our experience, intrathecal neurolytics are most suitable for pain localized in the sacrum and coccyx, e.g., in cases of rectal carcinoma. However, percutaneous cordotomy and intrathecal application of morphine are rival techniques that will be preferred in many cases.

Anterolateral Cordotomy

Since its introduction by Spiller and Martin (1912), surgical interruption of the ascending tract systems in the anterolateral part of the spinal cord has become the most widespread and most effective neurosurgical method in treatment of carcinoma pain. The development of the technique of percutaneous cordotomy by Mullan (1963) enabled this operation also to be carried out in those cancer patients who are regarded as inoperable because of their poor general condition. This operation is characterized by a minimum of operation trauma and stress and is performed under local anesthesia which gives immediate control of the pain relief attained. The anterolateral cord is punctured laterally between C1 and C2 under X-ray image intensifier control. The correct position of the electrode tip in the anterolateral cord outside the pyramidal tract is controlled by electric stimulation through the electrode used for coagulation. A lesion made in a somatotopically correct position produces analgesia, i.e., elimination of pain sensation with preserved tactile sensitivity. The reviews of large-scale results (Lorenz 1976; Piscol 1975) and the results obtained by the Heidelberg and Zürich University Departments of Neurosurgery can be designated as excellent in 75% of the cases. Unfortunately, the pain relief attained is mostly limited. Pain recurs frequently as early as 6 to 12 months after the operation. After 3 years, only 24% of the patients are still free of pain (Rosomoff 1971). For these reasons, cordotomy should be primarily employed in patients with limited life expectancy.

Usually, failures are due to technical difficulties, e.g., in some cases, it is not possible to introduce the electrode into the anterolateral cord. By electric test stimulation, the electrode position and thus the site of the thermolesion can be exactly localized topographically. Severe complications, for example, homolateral hemiplegia, are extremely rare and are likely to be due to a lesion of the vessels supplying the pyramidal tract (Kühner 1981). High cervical percutaneous cordotomy (at C1–C2 level) is the method of choice for unilateral pain below C5. Bilateral high cervical cordotomy for bilateral pain is dangerous even when the second operation is performed with a latency of a few weeks, since severe respiratory disorders with nocturnal apnea can occur (Krieger and Rosomoff 1974; Kuperman et al. 1971). In cases of bilateral pain below T5, bilateral open high thoracic cordotomy might be considered. However, the risk of definitive sphincter paralysis is high, so that the necessity for this operation should be carefully evaluated. The combination of unilateral high cervical percutaneous cordotomy with a stereotactic interruption of the spinothalamic tract of the other side at the mesencephalic level or a stereotactic lesion in the nonspecific nuclei of the thalamus is less problematic.

Myelotomy

Myelotomy or spinal commissurotomy, in which the decussating pain pathways in the spinal cord are interrupted after laminectomy, has been performed especially in midline pain and pain in the pelvic region. However, the relatively poor results and the introduction of other techniques have long rendered this method relatively unimportant.

Medullary Tractotomy

Medullary tractotomy is the interruption of the descending tract of the trigeminal nerve in the region of the medulla oblongata. It is noteworthy that here predominantly the pain-conducting afferent fibers are interrupted, producing analgesia but no anesthesia. In addition, analgesia in the areas innervated by the caudal cranial nerves, i.e., in the pharynx, can be attained. This operation is thus an alternative to coagulation of the trigeminal ganglion or the glossopharyngeal nerve for pain in the face or pharynx, and also has the advantage of selective analgesia. The first operation of this kind was performed by Sjöqvist (1938) after opening the posterior cranial fossa. However, this is a relatively burdensome microsurgical operation which cannot be carried out in most cancer patients. As an alternative, Crue (Crue et al. 1967) developed a percutaneous stereotactic technique in which the tractotomy is carried out by high-frequency thermocoagulation. This lighter operation is feasible in many cancer patients, but it requires a high technological standard and is not performed in all departments of neurosurgery. The results reported in the literature (Crue et al. 1971; Fox 1973; Hitchcock 1970; Hitchcock and Schvarcz 1972) are excellent. The incidence of complications is low and deaths have not been reported. Medullary tractotomy might thus be considered for treatment of carcinoma pain in the region of the face and nasopharynx.

Mesencephalotomy and Thalamotomy

Before spinal and intracerebral neurostimulation were introduced, stereotactic destruction (particularly within the thalamus) was frequently performed. With the aid of the stereotactic operation technique, it is possible to reach any point in the brain with high accuracy using an appropriate instrument. Exactly localized lesions in the pain system can be achieved by high-frequency thermocoagulation. The technique is characterized by a very slight burden for the patients. Stereotactic destruction of the spinothalamic and spinoreticulothalamic tracts at the level of the mesencephalon on one side only was carried out in bilateral pain, especially in the pharynx region (Nashold 1972; Whisler and Voris 1978) with good pain relief. However, complications such as Parinaud syndrome or contralateral hemiparesis or even persistent dysesthesias are very frequent (Nashold et al. 1977), so that this technique is hardly used nowadays.

In the thalamus, the destructive operations have the following targets: (a) the specific somatosensory thalamic nuclei (ventroposterolateral and ventroposteromedial nucleus); (b) the nonspecific thalamic nuclei such as the intralaminar nucleus, the centrum medianum, the parafascicular nucleus and the nucleus limitans; (c) the frontothalamic system with the group of the dorsomedian nuclei; and (d) the pulvinar nucleus, the function of which in pain processing is not yet clear. The targets most often used were the nonspecific thalamic nuclei and the pulvinar nucleus. The results of these operations are difficult to evaluate, so that there are contradictory data in the literature (Pagni 1974). In our experience, there is 60% relapse of pain after 6 months and 70% relapse is to be expected after 1 year (Siegfried and Krayenbühl 1972). The indication for application of these techniques should be cautiously examined, especially since they can be replaced by neurostimulation techniques in many cases.

Hypophysectomy

The first hypophysectomies in cancer-pain patients were performed in the early 1950's (Huggins and Bergenstal 1952; Luft and Olivecrona 1953; Perrault et al. 1952). By elimination of the hypophysis, both the growth of bone metastases and the associated pain can be favorably influenced in cases of hormone-dependent carcinomas (mammary carcinoma, prostate carcinoma). Carcinoma pain is the most important indication for hypophysectomy. As early as 1967, the results of 3,400 hypophysectomies were available from various clinics (Dargent and Romieu 1967). The first hypophysectomies were performed transcranially, then by transsphenoid microsurgery with a transnasal approach or stereotactically with implantation of radioactive substances, by cryosurgical measures or high-frequency coagulation. In the experience of the Zürich University Medical School (Landolt and Siegfried 1970), relief of bone pain persisted for up to 8 months in almost 80% of the cases after stereotactic transnasal high-frequency coagulation of the hypophysis. The experience of the Heidelberg University Department of Neurosurgery with hypophysis elimination by means of radiogold was less favorable: in 672 patients with mammary or prostate carcinoma, the bone pain could be reduced or abolished in only 42% of the cases by eliminating the hypophysis. Gros et al. (1975) observed an influence on pain in 65% of the cases after elimination of the hypophysis with yttrium 90. After transsphenoid microsurgical hypophysectomy, Hardy (1975) was able to influence the pain in 92% of the cases.

The introduction of alcohol injection into the hypophysis, introduced by Moricca in 1963 but published in 1974 once more aroused interest in hypophysis elimination. Moricca (1974) reported excellent results: thus, 687 cancer-pain patients attained immediate and long-lasting relief from pain following hypophysis elimination by means of alcohol injection. However, in a large number of cases the injection had to be repeated several times; thus, 1,600 injections were performed in 687 patients. In 1976, Moricca reported attaining pain relief in 1,139 patients with 2,775 injections in 86.5% of the cases. However, less favorable results were also reported: Miles (1979) attained pain relief in only 42.5% of these patients. Miles and Lipton (1976) postulated that the effect of the alcohol injection might be due to diffusion of the alcohol into the hypothalamus. This would explain why the alcohol injection into the hypophysis is also effective in carcinomas that are not hormone-dependent and why this method provides better results than most other procedures for the elimination of the hypophysis. However, highly divergent results are also found in the literature for alcohol injections (Lipton 1978; Madrid 1979; Swerdlow 1980). The typical complications of hypophysis elimination include CSF fistulae, diabetes insipidus, and oculomotor disorders. The mortality is reported to be 4% (Lipton 1978).

There is no doubt that elimination of the hypophysis by whatever technique can influence cancer pain, especially bone pain in hormone-dependent carcinomas, such as mammary and prostate carcinoma. However, as a rule the results obtained do not last for very long and the rate of complications cannot be ignored. This is one of the reasons hypophysectomies are performed in only a few centers. Furthermore, there has been a change since the introduction of bromocriptine (Pravidel). Drastic and long-lasting improvements of metastasis pain were attained with bromocriptine in prostate carcinomas (Jacobi et al. 1980) and in mammary carcinomas (Frantz 1978).

Neurosurgical Methods of Neurostimulation

The postulation of the gate-control theory (Melzack and Wall 1965) was a major incentive for the development of the neurostimulation technique. According to this physiologic working hypothesis, the pain signals which are conducted via the nonmyelinated and the thin myelinated afferent fibers are inhibited in the spinal dorsal horn by the sensory stimulations conducted via the large caliber medullated fibers. The technique was first applied clinically by Sweet and Wepsic (1968). These authors attained pain relief by electric stimulation of a peripheral nerve. The gate-control theory has been criticized in the meantime from various sides and the mechanisms by which stimulation of the spinal cord and midbrain in man may relieve pain are still open to discussion. Antidromic activation of large diameter primary afferents in the posterior columns, which inhibits activation of second order neurons, blockade of conduction of pain pathways in the spinothalamic tract, activation of descending inhibitory systems, coding at supraspinal levels, and liberation and/or accumulation of opioid substances are among the most frequently suggested theories. However, even in the absence of a definite convincing pain-inhibiting mechanism, clinical data have proved that neurostimulation can produce analgesia.

The largest accumulation of afferent fibers is found in the dorsal columns of the spinal cord, which suggests that neurostimulation could also be carried out at this level. Shealy et al. (1967) were the first to perform such a stimulation of the dorsal columns. The results of neurostimulation of the specific sensory thalamic nuclei (Mazars et al. 1976), as well as the results of animal experiments in which analgesia could be produced by stimulation of the central gray matter in the midbrain (Reynolds 1969), encouraged further development and spread of central stimulation methods. More recently developed systems enabled the effect of neurostimulation to be tested over long periods of time with a percutaneously implanted electrode before the actual stimulation instrument was actually implanted. Whereas up to now stimulation has been controlled from outside via a kind of transmitter-receiver system, the development of programmable stimulation instruments independent of external control is progressing. The destructive techniques like nerve, root or cord section, as well as stereotactic lesions in the midbrain as described above may give excellent initial results with complete pain relief; however, pain recurrence increases progressively as time passes. The results in patients with malignant disease are only seen to be good because they succumb to their disease before the percentage of pain recurrence reaches high values. For patients suffering from chronic persistent pain of benign origin, the introduction of neurostimulation, i.e., the nondestructive or nonablative methods, open a new attractive path. For pain of malignant origin, the use of these sophisticated and expensive methods can be an alternative only in patients with a relatively long life expectancy or when the other conventional techniques fail or are not indicated. This is particularly true for deafferentation pain, i.e., pain concomitant to loss or decrease of sensation by tumorous infiltration of nerve plexus or after nerve damage by radiation.

Dorsal Column Stimulation

Since the introduction of the percutaneous implantation technique in which flexible electrodes are implanted in the epidural space, this technique has become widerspread. It is an operation which produces little or no trauma with only slight complications. One electrode is introduced percutaneously into the dorsal epidural space of the vertebral canal cephalad to the site of the pain for monopolar stimulation. We have found no advantage in bipolar stimulation. If the patients obtain satisfactory pain relief with repetitive stimulation, the electrode is connected to a radio receiver placed in a subcutaneous pocket over which the patient can conveniently apply an externally transmitted signal (usually in the right abdominal region). In 146 patients suffering from chronic pain of both benign and malignant origin treated in this way at the Zürich clinic, good pain relief was obtained in 54% of the cases with deafferentation pain and in 43% of the cases with somatic pain, both with a 4-year follow-up. When one takes the pain of malignant origin separately, the results are better since the follow-up is shorter.

Intracerebral Stimulation

Since 1962 (first published in 1973), Mazars et al. have advocated intermittent stimulation with implanted electrodes in the sensory thalamic nuclei for pain relief, as have Hosobuchi and Adams (Hosobuchi et al. 1973), who also included the internal capsule as target. Richardson and Akil, starting in 1973, reported in 1977 that pain could be reduced by electric stimulation of periventricular and periaqueductal gray matter in humans. Over the years, experience has shown that deafferentation pain is best improved with intermittent stimulation of the sensory nuclei and somatic pain by intermittent stimulation of periaqueductal gray matter. The monopolar electrodes are introduced stereotactically and fixed to the skull with a screw. The connection to a subcutaneously implanted receiver is performed in the second stage, when the intermittent stimulation elicits satisfactory pain relief. The indication is limited to pain in the face and in the throat or to pain elsewhere, when other neurosurgical procedures, especially spinal cord stimulation have failed. In a series of 50 definitive implantations of intracerebral electrodes in Zürich, few cases of cancer pain have been operated on. The target point for deafferentation pain in a series of five cases was the sensory thalamic nucleus with very good to excellent pain relief in two cases and good relief in three cases. In three cases of somatic pain the target was the periaqueductal gray matter with good to excellent results in two cases and good relief in one case.

Summary

Neurosurgical pain operations in carcinoma patients should always be considered when conservative treatment methods fail or pain relief can be attained only at the cost of undesired side effects. The therapeutic spectrum of neurosurgery has been appreciably extended in recent years. Due to the introduction of percutaneous surgery methods, the operations have become less burdensome, so that carcinoma patients who were formerly regarded as inoperable can also be given neurosurgical pain treatment. The advances in neurophysiology have led to a better understanding of pain mechanisms, in consequence of which the various possibilities of treatment can be employed more specifically with prospects of better treatment results. The spectrum of neurosurgical treatment extends from destructive measures (rhizotomies, cordotomies, thalamotomies, neurolytics) via intrathecal administration of morphine-like substances to the augmentative nondestructive neurostimulation techniques. Despite the advances in conservative therapy of cancer pain, in many cases, a neurosurgical procedure is most efficacious in controlling carcinoma pain.

References

Broggi G, Siegfried J (1979) Percutaneous differential radiofrequency rhizotomy of glossopharyngeal nerve in facial pain due to cancer. In: Bonica JJ, Ventafridda V (eds) Advances in pain research and therapy, vol 2. Raven, New York, pp 469–473

Crue BL, Todd EM, Carregal EJA, Kilham O (1967) Percutaneous trigeminal tractotomy – case report utilizing stereotactic radiofrequency lesion. Bull Los Angeles Neurol Soc 32: 86–92

Crue BL, Carregal EJA, Felsoory A (1971) Percutaneous stereotaxic radiofrequency trigeminal tractotomy with neurophysiologic recordings. Am Assoc Neurol Surg Houston, Texas, April 18–21

Dargent M, Romieu C (eds) (1967) La chirurgie endocrinienne majeure dans le traitement du cancer du sein en phase avancée. Simep, Lyon

Fox JL (1973) Percutaneous trigeminal tractotomy for facial pain. Acta Neurochir (Wien) 29: 83–88

Frantz AG (1978) Prolactin. Physiol Med 298: 201–207

Gros C, Frerebeau Ph, Privat JM, Benezech J (1975) Place of hypophysectomy in the neurosurgical treatment of pain. Adv Neurosurg 3: 264–273

Hardy J (1975) Le traitement du cancer du sein metastasique par l'hypophysectomie transphenoidale. Union Med Can 104: 1557–1562

Hitchcock ER (1970) Stereotactic trigeminal tractotomy. Ann Clin 2: 131–135

Hitchcock ER, Schvarcz JR (1972) Stereotaxic trigeminal tractotomy for postherpetic facial pain. J Neurosurg 37: 412–417

Hosobuchi Y, Adams JE, Rutkin B (1973) Chronic thalamic stimulation for the control of facial anesthesia dolorosa. Arch Neurol 29: 153–169

Huggins C, Bergenstal DM (1952) Inhibition of human mammary and prostatic cancers by adrenalectomy. Cancer 12: 131–141

Jacobi GH, Altwein JE, Hohenfellner R (1980) Adjunct bromocriptine treatment as palliation for prostate cancer. Scand J Urol Nephrol [Suppl] 55: 107–112

Krieger AJ, Rosomoff HL (1974) Sleep induced apnea. I. respiratory and anatomic dysfunction syndrome following bilateral percutaneous cordotomy. J Neurosurg 39: 169–180

Kühner A (1981) La cordotomie percutanée. Sa place actuelle dans la chirurgie de la douleur. Anesth Analg (Paris) 38: 357–359

Kuperman AS, Krieger AJ, Rosomoff HL (1971) Respiratory function after cervical cordotomy. Chest 59: 128–132

Landolt AM, Siegfried J (1970) Zur Behandlung maligner metastasierender Tumoren mit der stereotaktischen transsphenoidalen Elektrokoagulation der Hypophyse. Schweiz Med Wochenschr 30: 1297–1306

Lipton S (1978) Percutaneous cervical cordotomy and the injection of the pituitary with alcohol. Anaesthesia 38: 953–957

Lorenz R (1976) Methods of percutaneous spino-thalamic tract section. Adv Tech Standards Neurosurg 3: 123–145

Luft R, Olivecrona H (1953) Experiences with hypophysectomy in man. J Neurosurg 10: 301–316

Madrid JL (1979) Chemical hypophysectomy. In: Bonica JJ, Ventafridda V (eds) Advances in pain research and therapy, vol 2. Raven, New York, pp 381–391

Mazars G, Merienne L, Cioloca C (1973) Stimulations thalamiques intermittentes antalgiques. Rev Neurol 128: 273–279

Mazars G, Merienne L, Cioloca C (1976) Etat actuel de la chirurgie de la douleur. Neurochirurgie [Suppl] 1: 22

Melzack R, Wall PD (1965) Pain mechanisms: a new theory. Science 150: 971–979

Miles J (1979) Chemical hypophysectomy. In: Bonica JJ, Ventafridda V (eds) Advances in pain research and theory, vol 2. Raven, New York, pp 373–380

Miles J, Lipton S (1976) The mode of action by which pituitary alcohol injection relieves pain. In: Bonica JJ, Albe-Fessard D (eds) Advances in pain research and therapy, vol 1. Raven, New York pp 867–869

Moricca G (1974) Chemical hypophysectomy for cancer pain. Adv Neurol 4: 707–714

Moricca G (1976) Neuroadenolysis (alcoholization of the pituitary). In: Anaesthesiology. Proceedings of the VI World Congress on Anaesthesiology. Excerpta Medica, Amsterdam

Mullan S, Harper PV, Hekmatpanah J, Torres H, Dobben G (1963) Percutaneous interruption of spinal pain tracts by means of a Strontium-90 needle. J Neurosurg 20: 931–939

Nashold BS Jr (1972) Extensive cephalic and oral pain relieved by midbrain tractotomy. Confin Neurol 34: 382–388

Nashold BS Jr, Slaughter DG, Wilson WP, Zorub D (1977) Stereotactic mesencephalotomy. Prog Neurol Surg 8: 35–49

Pagni A (1974) Place of stereotaxic treatment in surgery for pain. Adv Neurol 4: 699–706

Perrault M, Le Beau J, Klotz B, Sicard J, Clavel B (1952) L'hypophysectomie totale dans le cancer du sein. Thérapie 7: 290–301

Piscol K (1975): Open surgery for intractable pain. Adv Neurosurg 3: 157–169

Reynolds DV (1969) Surgery in the rat during electrical analgesia induced by focal brain stimulation. Science 164: 444–445

Richardson DE, Akil H (1977) Pain reduction by electrical stimulation in man. J Neurosurg 47: 178–194

Rosomoff HL (1971) Communication at the 39th Meeting of American Association of Neurological Surgeons, Houston

Shealy CN, Mortimer JT, Reswick J (1967) Electrical inhibition of pain by stimulation of the dorsal column: preliminary clinical reports. Anesth Analg (Cleve) 46: 489–491

Siegfried J, Krayenbühl H (1972) Clinical experience in the treatment of intractable pain. In: Janzen R, Kreidel WD, Herz A, Steichele C (eds) Pain. Thieme, Stuttgart, pp 216–218

Sindou M, Fischer G, Mansuy L (1976) Posterior spinal rhizotomy and selective posterior rhizidiotomy. Prog Neurol Surg 7: 201–250

Sjöqvist O (1938) Eine neue Operationsmethode bei Trigeminusneuralgie: Durchschneidung des Tractus spinalis trigemini. Zentralbl Neurochir 2: 274–281

Spiller WG, Martin E (1912) The treatment of persistent pain of organic origin in the lower part of the body by division of the antero-lateral column of the spinal cord. JAMA 58: 1489–1490

Sweet WH, Wepsic JG (1968) Treatment of chronic pain by stimulation of fiber of primary afferent neuron. Trans Am Neurol Assoc 93: 103–105

Swerdlow M (1980) Traitement de la douleur d'origine cancéreuse. Bull Cancer 67: 217–221

Tew J Jr (1977) Percutaneous rhizotomy in the treatment of intractable facial pain (trigeminal, glossopharyngeal and vagal nerves). In: Schmiedek HH, Sweet WH (eds) Current techniques in operative neurosurgery. Grune and Stratton, New York, pp 409–426

Whisler WW, Voris HL (1978) Mesencephalotomy for intractable pain due to malignant disease. Appl Neurophysiol 41: 52–56

Orthopedic Surgery for Management of Tumor Pain

A. Braun and K. Rohe

Orthopädische Klinik und Poliklinik, Universität Heidelberg, Schlierbacher Landstrasse 200a, 6900 Heidelberg 1, FRG

Orthopedic surgery for the management of pain in musculoskeletal tumors involves interdisciplinary cooperation. Chemotherapy, radiotherapy, and surgery are equally involved and require a critical analysis of the different therapeutic methods in order to cure the patient from the disease or to improve his quality of life and relieve his pain discomfort. Frequently, pain is an early symptom in bone tumors – even before X rays or bone-scan show any relevant signs. In many cases, a painful minor injury is the acute incident leading to early diagnostic information on a bone or soft tissue tumor that otherwise would have been overlooked at this stage.

Tumor pain is caused by *primary* or *secondary* musculoskeletal *tumors:* (I) primary bone tumors include benign bone tumors, tumor-like lesions, semimalignant bone tumors, and malignant bone tumors; (II) secondary bone tumors are metastases. Pain is caused by *intra-* or *extraosseous tumor growth.* Destruction or expansion irritates musculoskeletal nociceptors.

Surgical Management of Pain in Primary Bone Tumors

Benign Primary Bone Tumors

Intraosseous Tumor Growth. Painful benign bone tumors with intraosseous tumor growth are basically an indication for surgical treatment. Marginal excision removes the tumor and the cause of pain. The *osteoid osteoma,* a benign osteoblastic lesion with the typical well-demarcated nidus (Fig. 1a, b), shows intraosseous growth with a special pattern of clinical discomfort. Pain occurs mainly at night and can be temporarily relieved normally by acetylsalicylic acid.

Permanent relief of pain can only be achieved by surgical excision of the nidus, which has to be removed completely in order to avoid a recurrence. If the nidus can be identified intraoperatively by image intensification, a K wire is drilled into the center of the nidus and a bone cylinder 1.0 to 1.2 cm in diameter is removed with a hollow drill (Fig. 1c, d). One must then reconfirm that the nidus has been removed completely. The characteristic pain from an osteoid osteoma disappears immediately after the operation.

Extraosseous Tumor Growth. Benign bone tumors with expansive extraosseous growth should only be operated on if they cause pain or if benignancy cannot be verified. Exostosis cartilaginea is the most common tumor with expansive extraosseous growth.

In our patient V. M., large *osteochondroma* (Fig. 2a, b) originates from the dorsal pertrochanteric femur. The extraosseous expansion causes pressure on the musculoskeletal

Recent Results in Cancer Research. Vol. 89

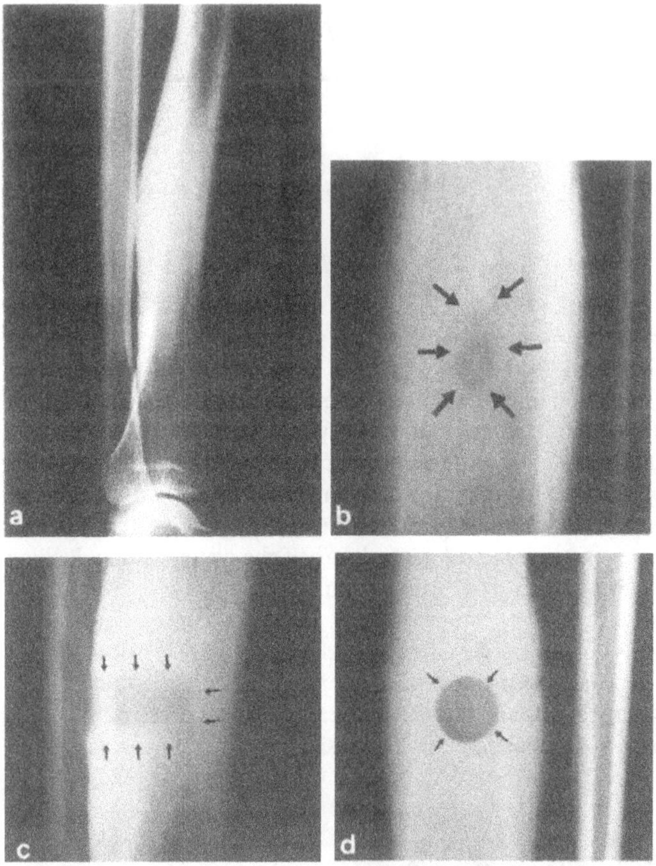

Fig. 1a–d. B. M., a 17-year-old male. Diagnosis: osteoid osteoma. Two years of pain in left lower leg; lateral X ray (**a**) shows spindle-shaped sclerosis of the cortex; ap tomogram (**b**) shows the nidus; postoperative X rays, lateral (**c**) and ap (**d**). The nidus has been excised with a hollow drill. No pain since operation

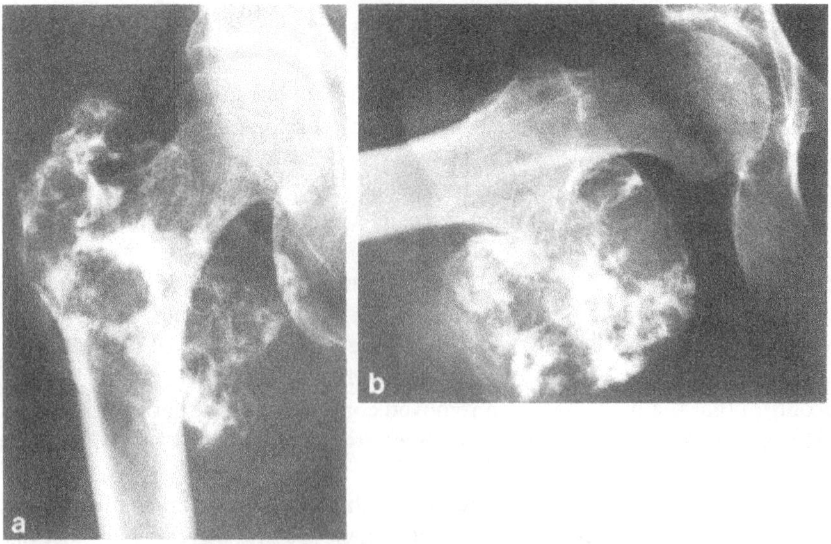

Fig. 2a, b. V. M., a 62-year-old female. Diagnosis: osteochondroma. Severe pain for approximately 3 months when sitting. A large osteochondroma originates from the dorsal pertrochanteric femur (**a, b**). No more pain after marginal excision

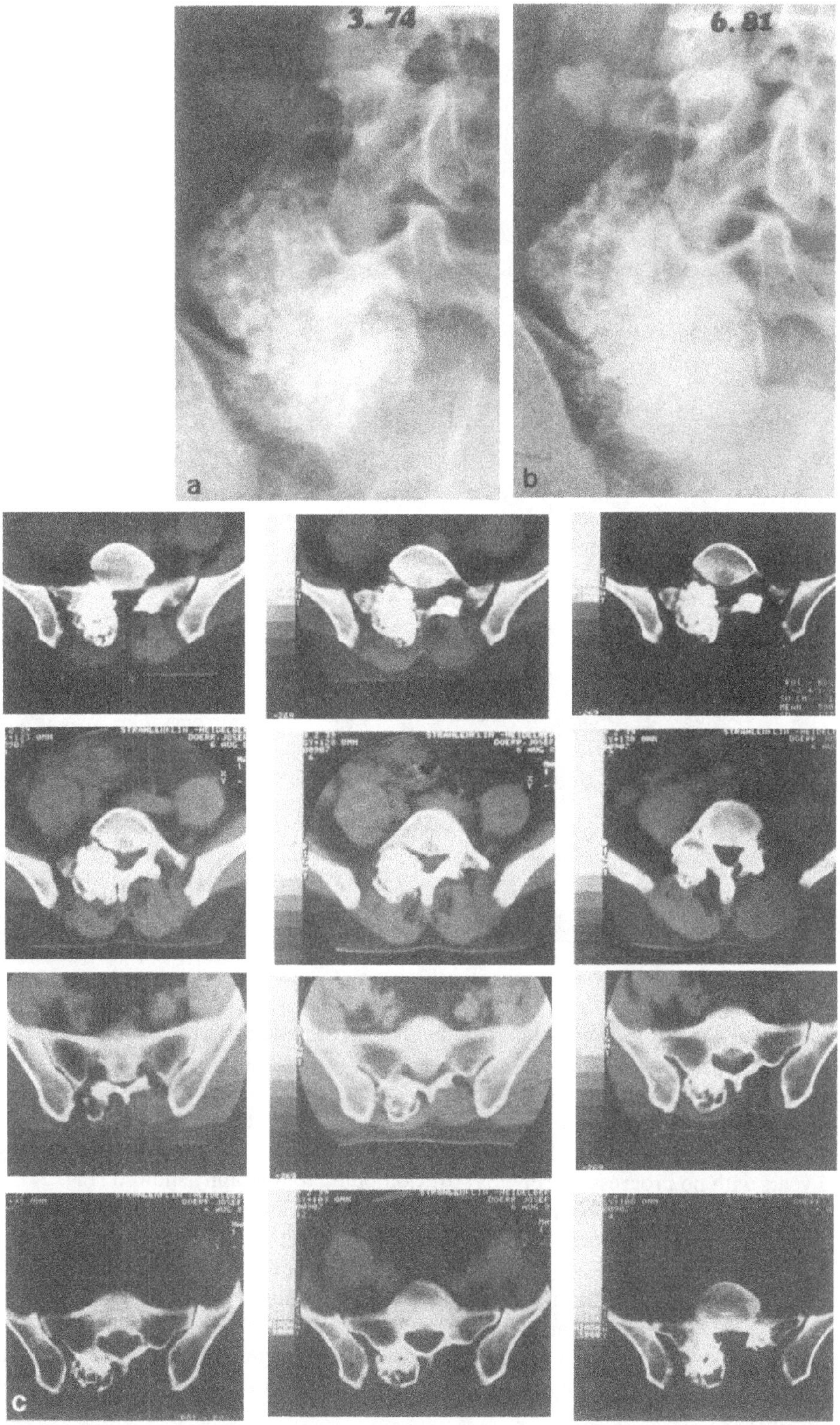

Fig. 3a–c. D. J., a 48-year-old male. Diagnosis: osteochondroma L4–S1. Ten years slight to moderate lumbar pain, no nerve-root irritation. X rays: ap 1974 (**a**) and 1981 (**b**) with no evidence of progression. In computerized tomography (**c** Universitäts-Strahlenklinik, Heidelberg), the pedicle and lateral vertebral body is involved. At this stage *no* indication for surgery

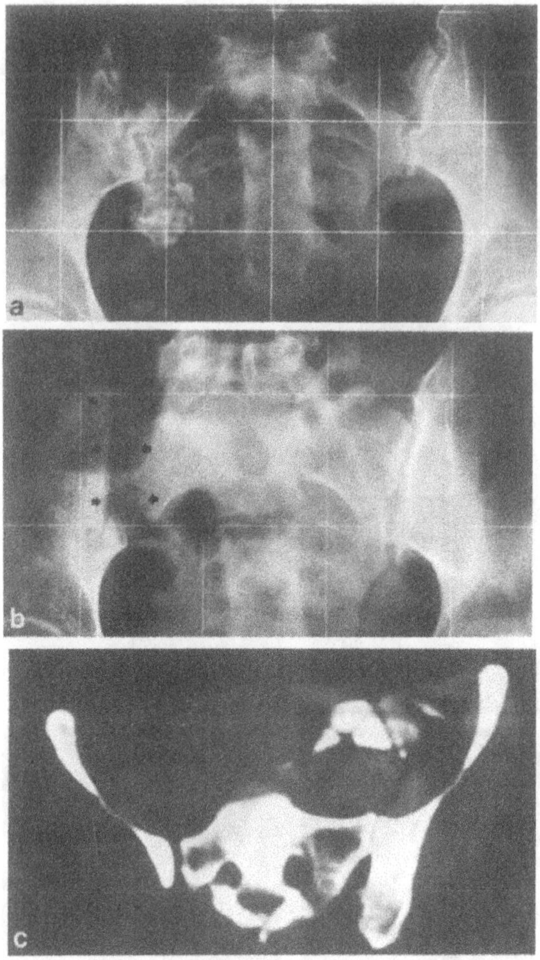

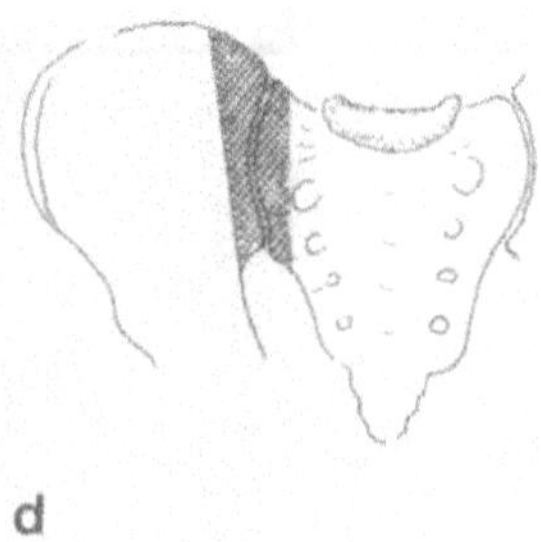

Fig. 4a–d. R. U., a 38-year-old female. Diagnosis: low-grade chondrosarcoma. One year severe pain with irritation of the lumbosacral plexus and the sciatic nerve. Tumor recurrence in right sacroiliac joint (**a**). Partial internal hemipelvectomy (**b, d**). In computerized tomography (**c** DKFZ, Heidelberg) the postoperative result. No recurrence, occasional slight pain

nociceptors particularly when the patient is sitting. The tumor was removed operatively by marginal excision and there was no history of postoperative pain.

According to the kind of tumor and to the anatomic site, benign extraosseous tumors with pain may only have a relative indication for surgery. Slight to moderate lumbar pain caused by an osteochondroma L4–S1 was followed up in patient D. J. radiographically for almost 7 years with no progression (Fig. 3a, b). Computed tomography showed (Fig. 3c) that the pedicle and even the lateral part of the vertebral body was affected by the tumor. Postulating that an osteochondroma – and, on the X ray, it looks very much like one – has to be removed marginally to prevent low-grade malignant degeneration, the spine would be exposed to instability and neurologic complications might occur after surgical excision. Based on the patient's history of slight pain, the fact of its being obviously a benign tumor, and the anatomic site making marginal excision difficult, there is no indication for surgery, but regular control in the bone tumor clinic with regard to malignant degeneration should be carried out.

After biopsy and obvious partial resection in patient R. U., an osteochondroma of the sacroiliac joint recurred. With insufficient prior surgery, the tumor was classified as a

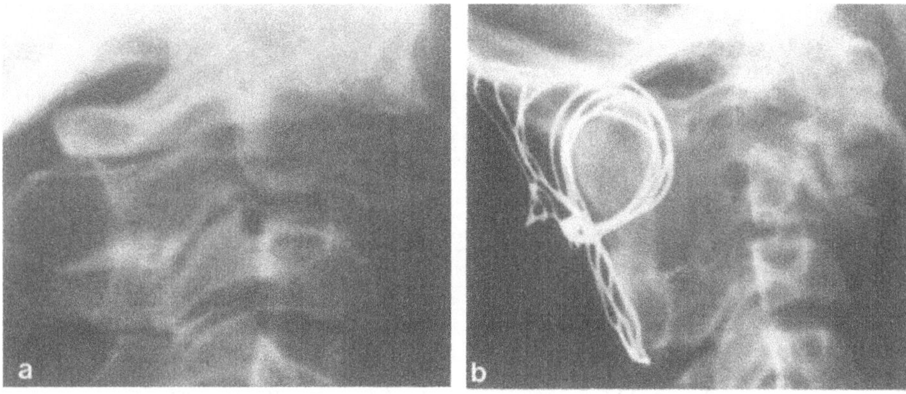

Fig. 5a, b. K. D., a 14-year-old female. Diagnosis: aneurysmal bone cyst. One year pain in the upper cervical spine. Lateral X ray shows destruction of C2 (**a**). Dorsal fusion from occiput to C3. Two years post operation (**b**). Limited motion in the upper cervical spine, no pain, no recurrence

low-grade chondrosarcoma. Severe pain was caused by the extraosseous tumor mass irritating the lumbosacral plexus and the sciatic nerve (Fig. 4a). By partial internal hemipelvectomy (Fig. 4b, c), a wide tumor excision was performed and a low-grade chondrosarcoma was histologically confirmed. Now, 2 years after the operation, there is no evidence of recurrence and slight pain occurred only occasionally.

Tumor-like Lesions

Radiologically, "tumor-like lesions" often look very similar to benign bone tumors, but they may show local recurrence and the diagnosis has to be made histologically. Pain is one indication for surgery. The tumor has to be marginally removed, and the indication for primary or secondary cancellous bone grafting often depends on whether the diagnosis could be determined pre- or intraoperatively. Most common is the *aneurysmal bone cyst* (Fig. 5a, b).

Semimalignant Bone Tumors

For semimalignant bone tumors, the indication for surgical treatment of pain is not as important as the grade of malignancy which requires marginal, wide, or radical tumor surgery.

The *benign giant-cell tumor* of the femoral head and neck (Fig. 6a) in patient K. H. had caused pain in the hip for almost 3 years. After biopsy, the tumor was marginally excised in the same session through a window in the anterior femoral neck. The cavity was filled with cancellous bone fixed with the fibrin-adhesion system (Tissucol) to promote ingrowth of granulation tissue and to keep the bone chips temporarily immobile so they would not fall into the joint (Fig. 6b). After the operation, there was no more pain but a slight limitation of hip movement. The regular radiologic follow-up of the tumor area is very important because of the danger of local recurrence.

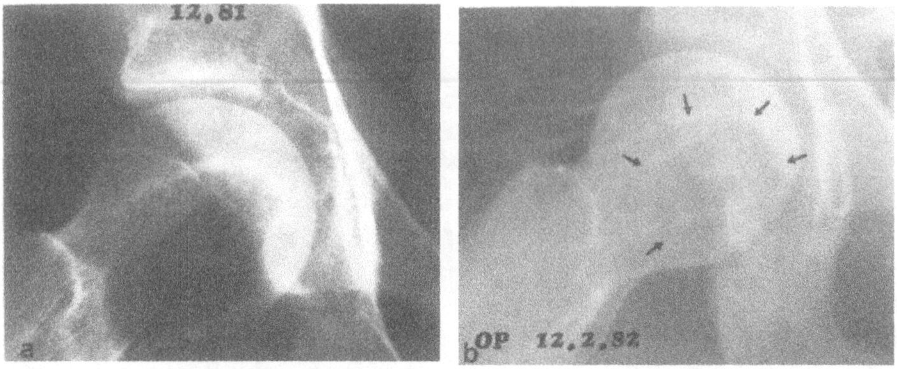

Fig. 6a, b. K. H., a 19-year-old female. Diagnosis: benign giant-cell tumor. Three years pain in right hip. Osteolytic area in the femoral head and neck (**a**). Excochleation and cancellous bone grafting with fibrin adhesion (**b**). No postoperative pain, no recurrence

Benign bone tumors, tumor-like lesions, and semimalignant bone tumors with a history of pain are in most cases an indication for surgery with marginal or wide excision. According to the expansion and localization of the tumor, cancellous bone grafting was necessary, but amputation or radical tumor resection could be avoided in almost every case.

Malignant Primary Bone Tumors

The histologic findings in malignant primary bone tumors determine further therapeutic procedures. In any case, the aim is – quoad vitam – curative treatment and so the relief of pain does not have primary importance in the therapeutic concept. Malignant bone tumors, which are hardly or not at all sensitive to radiotherapy or chemotherapy in particular, require early radical treatment. *Chondrosarcomas* (Fig. 7a, b), malignant *giant-cell tumors* (Fig. 8a–c), *fibrosarcomas,* and *malignant fibrous histiocytomas* (Fig. 9a–d) are the most common primary bone tumors that have to be treated surgically. With en bloc tumor resection or amputation the cause of cancer pain is eliminated. Amputations should only be performed if there is adequate hope of curative treatment.
Primary malignant bone tumors that are sensitive to chemotherapy, like *osteogenic sarcoma* or *Ewing sarcoma,* should receive preoperative chemotherapy. In many cases, aggressive chemotherapy reduces, eliminates, or prevents macroscopic occult metastases, especially in the lung, from becoming clinically manifest. Even the size of the primary tumor could be reduced and tumor pain initially relieved. In osteogenic sarcomas, combined chemotherapy and surgery has lowered the mortality rate by approximately 50% in comparison with radical surgery alone in a 5-year follow-up period (Kotz 1978).
Depending on the age of the patient and the sensitivity of the tumor to chemotherapy, we have three possibilities for radical surgical procedures: (1) Amputation: After amputation (Fig. 8c), no more pain is expected from the primary tumor. Although amputations might cause severe phantom and/or stump pain (Siegfried and Zimmermann 1982), radical, curative tumor resection is the most important concept for treatment. (2) Resection-plasty: Phantom and stump pain can be avoided and better function can be restored after resection-plasty. The resection-rotation-plasty described by Borggreve (1930) and Van Nes

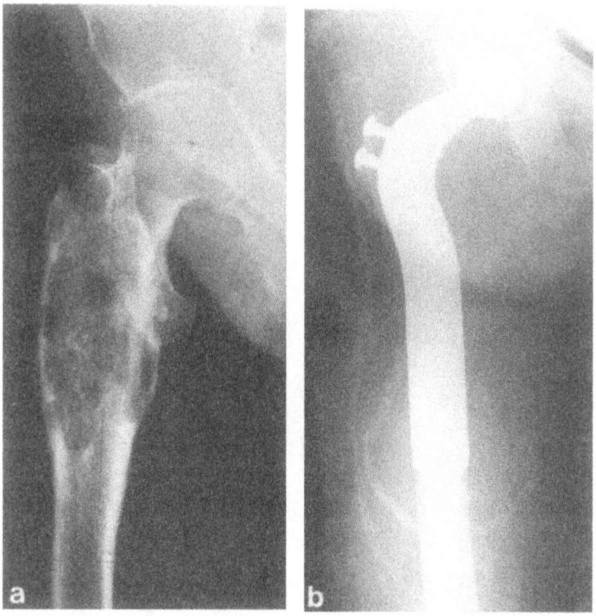

Fig. 7a, b. L. G., a 67-year-old female. Diagnosis: chondrosarcoma. Three years slight, 1 year severe pain in right thigh. Ap X ray shows destruction of the subtrochanteric femur (**a**). En bloc resection and endoprosthetic replacement (**b**). No more postoperative pain, good function, no recurrence

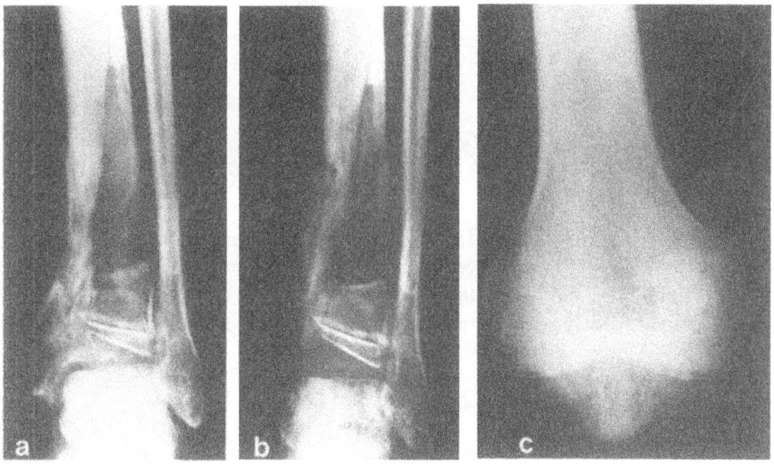

Fig. 8a–c. K. E., a 39-year-old male. Diagnosis: malignant giant-cell tumor. Ten years pain, malignant degeneration, ulceration, third recurrence. Two months pre operative (**a**), pre operative (**b**), knee exarticulation (**c**). Full stump function, no stump or phantom pain

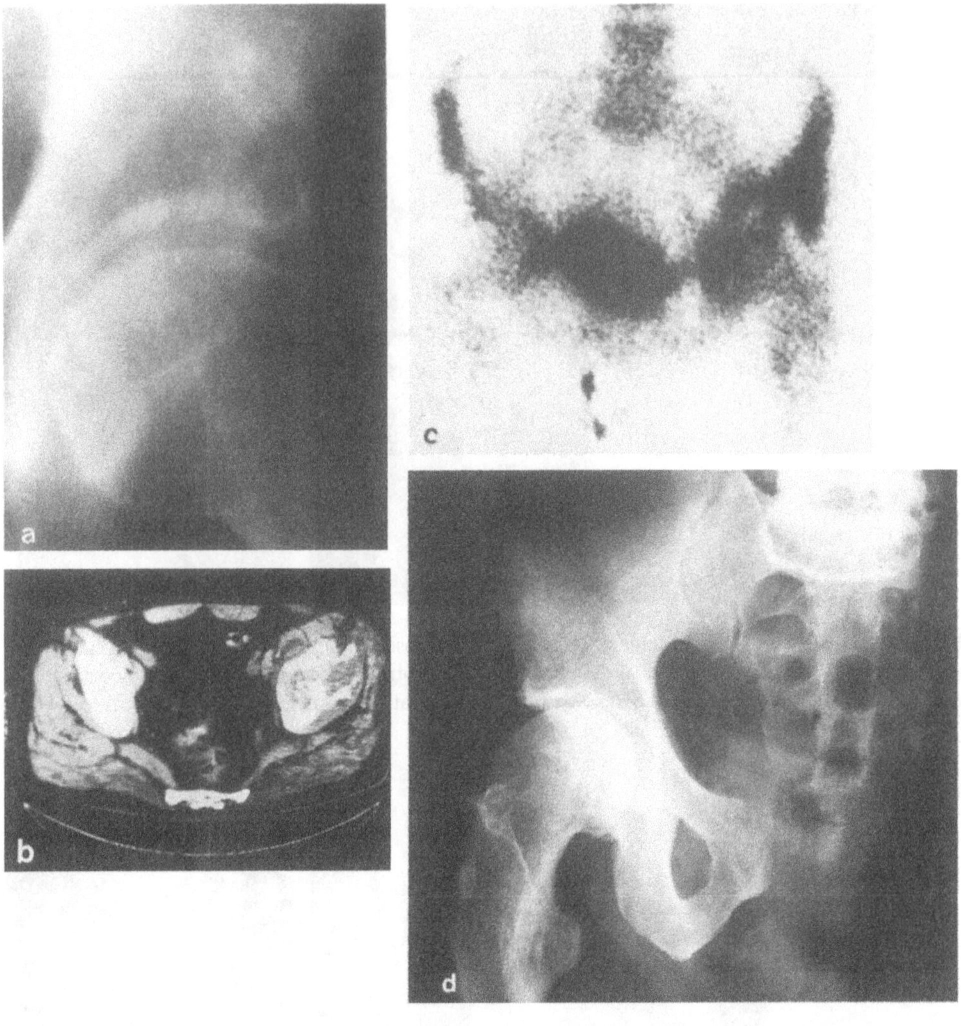

Fig. 9a–d. P. O., a 54-year-old male. Diagnosis: malignant fibrous histiocytoma. Pain for 6 months. Destruction of left supraacetabular region. X ray (**a**), computerized tomography (**b**) (Universitäts-Strahlenklinik, Heidelberg), bone scan (**c**), hemipelvectomy (**d**). Slight postoperative phantom pain, no local pain, pulmonary metastasis occurred

(1950) can be used for surgical treatment of osteogenic sarcoma of the distal femur (Salzer et al. 1981). The tumor is resected with two-thirds of the femur including the knee joint. The sciatic nerve, femoral artery, and two veins are preserved to guarantee nerve and blood supply of the lower leg. The foot is rotated through 180° and the lower leg osteosynthesized to the subtrochanteric femur (Fig. 10a). With the foot pointing backward, dorsiflexion and plantarflexion in the ankle (Fig. 10 b–d) simulate flexion and extension in the knee. This allows active knee movement in the orthoprosthesis (Fig. 10e).

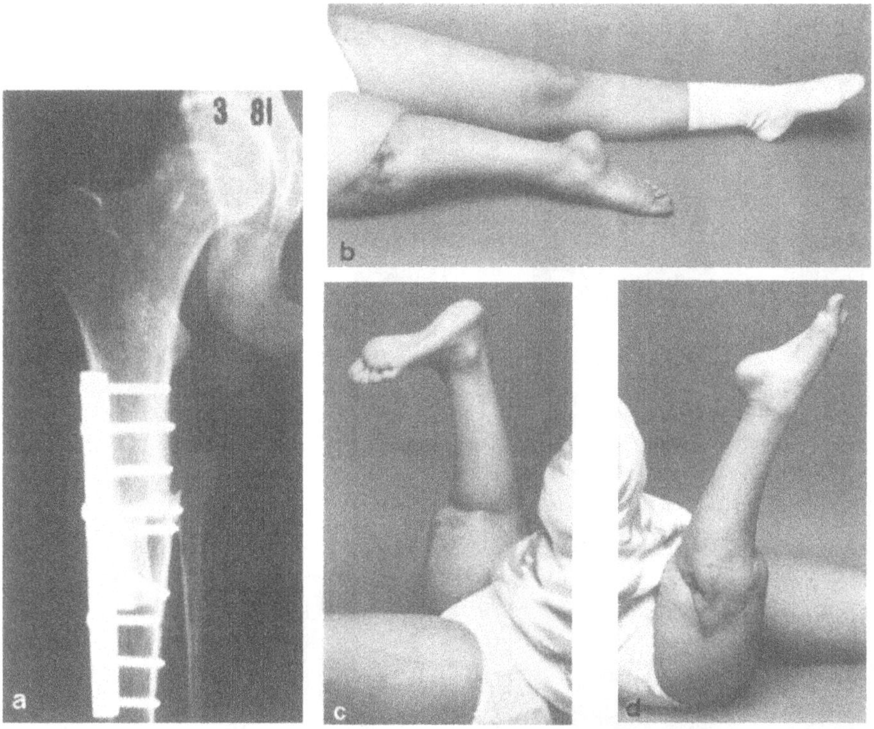

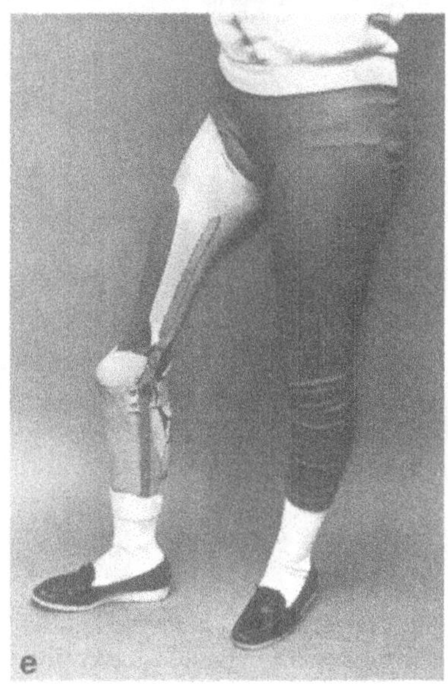

Fig. 10a–e. M. S., a 20-year-old female. Diagnosis: Osteogenic sarcoma distal femur. Three months pain in right knee. Rotation-plasty (Borggreve 1930; Van Nes 1950), X ray 4 months post operation (**a**), clinical result (**b**), dorsi- and plantarflexion (**c, d**) of the ankle for knee movement, orthoprosthesis with active knee movement (**e**)

(3) Endoprosthetic replacement: In the hip, knee, and shoulder joint, endoprosthetic replacement can be considered if radical tumor resection is possible (Fig. 11a–e). This is a limb salvage procedure. With the primary tumor, the cause of pain is removed and phantom and/or stump pain is not to be expected. Tumor resection and endoprosthetic

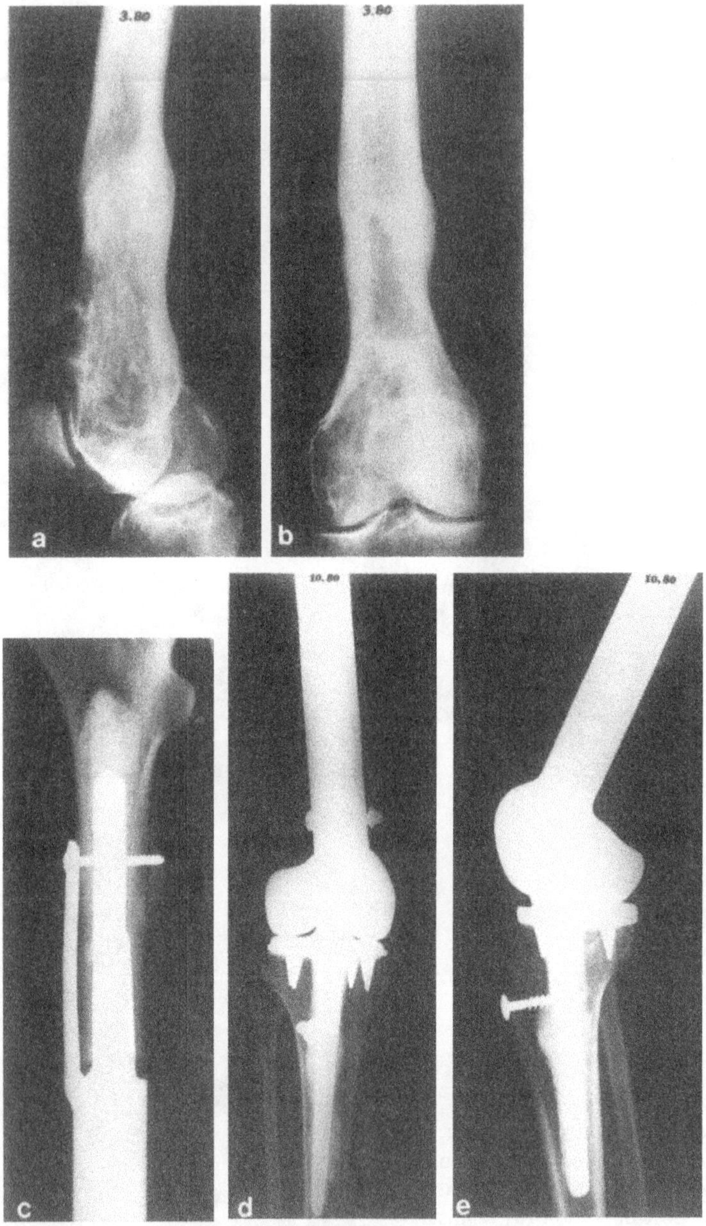

Fig. 11a–e. W. M., a 38-year-old female. Diagnosis: juxtacortical osteogenic sarcoma. History of pain for 8 years, previous surgery with recurrence (**a, b**), knee endoprosthetic replacement (**c–e**). No postoperative pain, adequate function, no recurrence

replacement is often difficult and mistakes can be made in radical tumor resection. On the other hand, limb salvage with a secure removal of the tumor and relief of pain could mean a tremendous improvement in the patient's way of life. Deep infection and loosening of the endoprosthetic replacement must be considered.

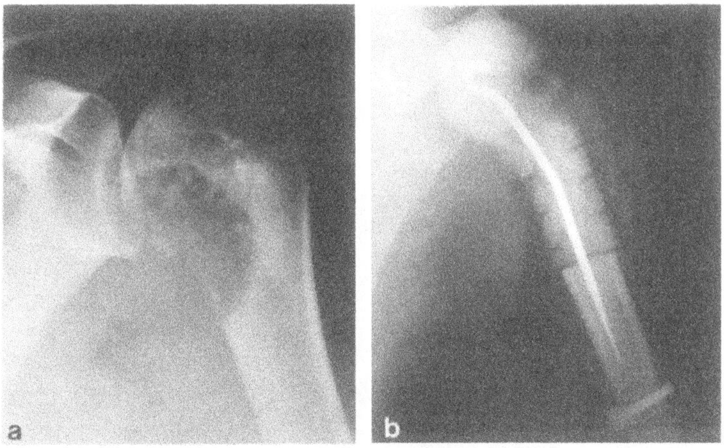

Fig. 12a, b. R. W., a 50-year-old female. Diagnosis: carcinoma of breast, multiple bone metastases. Persisting severe shoulder pain after maximal irradiation with progressive brachial plexus irritation. Metastatic destruction in proximal humerus (**a**), en bloc resection, and isoelastic-prosthetic replacement (**b**). Postoperatively, obvious relief of pain

Surgical Management of Pain in Secondary Bone Tumors (Metastases)

Skeletal metastases occur more often than primary bone tumors, especially in breast, prostate, thyroid, kidney, and lung cancer. However, almost every malignant tumor might show bone metastases, which can be very painful owing to osteolytic or osteoblastic bone destruction, expansive growth, and consecutive pathologic fractures. Radiotherapy, orthopedic surgery, bracing, and sometimes chemotherapy are individually important for the treatment of pain as a symptom of metastatic bone disease.

The *indications for orthopedic surgery* in skeletal metastases are as follows:

1) The general condition of the patient and the prognosis of the disease in general
2) The operability of the tumor
3) To *relieve pain* and to improve the quality of life by early mobilization and rehabilitation
4) Little or no sensitivity of the tumor to radiotherapy and/or chemotherapy
5) If the maximum dose of irradiation is applied and pain or instability are still present (Fig. 12a, b)
6) Pathologic fractures, particularly in the lower extremities (Fig. 13a, b)
7) If the advantages and intra- and postoperative complications have been discussed with the patient

Surgical treatment means resection or excochleation of the metastatic disease and implantation of an endoprosthetic replacement (Fig. 13a, b) or combined osteosynthesis with polymethylmethacrylate (PMMA; Palacos) and metallic implants (Fig. 14a, b, Fig. 15a–c). Most cases of metastases in the spine should preferably receive *non*surgical treatment, such as radiotherapy, orthotic bracing, and chemotherapy (Hupfauer 1981). Exceptions are solitary nonradiosensitive metastatic destructions of vertebrae with initial paraplegia and/or severe pain (Fig. 15a–c).

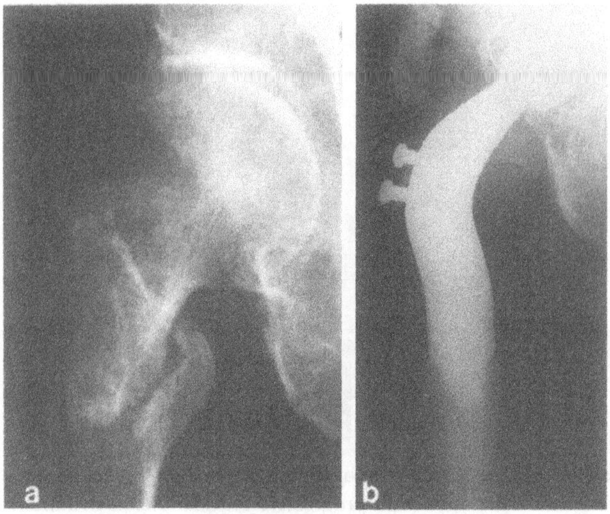

Fig. 13a, b. S. G., a 62-year-old female. Diagnosis: carcinoma of breast, multiple bone metastases, pathologic fracture. Severe pain after pathologic pertrochanteric fracture (**a**), en bloc resection and endoprosthetic replacement (**b**). No more pain post operation, fair hip motion

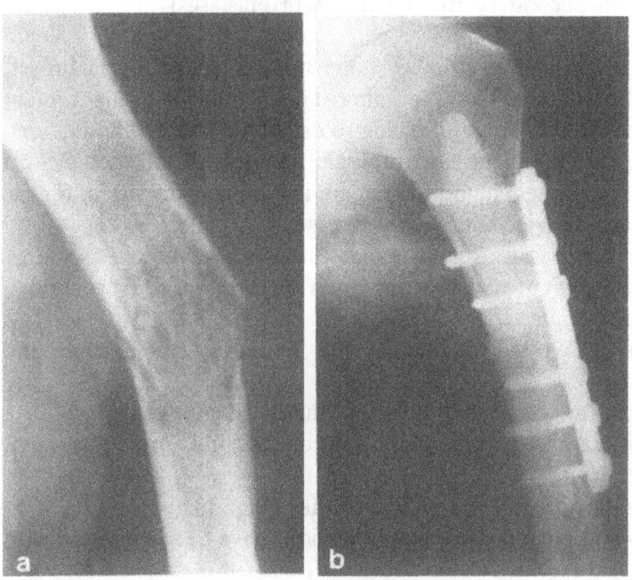

Fig. 14a, b. S. R., a 61-year-old male. Diagnosis: hypernephroma, bone metastasis, pathologic fracture. Severe pain after pathologic fracture of proximal humerus (**a**), treated surgically by combined osteosynthesis with PMMA and plate (**b**). No postoperative pain, early mobilization

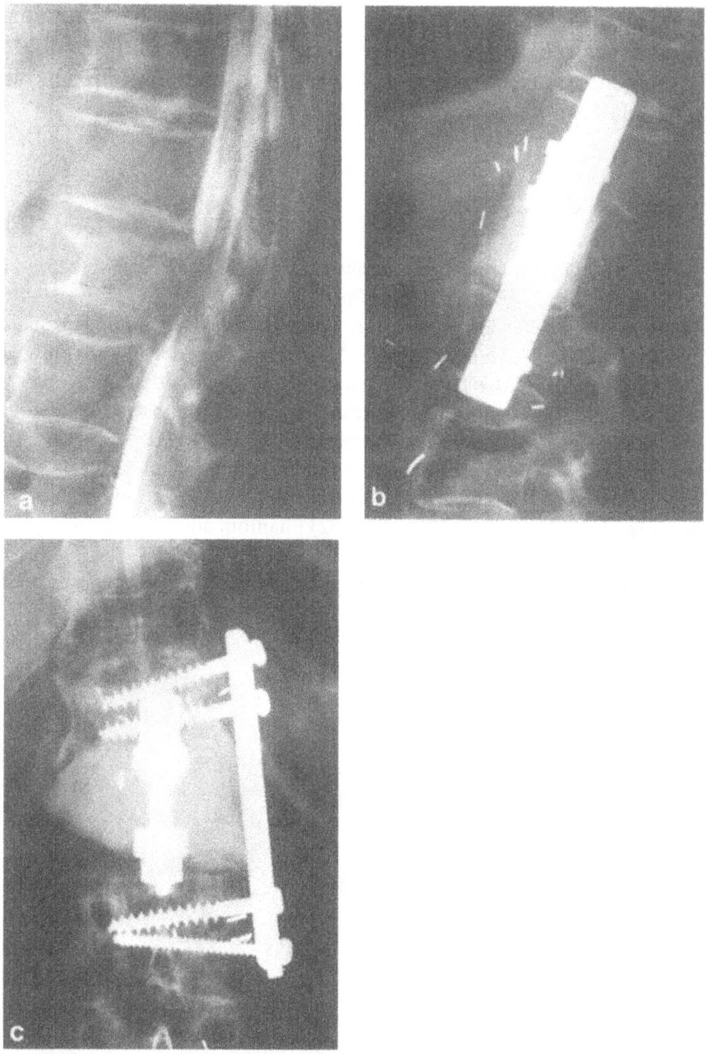

Fig. 15a–c. Z. K., a 61-year-old male. Diagnosis: hypernephroma, bone metastasis, pathologic fracture L1. Severe pain and initial paraplegia after pathologic fracture L1. Myelogram (**a**). Resection of metastatic L1 and replacement with combined osteosynthesis (Polster's device, PMMA, and plate) (**b, c**). Postoperative obvious relief of pain, no more spinal cord and nerve root compression, patient walking on crutches

Summary

Benign primary bone tumors, tumor-like lesions, and semimalignant bone tumors with pain are in most cases an indication for surgery with marginal or wide excision. In malignant primary bone tumors, the relief of pain does not have primary importance in the therapeutic concept. With en bloc resection or amputation, the cause of cancer pain is eliminated. Limb salvage procedures can be performed by endoprosthetic replacement, and phantom or stump pain will not occur. Skeletal metastases can be very painful owing to bone destruction, expansive growth, and consecutive pathologic fractures. Orthopedic surgery can relieve pain and improve the quality of life. Endoprosthetic replacement and combined osteosynthesis with PMMA and metallic implants are used to achieve early rehabilitation.

References

Borggreve J (1930) Kniegelenksersatz durch das in der Beinlängsachse um 180° gedrehte Fußgelenk. Arch Orthop Unfall Chir 28: 175–178

Hupfauer W (1981) Ergebnisse der kombinierten Behandlung primärer und sekundärer Wirbelsäulentumoren (Sammelstudie). 12. Arbeitstagung der Gesellschaft für Wirbelsäulenforschung – Tumoren der Wirbelsäule – Diagnose und Therapie, Tübingen

Kotz R (1978) Osteosarkom 1978. Die Wende der Prognose durch adäquate Chirurgie und adjuvante Chemotherapie. Wien Klin Wochenschr 90 (22): 1–25

Salzer M, Knahr K, Kotz R, Kirsten H (1981) Treatment of osteosarcomata of the distal femur by rotation-plasty. Arch Orthop Traumat Surg 99: 131–136

Siegfried J, Zimmermann M (eds) (1982) Phantom and stump pain. Springer, Berlin Heidelberg New York

Van Nes CP (1950) Rotation-plasty for congenital defects of the femur. J Bone Joint Surg 32-B: 12–16

Chemotherapy for the Treatment of Cancer Pain

W. Queißer

Onkologisches Zentrum Mannheim, Fakultät für klinische Medizin, Universität Heidelberg, Postfach 23, 6800 Mannheim 1, FRG

In Germany, we hear frequent complaints that no significant improvement of the cancer cure rate has been achieved during the past 30 years. At the National Cancer Institute (USA), cancer mortality rates have been documented since 1940 and a positive trend in the 5-year survival rates for different types of cancer has been observed (Cutler et al. 1975). The decreasing tendency of the mortality curve is evident for tumors occurring predominantly during the fourth and fifth decades of life, including the frequent breast cancer, other gynecologic cancers, various solid tumors, acute and chronic hemoblastoses, and malignant lymphomas. These cancers are treated not only by surgery and radiotherapy, but also by cytostatic and hormonal drugs, and different „combined modality procedures" have been developed. In this way, the medical oncologist (chemotherapist) has taken on an increasing responsibility not only for hematologic neoplasias, but also for different solid tumors.

The field of chemotherapy first developed in 1946 with the discovery of the antineoplastic effect of nitrogen mustard and, during the following 36 years, a total of 42 cytostatic agents have been introduced into clinical medicine (Fig. 1). One can assume that an average of one or two new drugs per year becomes available and this development will continue, as about the same number of substances are presently undergoing preclinical and clinical evaluation. Up to now, chemotherapeutic treatment has mainly been used for patients with tumor recurrence or distant metastases and for the palliative care of tumor-related symptoms. The management of intractable pain due to malignant diseases at first requires reduction or elimination of the tumor with anticancer modalities (Bonica 1980). The symptomatology of cancer pain is the outcome of organ-infiltrating tumor growth, on the one hand, and tumor-related organ destruction, lesion, and obstruction on the other (Table 1). By systemic antineoplastic therapy (cytostatic and hormonal therapy), a reduction of the tumor mass is attainable and, in this way, a decrease of cancer pain is frequently possible. However, the different types of organ destruction and lesions resulting from tumor growth usually cannot be sufficiently influenced by antineoplastic chemotherapy alone. Thus, the pain caused by bone metastases may well be influenced by chemotherapy if the tumor proves to be drug-responsive. However, if pathologic fractures or compression fractures of the vertebra have occurred, sufficient care of cancer pain by this method alone is no longer possible. The complaints caused by a compression of peripheral nerves, nerve plexus or spinal cord may be successfully influenced by cytostatic agents; paralysis, however, mostly proves to be irreversible.

From these instances, one may conclude that antineoplastic hormonal and cytostatic therapy cannot be regarded as "analgetic therapy." It can only be successfully used in the treatment of cancer pain if a reduction of the tumor size can be expected. Moreover, for analgetic therapy its side effects are too severe and, finally, it is too expensive. However, it

Recent Results in Cancer Research. Vol. 89

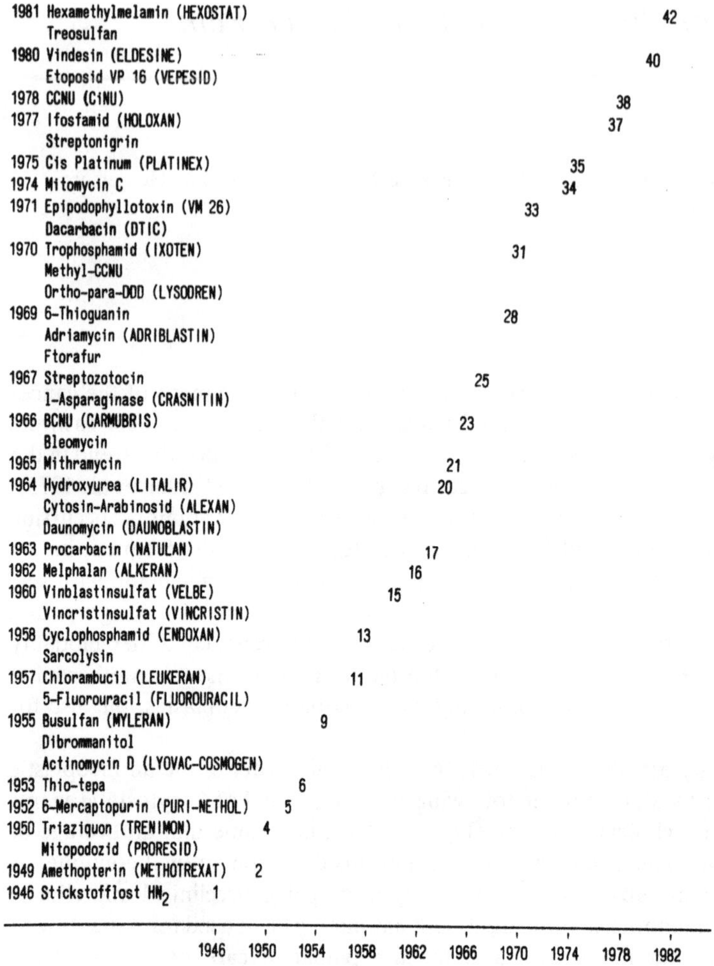

Fig. 1. The developing pace of new cytostatic agents from 1946–1982

Table 1. Symptomatology of cancer pain influenced or not influenced by cytostatic chemotherapy

Influenced	Not influenced
Primary or metastatic bone infiltration	Pathologic fractures, vertebra compression fracture, fracture of rib
Compression of nerves, nerve plexus, and spinal cord	Nerve destruction, paralysis
Compression of blood and lymph vessels	Destruction, lymph edema
Infiltration of parenchymatous organs (liver, spleen, kidney)	Organ lesions, destruction of contiguous tissues
Mucous infiltration of small and large bowel	Stenosis, ileus
Compression of ureter and urethra	Destruction, urinary congestion
Metastatic brain compression, cerebral edema	Apoplexy

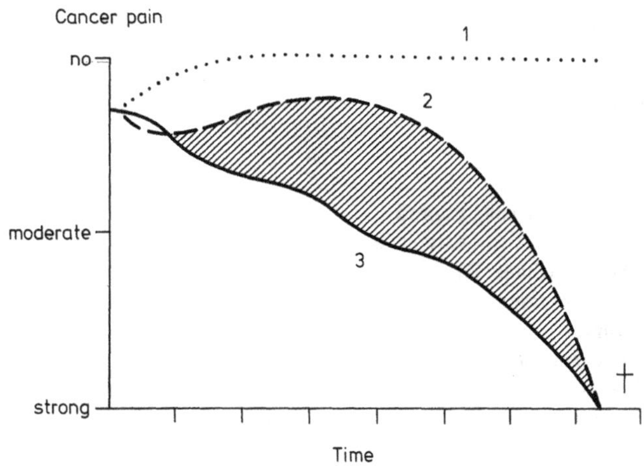

Fig. 2. Effect of antineoplastic chemotherapy on cancer pain. 1. Curative treatment. 2. Palliative treatment. 3. No treatment

may be suitable for the treatment of painful paraneoplastic syndromes (polyneuropathies, rheumatoid syndromes), which frequently disappear after effective cancer reduction. In this respect, the treatment of cancer pain is an important aim of palliative tumor chemotherapy. Figure 2 demonstrates graphically the intensity of cancer pain during the course of malignant disease. Line 1 shows the prompt disappearance of some initial cancer pain after curative treatment of the cancer. Line 3 shows the continuous increase of pain in untreated cancer. Line 2 demonstrates the intensity of pain following sufficient antineoplastic therapy. The area between lines 2 and 3 shows the advantage of palliative chemotherapy in pain reduction. However, this "quality of life" must be purchased by binding the patient to continuous ambulatory or repeated inpatient treatment and by different side effects of the antineoplastic drugs.

Up to now only a few clinical trials concerning the quality of life of cancer patients have been performed comparing the advantages of antineoplastic chemotherapy (freedom from disease) with the disadvantages of drug toxicity. It may not be fully realized that a number of cytostatic agents show only slight or even no subjective toxicity, e.g., some alkylating agents (melphalan, busulfan, chlorambucil), plant alkaloids (vincristine, vinblastine, VP_{16} except neurotoxicity), and antimetabolites (amethopterin). Among the hormonal therapies, tamoxifen and high-dose medroxyprogesterone acetate are also well tolerated. In each clinical situation, the expected benefit has to be carefully balanced against the specific side effects of antineoplastic chemotherapy. The efficacy of cytostatic therapy must not be measured by the disappearance of cancer-related pain alone, even if freedom from pain is a substantial aim of this therapy. A possible placebo effect of these agents has to be considered. Further cancer pain originating from organ destruction may continue even after a good objective response. In patients showing far advanced necrotic tumor masses, the cancer-related pain may eventually decrease. There is broad accordance with cooperative study groups that the response to chemotherapy has to be evaluated not by an improvement of subjective symptoms, but by objective measurable parameters. The criteria are a reduction of measurable disease (complete and partial remission), duration of response, and survival, which can only be sufficiently assessed within clinical trials (Muggia et al. 1979).

Table 2. Response rate of solid tumors following treatment with cytostatic agents (from De Vita et al. 1982)

Cancer site	Response (%) CR + PR	CR
Lung, small cell, limited	81	52
extensive	71	29
Chorion (Stage II)	80	70
Testis, not seminomatous	70	68
Ovary	70	30
Head and neck, squamous type	65	?
Breast	50	20
Stomach	42	0
Soft tissue	40	4
Prostate	40	?
Lung, non-small cell	34	?
Pancreas	30	?
Colon, rectum	20	?
Esophagus	20	?
Anus	?	?
Gallbladder	?	?
Kidney	?	?

CR, complete remission; *PR*, partial remission

In Table 2, the response rates to cytostatic therapy of the most important solid tumors are listed. These data should be taken into consideration when chemotherapeutic treatment of cancer pain is planned. If, for instance, bone pain appears in a patient suffering from small-cell bronchogenic carcinoma, freedom from complaints after chemotherapy may be expected earlier than in non-small-cell bronchogenic carcinoma or hypernephroma. The efficacy of the treatment of cancer pain by chemotherapy is strongly dependent on the specific response rates. In Table 3, the responses to hormonal therapy are summarized. With regard to hormonal management of cancer, ablative (ovarectomy, castration) and additive modalities have to be distinguished, both being important for sufficient treatment of advanced breast and prostatic carcinoma. Cases of breast carcinoma showing positive estrogen receptor (ER^+) have proven to be more sensitive to hormonal management than all other cases (including ER^-). Cases of carcinoma of the corpus uteri with positive progesterone receptor (PR^+) yield a better response to progestational agents than PR^- cases. As regards the therapeutic efficacy, tumors can be divided into three groups, the first being accessible to curative treatment, the second being influenced palliatively, and the third showing not treatment success up to now. Today twelve different tumors can be potentially cured by cytostatic agents (Table 4), but these tumors account for less than 10% of all cancers per year. Another 15 tumors show objective responses and a significantly prolonged survival (Table 5), accounting for about 40% of all cancers per year. In other tumors, a response is sometimes achieved but up to now prolonged survival has not been reported (Table 6). Thus, at present, about 50% of all cancer patients may benefit from antineoplastic drug therapy (De Vita 1982).

Table 3. Response rates of solid tumors following hormonal treatment (from De Vita et al. 1982)

Cancer type/treatment	Response (%)
Breast, all types	
Ovarectomy	30–40
Progestational agents (high dose)	50
Antiestrogens (tamoxifen)	40
Aminoglutethimide	35
Breast, ER^+	
Ovarectomy	50–60
Progestational agents (high dose)	70
Antiestrogens (tamoxifen)	75
Aminoglutethimide	50
Corpus uteri	
Progestational agents	30–37
Corpus uteri, PR^-	
Progestational agents	13
Kidney (hypernephroma)	
Progestational agents	6
Ovary	
Progestational agents	10
Prostate	
Castration	90
Estrogenes	50

Table 4. Cancers in which a fraction of patients with advanced disease can be cured with chemotherapy

Choriocarcinoma	Ovarian carcinoma
Acute lymphocytic leukemia in children	Acute myelogenous leukemia
Hodgkin's disease	Wilms tumor
Diffuse histiocytic lymphoma	Burkitt's lymphoma
Nodular mixed lymphoma	Rhabdomyosarcoma
Testicular carcinoma	Ewing's sarcoma

Table 5. Advanced cancers in which a fraction of patients respond to chemotherapy and improved survival is demonstrable

Breast carcinoma	Gastric carcinoma
Chronic myelogenous leukemia	Malignant insulinoma
Chronic lymphocytic leukemia	Endometrial carcinoma
Nodular poorly differentiated lymphocytic lymphoma	Adrenal cortical carcinoma
Multiple myeloma	Medulloblastoma
Small-cell carcinoma of the lung	Neuroblastoma
Soft-tissue sarcomas	Polycythemia vera
Prostatic carcinoma	

Table 6. Advanced cancers in which a fraction of patients respond but no improvement in survival has yet been demonstrated

Adenocarcinoma of the lung	Malignant carcinoid tumors
Bladder carcinoma	Malignant melanoma
Carcinoma of cervix	Thyreoid carcinoma
Colon carcinoma	Rectal carcinoma
Head and neck carcinoma	Hepatocellular carcinoma
Hypernephroma	Carcinoma of the penis

To improve the palliative effect of chemotherapy some application forms may be used other than oral and intravenous administration. For metastatic skin ulcerations, ointments containing cytostatic agents (e.g., 5-fluorouracil) can be applied. For the intracavitary (intrapleural, intraperitoneal) treatment of malignant effusions, drugs showing a limited resorption are available (e.g., thiotepa). For the intrathecal treatment of meningeal infiltration (meningiosis leukemica or carcinomatosa), cytostatic drugs can also be used (e.g., amethopterin). For the palliative treatment of cancer pain originating from liver metastases or metastatic infiltration of the small pelvis, the intra-arterial perfusion technique is used. A teflon catheter is introduced under X-ray control into the artery supplying the tumor. The infusion of cytostatic drugs (e.g., 5-fluorouracil, adriamycin, mitomycin C, nitrosoureas) results in an increased tissue concentration. This technique has also been used for treatment of malignant melanoma of the extremities. However, there is still no evidence for the superiority of intra-arterial over intravenous administration (Grage et al. 1979; Heim et al. to be published).

Summary

First, the cystostatic and hormonal therapy of cancer primarily affects the tumor mass and in this way also the cancer pain. If chemotherapy is effective, malignant organ infiltrations may be sufficiently treated. However, the pain resulting from malignant organ destruction cannot usually be influenced by chemotherapy alone. Second, paraneoplastic syndromes showing pain symptomatology (e.g., polyneuropathies, rheumatoid symptoms) may be affected positively in chemotherapy-sensitive tumors. Third, the alleviation of cancer pain by palliative chemotherapy must be purchased by the specific drug toxicity. Detailed trials comparing the advantages and disadvantages of cancer chemotherapy are still lacking. Fourth, the efficacy of cancer chemotherapy should not be evaluated by subjective improvement (reduction of cancer pain) alone, but by objective response criteria (remission rate, response duration, survival). Fifth, at present about 50% of all cancers can potentially be influenced by chemotherapy (10% curative, 40% palliative). And, sixth, besides oral and intravenous administration, local, intrathecal, intracavitary, and intra-arterial administration of cytostatic agents is also used in the palliative care of cancer pain.

References

Bonica JJ (1980) Cancer pain. In: Bonica JJ (ed) Pain. Raven, New York, pp 335–362

Cutler SJ, Myers MH, Green SB (1975) Trends in survival rates of patients with cancer. N Engl J Med 293: 122–124

De Vita VT Jr (1982) Principles of chemotherapy. In: De Vita VT Jr, Hellman S, Rosenberg SA (eds) Cancer – principles and practice of oncology. Lippincott, Philadelphia, pp 132–155

De Vita VT Jr, Hellman S, Rosenberg SA (eds) (1982) Cancer – principles and practice of oncology. Lippincott, Philadelphia

Grage TB, Vassilopoulos PP, Shingleton WW, Jubert AV, Elias EG, Aust JB, Moss SE (1979) Results of a prospective randomized trial study of hepatic artery infusion with 5-fluorouracil versus intravenous 5-fluorouracil in patients with hepatic metastases from colorectal cancer: a central oncology group study. Surgery 86: 550–555

Heim ME, Eberwein S, Georgi M (to be published) Palliative therapy of pelvic tumors by intraarterial infusion of cytotoxic drugs. International symposium on vascular perfusion in cancer therapy, Giessen

Muggia FM, McGuire WP, Rozencweig M (1979) Rationale, design, and methodology of phase II clinical trials. In: Busch H, De Vita VT Jr (eds) Methods of cancer research, vol 17. Academic, Press, New York, pp 199–214

Calcitonin: Analgesic Effects

R. Ziegler

Ruprecht-Karls-Universität Heidelberg, Medizinische Poliklinik, Abteilung für Innere Medizin VI (Endokrinologie), Luisenstrasse 5, 6900 Heidelberg 1, FRG

Historical Development

Calcitonin was discovered 20 years ago and was first regarded as an osteotropic hypocalcemic hormone, antagonizing parathyroid hormone (Copp 1969). Later, the stimulation of calcitonin secretion by gastrointestinal hormones and the inhibition of the function of several gastrointestinal organs were described (for review, see Ziegler 1981). Presumably, calcitonin is a calcium-conserving hormone at least in mammals. Calcitonin was detected not only in the thyroid C cells, originating from the terminal branchial pouch, but also in the thymus, adrenals, lungs, and the brain (MacIntyre and Stevenson 1981), depending on the species investigated. The hormone is found in primitive prevertebrate organisms, such as *Ciona intestinalis,* and it is possible that, primarily, it exerts neuroendocrine functions. Later in phylogenesis, it becomes involved in the regulation of bone metabolism after the development of mineralized hard tissue.

The Italian researchers Pecile et al. (1975) demonstrated that the administration of salmon calcitonin into the cerebral ventricles of the rabbit increases the threshold of nociceptive reflexes evoked by electrical stimulation of the tooth pulp. Obviously not much attention was paid to these observations until Yamamoto et al. (1978) confirmed the phenomenon: the intraventricular administration of porcine as well as salmon calcitonin produced analgesic effects in mice and rabbits and a central nervous system mechanism for analgesia by calcitonin was proposed. Further studies were devoted to the investigation of this question and Braga et al. (1978) showed in the rabbit that calcitonin analgesia was not reversible by naloxone. Yamamoto et al. (1979) found that the opiate antagonist levallorphan had no influence upon the analgesic effect of calcitonin. In brain opiate-receptor preparations, ^{3}H-dihydromorphine could not be displaced by the addition of calcitonin. If a combination of calcitonin and morphine was injected into the brain ventricles, the resulting pain threshold was higher than after single injection of either substance.

The administration of calcitonin is not accompanied by changes in β-endorphin levels. After IV injection of salmon calcitonin in man, no changes in β-endorphin and β-lipotropin concentrations occurred either in peripheral plasma or in cerebrospinal fluid (Fabbri et al. 1981). In contrast, Gennari (1981) reported an increase in plasma β-endorphins after administration of salmon calcitonin. Thus, until now the mechanism of analgesic calcitonin action is not known. The authors of further studies discuss intracellular calcium movements, the modification of the prostaglandin system (Chiarini et al. 1978; Ceserani et al. 1979), and of the kinins. The demonstration of binding sites for calcitonin in the brain supports the assumption of a centrally acting mechanism (Nakamuta et al. 1981).

Recent Results in Cancer Research. Vol. 89

Calcitonin Treatment: Retrospective Analysis

It is somewhat surprising that, although calcitonin was administered to many patients over years, most investigators did not suspect a specific analgesic potency beyond calcitonin's effects on the respective disease. Therefore, it is worth analyzing the data on calcitonin treatment with respect to the documentation of pain relief before the analgesic effectiveness of the hormone was considered.

Calcitonin is a drug of choice (beside the diphosphonates) in the treatment of patients with Paget's disease of the bone. Most of these patients suffer from bone and articular pains, which are the main indication for treatment. If one looks for the relief of symptoms during treatment, about two-thirds of the respective groups report a definite improvement in pain relief and reduced mobility – in general, pain relief parallels the improvement in biochemical parameters such as alkaline phosphatase in serum or hydroxyproline excretion (Kanis 1976; MacIntyre 1977). However, in the remaining patients, the complaints are hardly relieved at all, although the fall of the pathologically elevated parameters documents a response of the diseased bone (Ziegler et al. 1977). It is our impression that, in particular, secondary osteoarthritic changes in the joints adjacent to the affected bone produce pains which are not relieved by calcitonin. This clinical observation indicates that pain relief by calcitonin treatment is limited and not found in all patients.

Because calcitonin inhibits the secretion of pancreatic enzymes, its effectiveness as an adjuvant in the treatment of acute pancreatitis was studied and demonstrated in two parallel multicenter double-blind studies comprising 200 patients altogether (Goebell et al. 1979; Paul et al. 1979), of whom about 100 were given calcitonin and 100 a placebo. Although calcitonin had no influence on the mortality rate, it distinctly alleviated the course of the disease: the calcitonin-treated patients showed faster normalization of the amylases and leukocytes and pain intensity was reduced. This is documented by a diminished need for other analgesics, which could serve as a parameter for the analgesic potency of calcitonin (without considering that effects of calcitonin on enzyme secretion could also contribute to pain relief). Table 1 (Goebell et al. 1979) shows that the calcitonin-treated pancreatitis patients altogether needed less treatment with additional analgesics and increases in pain were only observed in 18% of patients (placebo: 25%). However, the differences were not statistically significant. The evaluation of the number of patients without pain during the 7 days of the study revealed trends in favor of calcitonin, but statistical significance was only observed once (day 3).

The data of Paul et al. (1979) yield the same result (Table 2): Calcitonin reduced the intensity of pain, but the difference between the calcitonin and the placebo group was only

Table 1. Calcitonin in pancreatitis (double-blind study of Goebell et al. 1979)

Abdominal pains	S–CT (50 patients)		Placebo (44 patients)
Total applications of additional analgesics	310		392
Average applications per patient	6 ± 9	N.S.	9 ± 12
Increase in pain (% of patients)	18		25

Effect of adjuvant treatment with synthetic salmon calcitonin (S–CT, 60 μg = 300 MCR units per day IV for 6 days) on abdominal pain in acute pancreatitis compared with placebo. For analgesia, all patients received procaine hydrochloride (2.0 g/24 h) and additional analgesics as required (pethidine, aminophenazone). The frequency of these applications is listed in the table

Table 2. Calcitonin treatment in pancreatitis, based on the double-blind study of Paul et al. (1979)

Abdominal pains	Day	S−CT (51 patients)	Placebo (52 patients)	Significance
Intensivity of pain (score)	1	2.29	2.23	N.S.[a]
	2	1.33	1.46	N.S.
	3	0.76	0.98	N.S.
	4	0.49	0.75	N.S.
	5	0.27	0.50	N.S.
	6	0.22	0.46	N.S.
	7	0.10	0.37	p 0.05
Increase in pain intensity during study (% of patients)		13	31	$p<0.05$
Percentage of patients without pain	2	20	19	N.S.
	3	43	37	N.S.
	4	61	52	N.S.
	5	75	65	N.S.
	6	80	69	N.S.
	7	90	77	N.S., $p<0.1$
Days without analgesics (per patient)		2.3	3.0	N.S.
Single applications of analgesics (per patient)		4.3	7.3	N.S., $p<0.1$

Effect of adjuvant treatment with synthetic salmon calcitonin (S−CT, 60−120 μg = 300−600 MRC units per day IV for 6 days) on abdominal pain in acute pancreatitis compared with placebo. Analgesics (pentazocine, pethidine) were administered as required

[a] NS, not significant

statistically significant on 1 day (7th day) of 7. Fewer patients report an increase in pain intensity when receiving calcitonin (13% versus 31%) and the (not significant) diminished need for analgesics might reflect the analgesic potency of calcitonin.

Intended Studies: Calcitonin for Pain Relief

Among the benign bone diseases other than Paget's disease, conditions such as Sudeck's algodystrophy and rheumatoid arthritis were treated with calcitonin and the respective reports describe improvement in pain relief (Vignon et al. 1977; Pietrogrande 1976). However, the evaluation of the effectiveness of calcitonin in such diseases is very complicated and one cannot draw general conclusions. During the treatment of hypercalcemia due to osteolytic bone metastases or multiple myeloma with calcitonin, it became evident that the patients not only profited from a drop in serum calcium and other biochemical parameters, but also from relief of bone pain (Behn and West 1977; di Silverio et al. 1977). The pain-relieving effect was reported to be manifested after 5 to 6 days of calcitonin administration and to last for 3 (minimum) to 7 (maximum) months. In part also radiologic improvements of the tumor lesions, e.g., remineralization, were reported (Favini et al. 1979). In a study on 61 patients, Barreca et al. (1979) found a mean pain relief of 50% of the initial pain score and this relief was maintained for up to 6 months. These authors saw no functional or radiologic improvement.

Schedel (1982) reported analgesic effects of calcitonin in patients with multiple myeloma. Analgesia outlasted the hormone administration by several days. The results of these studies seem to be encouraging, but the questions still open cannot be disregarded. The clinical details given in the reports are sometimes scarce, aspects of placebo effects are neglected, and the data on other types of therapy in these patients are limited. Therefore, the investigation of calcitonin as an analgesic drug under double-blind conditions was necessary and such studies have, in fact, begun. Admittedly it is difficult to study calcitonin in comparison with a placebo because many patients receiving calcitonin feel the effects of the hormone: they experience flushing of their ears or face, in some cases, nausea, and occasionally vomiting. Therefore, some of these patients might recognize the administration of the true preparation. In a double-blind controlled study of the effects of salmon calcitonin in patients with malignancy and associated pain, 200 IU salmon calcitonin were applied every 6 h for 48 h. Pain reduction was reported by five of 13 patients from the calcitonin group, whereas no patient from the control group ($n = 12$) showed improvement (Leyland and Hindley 1982).

An interesting study in patients without malignancy was performed by Welzel (1982). Sixty women undergoing vaginal hysterectomy received either calcitonin or placebo on the 1st day after the operation. The duration of complete pain relief in the calcitonin group was distinctly longer than in the placebo group. Placebo patients needed a second application sooner and the decrease in pain intensity after placebo was significantly smaller than after calcitonin. Thus, the analgesic effectiveness of calcitonin has been proven under double-blind trial conditions. What conclusions can be drawn?

Aspects of the Future Development

It can be assumed that calcitonin possesses analgesic potency obviously independent of its effect on bones or bone diseases and the intestine or intestinal diseases. This does not exclude the possibility that pain relief due to calcitonin is more pronounced if the pain is due to a disease which itself is influenced by calcitonin. For our physiologic and pathophysiologic understanding, one should be able to differentiate between a peripheral and central mechanism of calcitonin. Before calcitonin can be generally recommended as an analgesic drug, the following questions should be answered, at least in part.

Which Painful Diseases Respond to Calcitonin?

It is evident from the data presented here that it took some time before the analgesic quality of calcitonin was recognized, because not all patients respond. It would be desirable to identify specific subgroups of patients who might benefit from calcitonin treatment (Leyland and Hindley 1982), as otherwise the hormone might be administered to too many nonresponders.

What Are the Optimal Doses?

Until now, the doses used for hypercalcemia (which are higher than those for Paget's disease of bone) have been given empirically. However, it is possible that they are higher than necessary because other organ systems (pancreas, stomach) respond to much lower doses.

How Long Does the Analgesic Effect of Calcitonin Persist?

This is of importance because calcitonin may become ineffective due to two mechanisms: First, animal calcitonins, like the most commonly used salmon calcitonin, may result in the induction of neutralizing antibodies. In patients suffering from a disease that has a biochemical marker like alkaline phosphatase in Paget's disease of bone, this can be demonstrated by the renewed increase of alkaline phosphatase (Rojanasathit et al. 1974). Second, constantly elevated calcitonin levels in blood induce an escape phenomenon of many biologic effects of calcitonin, e.g., after several months of calcitonin treatment, glucose tolerance and insulin secretion are no longer impaired by calcitonin (Ziegler et al. 1980). This escape phenomenon is fully reversible after a certain time. Patients with hypercalcitoninemia due to C-cell carcinoma show the same inertness against endogenously elevated serum calcitonin and may suffer from severe and almost intractable bone pains in the case of diffuse metastases (our personal observations). Therefore, these phenomena of escape and/or resistance (tolerance) must be considered during all trials with calcitonin.

Are There Any Side Effects?

Fortunately, there are no serious side effects of calcitonin treatment. Some patients experience flushing etc. after calcitonin injections as described above, but the severity of the effects decreases rapidly. During long-term treatment, no toxic effects upon liver, kidney, bone marrow, or other organs became evident, which might be a consequence of the escape phenomenon discussed earlier. Thus, no contraindications against calcitonin treatment are known. Against this background, further studies would be useful in defining the suitable times and the limits of calcitonin treatment of painful diseases.

Summary

Animal experiments demonstrate that the intracerebro-ventricular administration of calcitonin induces analgesia. During the treatment of such diseases as osteitis deformans Paget and acute pancreatitis with calcitonin no spectacular pain-relieving effect was evident, but the application of calcitonin in hypercalcemic patients with bone tumors led to considerable pain relief. Recent double-blind studies document the analgesic effectiveness of calcitonin in malignant diseases, but also against postoperative pains in nontumor patients. Calcitonin as an analgesic drug deserves further investigation.

References

Barreca T, Cicchetti M, Magnani G, Sannia A, Rolandi E (1979) Effects of long-term treatment with porcine calcitonin in patients suffering from neoplastic osteolysis. Curr Ther Res 26: 644–649

Behn AR, West TET (1977) Emergency treatment with calcitonin of hypercalcemia associated with multiple myeloma. Br Med J 1: 755–756

Braga P, Ferri S, Santagostino A, Olgiati VR, Pecile A (1978) Lack of opiate receptor involvement in centrally induced calcitonin analgesia. Life Sci 22: 971–978

Cesarini F, Colombo M, Olgiati VR, Pecile A (1979) Calcitonin and prostaglandin systems. Life Sci 25: 1851

Chiarini P, Matassi L, Fabrizi G (1978) Calcitonin and somatic pain: effect of the hormone on the algogenic component of experimental skin inflammation induced by cantharidin. Curr Ther 86: 451–463 (abstract)

Copp DH (1969) Endocrine control of calcium homeostasis. J Endocrinol 43: 137–161

Di Silverio F, Giacobini S, Liberti M, Fragomeri R, Petrone U (1977) Impiego della calcitonia nelle metastasi ossie da carcinoma della prostata. Clin Ter 83: 3–15

Fabbri A, Santoro C, Moretti C, Cappa M, Fraioli F, Di Julio GP, Galluzi T, La Manna V (1981) The analgesic effect of calcitonin in humans: studies on the role of opioid peptides. Int J Clin Pharmacol Ther Toxicol 19: 509–511

Favini G, Arosio A, Libretti A (1979) Bone metastases from breast cancer treated with calcitonin. Case report. Tumori 65: 713–717

Gennari C (1980) Calcitonin and bone metastases of cancer. In: Pecile A (ed) Calcitonin 1980. Excerpta Medica, Amsterdam, pp 277–287

Goebell H, Amman R, Herfarth Ch, Horn J, Hotz J, Knoblauch M, Schmid M, Jaeger M, Akovbiantz A, Linder E, Abt K, Nüesch E, Barth EA (1979) A double blind trial of synthetic salmon calcitonin in the treatment of acute pancreatitis. Scand J Gastroenterol 14: 881–889

Kanis JA (1976) Bone disease and calcitonin. Armour, Eastbourne

Leyland MJ, Hindley A (1982) Calcitonin in the management of malignant bone pain. Clin Sci 62: 43P

MacIntyre I (1977) Human calcitonin and Paget's disease. Huber, Bern

MacIntyre I, Stevenson JC (1981) Calcitonin: a modern view of its physiological role and interrelation with other hormones. In: Pecile A (ed) Calcitonin 1980. Excerpta Medica, Amsterdam, pp 1–10

Nakamuta H, Furukawa S, Koida M, Yajima H, Orlowski RC, Schlueter R (1981) Specific binding of ^{125}I-salmon calcitonin to rat-brain: regional variation and calcitonin specificity. Jpn J Pharmacol 31: 53–60

Paul F, Ohnhaus EE, Hesch RD, Chemnitz G, Hoppe-Seyler R, Henrichts HR, Hartung H, Waldmann D, Kunzek K, Barth E, Nüesch E, Abt K (1979) Einfluß von Salm-Calcitonin auf den Verlauf der akuten Pankreatitis. Dtsch Med Wochenschr 104: 615–622

Pecile A, Ferri S, Santagostino A, Olgiati VR (1975) Effects of intraventricular calcitonin in the conscious rat. Experientia 31: 332–333

Pietrogrande V (1976) Il trattamento dell' osteoporosi con Calcitonina. Fondazione Carlo Erba, Milano

Rojanasathit S, Rosenberg E, Haddad JG (1974) Paget's bone disease: response to human calcitonin in patients resistant to salmon calcitonin. Lancet 2: 1412–1415

Schedel I (1982) Calcitonin bei Knochenschmerzen bei multiplem Myelom. Symposium Beeinflussung von Schmerzen durch Calcitonin, Heidelberg, 20 May 1982 (abstract)

Vignon E, Chapuy MC, Courpron P, Colombet P, Meunier P (1977) Effets cliniques et biologiques de la calcitonine synthétique de saumon dans les algodystrophies des membres. Lyon Med 237: 291–295

Welzel D (1982) Postoperative Schmerzen. Symposium Beeinflussung von Schmerzen durch Calcitonin, Heidelberg, 20 May 1982 (abstract)

Yamamoto M, Kumagai F, Tachikawa S, Murayama S (1978) Effects of porcine calcitonin on various analgesic responses in mice and rabbits. Ciba Med J 54: 27–33

Yamamoto M, Kumagai F, Tachikawa S, Maeno H (1979) Lack of effect of levallorphan on analgesia induced by intraventricular application of porcine calcitonin in mice. Eur J Pharmacol 55: 211–213

Ziegler R (1981) Calcitonin. Sandoz, Nürnberg

Ziegler R, Holz G, Raue F, Minne H, Delling G (1977) Therapeutic studies with human calcitonin. In: MacIntyre J (ed) Human calcitonin and Paget's disease. Huber, Bern, pp 167–178

Ziegler R, Raue F, Holz G, Minne H (1980) Calcitonin and the endocrine pancreas. In: Pecile A (ed) Calcitonin 1980. Excerpta Medica, Amsterdam, pp 314–325

*Treatment of Terminal Pain in Cancer Patients by Means of Iontophoresis of Vinca Alkaloids**

A. Szücs, B. Csillik, and E. Knyihár-Csillik

Department of Radiology, Department of Anatomy and Pain Control Unit at the Department of Clinical Neurology, University Medical School, Szeged, Hungary

Introduction

One of the most delicate tasks of the medical profession is caring for the terminal cancer patient suffering from intolerable pain with no prospect of recovery. However desperate the situation is, the physician is always bound by the Hippocratic oath to alleviate pain by all efforts, even when the inevitable end is approaching. A recently (re)discovered reaction of primary sensory neurons, transganglionic degenerative atrophy (see Discussion), offers a new, noninvasive technique of alleviating pain in terminal cancer patients by means of iontophoretic application of microtubule inhibitors to the skin. The result of this treatment in seven cancer patients is described and the possible mechanisms underlying these therapy results are discussed.

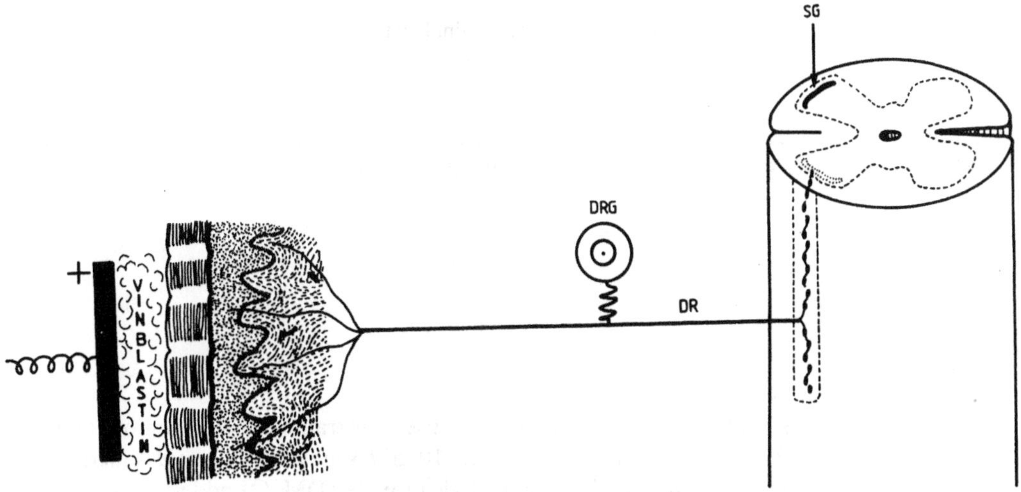

Fig. 1. Iontophoresis of a microtubule inhibitor (Vinblastin) to the skin induces transganglionic degenerative atrophy of central terminals of primary sensory neurons in the upper dorsal horn of the spinal cord

* Supported by Research Grants No. 06/4-01/449 from the Hungarian Ministry of Health and No. 375/82/3.2. from the Hungarian Academy of Sciences

Table 1. Pain relief by transcutaneous iontophoresis with Vinca alkaloids

Sex	Age	Diagnosis	Pain syndrome	Onset of intolerable pain prior to treatment
F[b]	33	Carcinoma of uterine cervix with metastases	Paresthesia dolorosa	9 weeks
M[c]	36	Abdominal chondrosarcoma	Causalgia	5 weeks
M	71	Bronchial carcinoma	Intercostal neuralgia Th3–5	8 weeks
M	34	Hypernephroma with metastases	Limb pain	3 months
M	55	Laryngeal carcinoma with metastasis in Th5	Dorsalgia	6 weeks
F	60	Plasmocytoma, multiple myeloma	Neuritis from compression; brachialgia post radiotherapy	1 year
M	50	Maxillary tumor	Trigeminal neuralgia V/2–3	6 weeks

[a] Minor tranquillants were used in various doses in all cases; not listed here
[b] *F*, female
[c] *M*, male

Methods

The Vinca alkaloids Vinblastin and Vincristin were used for transcutaneous iontophoresis in 0.01% and 0.001% concentrations, respectively; 10 m*M* Vinblastin or 1 m*M* Vincristin, dissolved in physiological saline, and 5% dimethylsulfoxide (DMSO) added to promote permeation were sprayed on a hydrophilic fabric (textile) cut to the size of the electrode. The wet fabric was placed upon the dermatomic area where pain was registered or reported by the patient (Fig. 1). The fabric was covered by a 20 × 40 cm, 0.5 mm thick flat and flexible lead electrode. An indifferent electrode was placed on a contralateral region, using a fabric soaked in tap water. A Nervostat therapeutic apparatus, set to dc ("Galvan") was used with the positive pole connected to the therapeutic electrode. The current was slowly increased to 10–30 mA and maintained for 1 h. At the end of the session, the current was

Analgesic drugs[a] prior to treatment	Dermatome(s) treated	Vinca alkaloid used	No. of session	Results
Morphine 0.08 g/day	L1–L2–L3 (left)	Vinblastin	8	100% Alleviation of pain without drugs (until death = 7 weeks)
Ethylmorphine 0.1 g/day	S1 (right)	Vincristin	24	100% Alleviation of pain without drugs (until death = 8 months)
Novamidazophen 4.5 g/day Ethylmorphine 0.02 g/day	Th3–5 (left)	Vinblastin	15	90% Alleviation of pain; Novamidazophen 0.5 g/day (for 6 months)
Ethylmorphine 0.06 g/day Bromacetocarbamide 0.7 g/day Pethidin 0.5 g/day	L3–5 (left)	Vinblastin	20	80% Alleviation of pain; Novamidazophen 3 g/day (for 2 months)
Novamidazophen 4.5 g/day Ethylmorphine 0.06 g/day	C4–Th7 dorsum (bilateral)	Vinblastin	19	100% Alleviation of pain for 1 month; but later new metastasis in vertebra L2 with new pain
Pethidin 0.3 g/day Novamidazophen 3 g/day	C5–Th2 (left arm)	Vinblastin	21	100% Alleviation of pain; Novamidazophen 1 g/day (for 2 months)
Ethylmorphine 0.06 g/day Carbamazepin 0.6 g/day	V/2–V/3 (right)	Vinblastin	9	No effect; discharged from hospital because of radioresistance of tumor

slowly decreased and the electrodes and the fabrics removed. Except for occasional local hyperemia, there was no visible alteration in the skin. The treatment was repeated daily for 7–20 days, depending on the extent of pain alleviation. As a rule, treatment was initially accompanied by 7–14 days of placebo iontophoresis in double-blind experiments; neither the patient nor the attending nurse knew whether saline was switched with Vinblastin or Vincristin. The blood cell count, ionograms (blood sodium, potassium, and calcium levels), and electrocardiograms were controlled weekly during the treatment and two-monthly afterwards. For a semiquantitative estimation of the efficacy of iontophoresis therapy, patients were requested to express any alterations in their pain state in percentages. In this scoring system, 100% means total relief of pain, 0% means no alteration, and negative percentages mean worsening of pain. Prior to the therapy, patients were informed of the essence of this technique and were requested to sign a statement giving their consent to be submitted to this new treatment.

Results

In seven patients suffering from various forms of incurable malignancy (Table 1), transcutaneous iontophoresis with Vinca alkaloids was used for pain relief. The number of daily 1-h sessions of iontophoresis with Vinblastin varied from 8 to 24, depending on the improvement of the pain state. The size of the electrodes varied according to the extent of the dermatomic area treated, but, in general, electrodes measuring 20 × 40 cm were used. The current (dc) was 30 mA in all but one case (KG), where we had to use much smaller electrodes (10 × 15 cm) and a less intense current (5 mA). Except for this single patient, who has been discharged from the university hospital for other reasons and in whom, therefore, iontophoretic therapy could not be concluded, this treatment resulted in pain relief in all subjects by 80% to 100%; consequently, the administration of pain-killing drugs could be either markedly reduced or even totally discontinued. There was no difference in effect between Vinblastin and Vincristin. None of the patients reported alteration of pain during placebo iontophoresis, but 5–7 days after saline was replaced by a Vinca alkaloid, they reported alleviation of pain.

Discussion

This noninvasive therapy proved to be entirely harmless, and no side effects were encountered in the skin or in the hemopoietic system. An important aspect of pain alleviation by transcutaneous Vinca iontophoresis is that the skin does not become either analgetic or anesthetized. Detailed clinical studies revealed normal skin sensitivity to light touch, cold and heat stimulation, as well as to pain from pinching (with forceps) or piercing (with needle). The chronic pain, however, is alleviated by this treatment, suggesting that the effect of Vinca alkaloids is exerted at a central rather than at a peripheral level.
It is now well established that Vinca alkaloids specifically bind to tubulin (Borgers and De Brabander 1975) and, in fact, this dimeric constituent of microtubules, consisting of two subunits, is regarded as a specific receptor for Vinca alkaloids (Dustin 1978). If administered systemically, tubulin binding of Vinca alkaloids results in the arrest of mitoses due to inhibiting microtubules in mitotic spindles, hence their use in tumor therapy. However, our experiments indicate that, in the case of iontophoretic application, Vinca alkaloids do not enter the circulation. In addition, animal tests prove that only 1% of the drug applied at the electrode infiltrates various layers of the skin (Knyihár-Csillik et al. 1982). It seems, therefore, safe to say that in the course of iontophoretic treatment of chronic pain syndromes, including terminal pain, Vinca alkaloids are bound to tubulin in peripheral axon arborizations within the skin.
The fact that the dermatome(s) treated iontophoretically become neither analgetic nor anesthetized rules out any direct effect upon peripheral nociceptors. It has been shown in animal experiments that a series of daily Vinblastin iontophoresis induces within 15 to 21 days histochemical and fine-structural alterations in the upper dorsal horn of the spinal cord producing transganglionic degenerative atrophy. These changes are similar to those observed after blockade of axoplasmic transport in a peripheral nerve by a perineural Vinblastin cuff (Knyihár-Csillik et al. 1982) and to structural alterations in central terminals of primary sensory neurons after peripheral nerve injury (Csillik and Knyihár 1975, 1978), first reported at the end of the last century but virtually forgotten since then (see Knyihár and Csillik 1976; Knyihár-Csillik and Csillik 1981). Transganglionic degenerative atrophy affects both thin (Aδ and C) and thick (Aβ) primary afferent axons (Knyihár-Csillik and

Csillik 1981). We therefore assume that descending inhibitory control systems become predominant over the impaired primary afferent input.

Atrophied primary central sensory terminals are later revived by a synaptoneogenetic process within the substantia gelatinosa (Csillik and Knyihár-Csillik 1981). If one supposes that this results in a proper wiring, these changes might explain the long-term beneficial effects of Vinca alkaloid iontophoretic therapy in pain syndromes. Thus, the effect of locally applied Vinca alkaloids differs considerably from that of systemically administered microtubule inhibitors (e.g., in cancer therapy) that not infrequently result in generalized Wallerian degeneration and demyelinization in the central nervous system (Borgers and De Brabander 1975). Though the underlying mechanism (blockade of axoplasmic transport) seems to be identical, demyelinization may result in increased pain sensation, whereas locally restricted transganglionic degenerative atrophy of primary afferent terminals, which is followed by a synaptoneogenetic process, alleviates chronic, intractable pain.

References

Borgers M, De Brabander M (eds) (1975) Microtubules and microtubule inhibitors. North-Holland, Amsterdam

Csillik B, Knyihár E (1975) Degenerative atrophy and regenerative proliferation in the rat spinal cord. Z Mikrosk Anat Forsch 89: 1099–1103

Csillik B, Knyihár E (1978) Biodynamic plasticity in the Rolando substance. Prog Neurobiol 10: 203–230

Csillik B, Knyihár-Csillik E (1981) Regenerative synaptoneogenesis in the mammalian spinal cord: dynamics of synaptochemical restoration in the Rolando substance after transganglionic degenerative atrophy. J Neural Transmission 52: 303–317

Dustin P (1978) Microtubules. Springer, Berlin Heidelberg New York

Knyihár E, Csillik B (1976) Effect of peripheral axotomy on the fine structure and histochemistry of the Rolando substance: degenerative atrophy of central processes of pseudounipolar cells. Exp Brain Res 26: 73–87

Knyihár-Csillik E, Csillik B (1981) FRAP: Histochemistry of the primary nociceptive neurons. Fischer, Stuttgart

Knyihár-Csillik E, Szücs A, Csillik B (1982) Iontophoretically applied microtubule inhibitors induce transganglionic degenerative atrophy of primary central nociceptive terminals and abolish chronic autochtonous pain. Acta Neurol Scand 66: 401–412

Radiotherapy of Cancer Pain

H. Kuttig

Abteilung für Allgemeine Radiologie, Radiologisches Zentrum, Universität Heidelberg, 6900 Heidelberg 1, FRG

The alleviation of cancer pain by ionizing radiation was observed early in the development of radiotherapy. In the first months of 1896 – on 28 December 1895 Roentgen had just presented his discovery of X-rays – Despeignes in Lyon reported a striking analgetic effect of X-ray therapy on a cancroid of the floor of the mouth and a stomach cancer and, at the end of 1896, Williams in Boston published a report of remarkable, fast regression of pain in a repeatedly operated patient with breast cancer (see Glasser 1958). Subsequently, the analgetic effect of ionizing radiation has also been utilized for a large number of benign diseases within the scope of the anti-inflammatory irradiation of acute and chronic processes inaugurated by Heidenhain and Fried in 1924. The effect has been explained by an influence on the autonomic nervous system, by electrolyte redistribution at the peripheral ends of the nerves, and a change of acidosis frequently present in the tissue toward neutral pH.

Today the analgetic influence of ionizing rays represents an important factor in radiologic cancer therapy as well as having great significance in the cure and palliative treatment of oncological diseases. Schlegel (1982) found that, among all the patients of a radiology hospital with a yearly admission of 1,200 new patients, the application of radiotherapy was to relieve pain in 37.5% of the cases. In Table 1 the various types of *indication* for radiologic therapy of pain are listed. Its application in primary therapy covers, in the first place, cases where the pain situation is directly conditioned by the tumor, especially by a progression of the tumor with infiltration into the surrounding tissues. The rationale for radiotherapy is a direct effect on tumor infiltration and a reduction of the tumor mass by

Table 1. Indications for radiologic pain therapy

1.	In primary treatment: Effect on tumor infiltration Reduction of tumor mass Infiltration of nerve tissue, plexus Meningeal carcinosis Epidural metastases Capsular pain (spleen, liver)
2.	Bone metastases Solitary – curative Multiple – palliative
3.	Palliation of localized symptoms of pain
Therapy aim:	Longer lasting analgesic effect or mitigation

Recent Results in Cancer Research. Vol. 89

influencing tumor growth. The radiologic effect manifests itself in a decompression of the nerve roots and nerve plexus. I shall take as an example the Pancoast syndrome with infiltration of the plexus brachialis and costal destruction. Further indications for radiologic therapy are, e.g., pain-producing meningeal carcinosis and epidural metastasis and primary and secondary brain tumors with severe headaches. Important applications of radiotherapy are in the treatment of compression of nerve roots with lumbago and of ischialgia with tumors of the testicles – mainly seminomas – with metastases in retroperitoneal lymph nodes. Other cases include pain caused by swelling and streching of tissue or organs surrounded by fasciae or capsules, e.g., the capsular pain with spleen and liver tumors that cannot be influenced by other types of therapy.

The second important group of symptoms indicating radiotherapy are bone metastases, in which pain is related to the irritation of nociceptors in the periosteum. The use of radiotherapy to produce a cure by remineralization is only justified in the case of solitary metastases or imminent or already existing fractures of important skeletal parts. In this case, relatively high doses of radiation often in combination with hormonal therapy or chemotherapy are required. Multiple symptomatic skeletal metastases are irradiated for a palliative effect. Methodology and results are discussed below.

The final indication for radiologic therapy is an advanced tumor stage when localized pain symptoms can frequently only be palliated. In all cases, the aim of therapy is a longer lasting relief from pain or at least pain mitigation to restrict the use of analgesics and psychotropic drugs as much as possible if not completely.

The available *methods of radiotherapy* for cancer pain are percutaneous irradiation with ultrahard rays, radionuclide therapy, radioresection of the pituitary gland, and stereotactical thalamotomy. *Percutaneous radiotherapy* is directed at the primary tumor, the region of metastases, or the site of recurrence. The dose is determined by whether the therapy aims at cure or palliation, the necessary dose being established by histology, tumor volume, and nearby organs at risk in the case of cure. The same applies to solitary metastases. Palliative irradiation can be administered at far lower doses. Thus, a longer lasting analgetic radiation effect, e.g., in the case of bone metastases, is attainable with a maximum of 40 Gy. An analgetic effect is attained earlier when higher single doses are given than with the usual fractionation of 2 Gy daily. The administration of higher single doses is especially recommended by American authors (Ambrad 1981; Allen 1981; Wizenberg 1981). At the end of 4 weeks, the results of long-term and short-term fractionation can be adjusted. Most patients remain without pain for the rest of their life. Short-term fractionation is well tolerated and avoids the need for a long stay in hospital. To obtain an analgetic effect by palliative irradiation, the radiation field should cover and even go beyond the site of metastases or recurrence.

Table 2 shows the *results* of percutaneous irradiation for pain relief in bone metastases of various organ tumors. Complete relief or at least mitigation of the pain was achieved in 74%–80% of the patients. The pain-free period lasts 14 (2–36) months on average

Table 2. Analgesia or pain mitigation after percutaneous irradiation

Source of pain	Percentage
Bone metastases	74 –80
Recurrence of rectum carcinoma	75

Recurrence of pain from bone metastases after reaction in nearly 14%

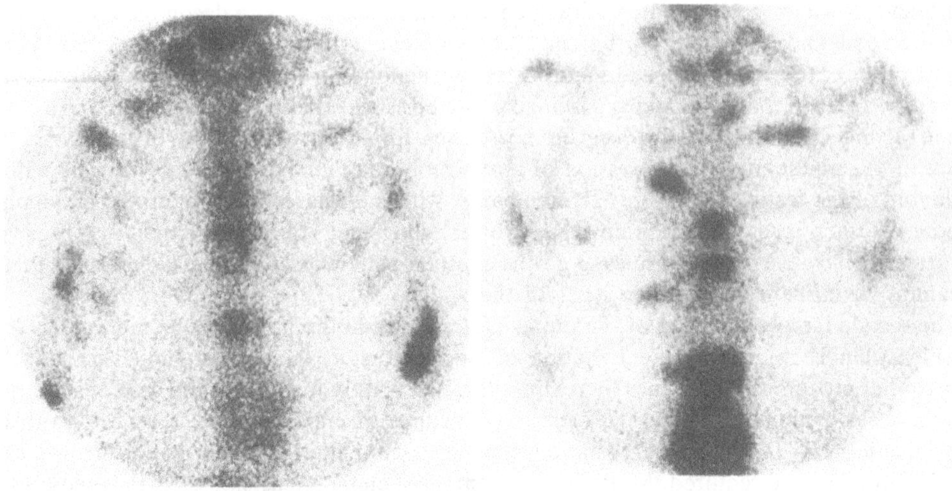

Fig. 1 (*left*) and **2** (*right*). Scintigram showing higher uptake of radionuclide in osteoblastic metastases of cancer of the prostate

(Gottwald and Szakolczai 1981). Pain recurrence after a period of analgesia occurs in approximately 14% of the surviving patients. The influence on pain of infiltration of the plexus sacralis, with recurrence of an inoperable rectum carcinoma, could be observed in 75% of the cases. However, the recurrence of pain is less easily influenced in gynecologic tumors. Pain, especially agonizing headaches, can be improved in 70% of patients with epipharyngeal tumors for different lengths of time. Other tumors in the otorhinologic region show a less significant analgesic reaction.

Radionuclide therapy is used in cases of painful multiple bone metastases of carcinomas of the breast and prostate. The beta emitters strontium 89 and yttrium 90 are suitable in this form of treatment. A diagnostically higher concentration of activity is found in regions of increased bone regeneration after administration of a ^{99m}Tc-phosphate complex. This also applies to the two therapeutically used radionuclides with bone affinity. The rate of uptake is higher in osteoblastic metastases than in osteolytic metastases with fewer blastic parts. For slowly progressing osteolyses and plasmocytoma, this method is less suitable. Figures 1 and 2 show the higher radionuclide uptake in bone metastases in a patient with carcinoma of the prostate. The uptake factor for metastases is 4 compared to 1 in the normal bone. The analgesic effect is felt within 24 to 48 h and lasts for 7 weeks on average (Kutzner et al. 1981).

Radioresection of the pituitary gland as an ablative measure by implantation of radioactive gold seeds was recommended by Bauer and Klar (1958) as a method of therapy for far advanced inoperable tumors. Forest et al. (1967) used radioyttrium. An analgetic effect on bone metastases due to breast cancer was obtained in 75% of 300 patients by Denoix (1970), while the results of Piotrowski (1971), who investigated the effect on a large number of tumors in 548 patients show pain relief in only 55.5% of patients. However, this method is not without risk. Piotrowski (1971) observed complications as diabetes insipidus in 2.9%, a liquor fistula in 4.7%, and sight disorders in 1.5% of cases. Denoix (1970) reported 3% brain nerve damage, 2% optic nerve damage, 8% liquor fistulas, 4% meningitis, 77% diabetes insipidus, and a mortality rate after operation of 2%. The

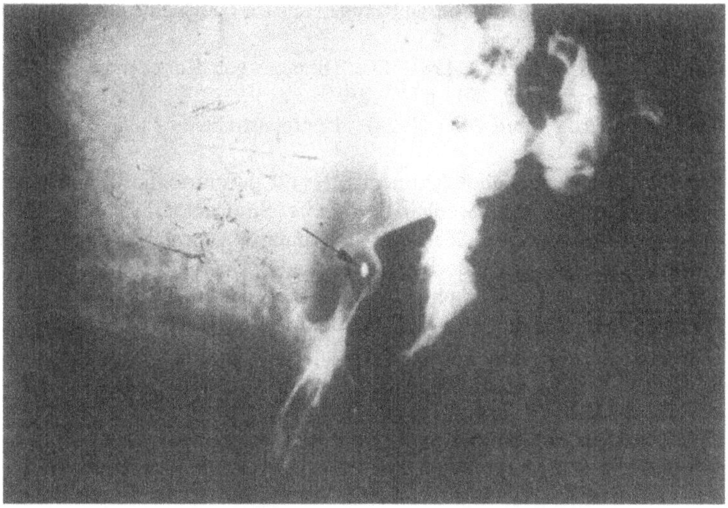

Fig. 3. Lateral roentgenogram of the skull of a patient showing implanted radiogold seeds in the hypophysis *(arrow)*

destruction of the pituitary anterior lobe is only partial and has no influence on the results.

Radiologic thalamotomy has so far only been performed in Stockholm. In this therapy, a single stereotactic irradiation of the centrum medianum of the thalamus was applied at a dose of 150–200 Gy, produced by 180 single cobalt 60 sources in a hemispheric array focused by radial channels in a lead shield. Indications for this form of intervention are intractable and severe pain. Considerable pain relief could be obtained in 85%–90% of 600 treated patients (Larsson 1982). However, there are still technical limits inherent to this rather expensive method.

Radiotherapy of cancer pain in its various forms is definitely an effective form of palliative treatment and should be taken into consideration in all cases within the scope of therapy planning. With the relevant indications and optimal doses, results can be obtained that avoid more risky operations and reduce long-term analgetic medication. In far advanced incurable tumor stages it may give the patient considerable relief from suffering and make his condition tolerable.

References

Allen KL (1981) Rapid palliation in private practice. In: Weiss L, Gilbert HA (eds) Bone metastasis. Hall, Boston, pp 457–468

Ambrad A (1981) Single-dose and short high-dose fractionation radiation therapy for osseous metastases. In: Weiss L, Gilbert HA (eds) Bone metastasis. Hall, Boston, pp 452–456

Bauer KH, Klar E (1958) Zur Technik der perkutanen Hypophysenausschaltung durch radioaktives Gold. Chirurg 29: 145

Denoix P (1970) Treatment of malignant breast tumors. Springer, Berlin Heidelberg New York (Recent results in cancer research, vol 31)

Forrest APM, Stewart HJ (1967) Technical problems and results of yttrium hypophysectomy. In: Dargent M, Romieu C (eds) Major endocrine surgery for the treatment of cancer of the breast in advanced stages. Simap, Lyon, p 89

Glasser O (1958) Wilhelm Conrad Röntgen und die Geschichte der Röntgenstrahlen. Springer, Berlin Göttingen Heidelberg

Gottwald G, Szakolczai I (1981) Die Therapie von Knochenmetastasen beim Mammakarzinom. Strahlentherapie 157: 801–807

Heidenhain L, Fried C (1924) Röntgenstrahlen und Entzündung. Klin Wochenschr 3: 1121–1122

Karageorgis P, Emmanuil E, Throuvalas N (1982) Contribution of the hyperdynamic radiotherapy in the treatment of the nasopharynx tumors. Strahlentherapie 158: 156–159

Kutzner J, Dähmert W, Schreyer T, Grimm W, Brod KH, Becker M (1981) Yttrium-90 zur Schmerztherapie von Knochenmetastasen. Nuclearmedizin 20: 229–235

Piotrowski W (1971) Hypophysenausschaltung mit Radioisotopen bei fortgeschrittenen Krebserkrankungen. In: Linder F, Ott G, Rudolph H (eds) Diagnostische und therapeutische Fortschritte in der Krebschirurgie. Springer, Berlin Heidelberg New York, pp 70–77

Schlegel G (1982) Die Therapie des Tumorschmerzes. Tumordiagnostik 3: 10–16

Wizenberg MJ (1981) The philosophy and economics of palliative radiotherapy for bone metastases. In: Weiss L, Gilbert HA (eds) Bone metastasis. Hall, Boston, pp 390–398

Psychological Treatment Modalities for Pain in Cancer Patients

R. H. Adler and W. Hemmeler

Abteilung für Medizin, C.-L.-Lory-Haus, Inselspital, 3010 Bern, Switzerland

Introduction

Psychological therapies such as hypnosis and autogenic training may be used to treat pain in the cancer patient. Some patients may draw relatively small benefit from these methods, while others benefit more significantly. These methods may result in the diminution of anxieties, hope for mitigation of pain, lessening of feelings of isolation, the experience of goal-directed medical therapy, as well as the feeling of belonging to a group. The more general effects apart from the goals of the specific therapy relate to emotional factors essential for the experience and tolerance of pain. Therefore, a more general psychological treatment should be based on the comprehension of and should deal with the psychological and social problems that appear in the course of a neoplastic disease.

We discuss the psychologically and socially appropriate care of cancer patients and the particular problems involved, such as the preconditions for this kind of therapy, the empathy and working alliance between the physician and the patient, the relationship with the patient at the time the diagnosis is established, the discussion with him about the prognosis, the assistance given to the patient during the various phases of illness, and the attitute toward the family.

Preconditions for the Care of the Cancer Patient: Empathy and the Working Alliance

Insight into his own emotions and problems concerning the treatment of cancer patients is a necessity for the therapist. The experiences of Sanes (1979), a pathologist suffering from a sarcoma who wrote about his personal experience for 5 years until his death, point to the fact that many physicians, in contrast to their own judgment, have difficulty in establishing a good relationship with the cancer patient. "Despite superior academic records in school, scientific and technical success in postgraduate education and practice, many lack the ability to relate personally to patients and their families" (Sanes 1979).

Even when we begin to gain an insight into our own emotions and problems concerning our relationship to cancer patients, we can never fully feel and comprehend what the patient really experiences. Medical students and physicians have their own – perhaps partially covered up – experiences of sadness, hopelessness, anger, etc. They may remember an accident which forced them to abandon their beloved sport forever; they may have experienced shock and disbelief after a failed examination, or felt emptiness and senselessness after the loss of a close relative. The gamut of such sentiments can neither be taught nor learned. However, the ability to become aware of them can be furthered (Adler

Recent Results in Cancer Research. Vol. 89

1981) either during psychotherapy or in a Balint group, etc. These emotions, experienced by the physician who puts himself into the position of the patient, are called "empathy" (Greenson 1978) and are one of the preconditions for the care of a cancer patient. Sanes repeatedly expresses in his book the need of a cancer patient to have a physician with empathy: "The cancer patient may adapt to the fact that his physician cannot cure him or prolong his life. He cannot accept being disregarded emotionally. It crushes his spirit. For palliation empathy ought to rank with medical and surgical measures" (Sanes 1979). He suggests that the medical student should be taught to develop a holistic and humane attitude toward the patient. This will then enable the physician to consider the cancer patient as a sick human being with a multitude of problems and needs. But he goes on to say that physicians have the same anxieties as the layman toward cancer and their one-sided technologic education is an obstacle for the development of empathy. He continues that it is, of course, impossible to incorporate into the study of medicine a learning process by which the student may himself experience what it means to suffer from cancer. But he suggests a procedure which could help the medical student to develop a holistic and humane approach to patients, enabling physicians to learn about the psychological, physical, social, and economic problems inflicted upon the patient suffering from an incurable disease such as cancer. "Wouldn't it be possible they might attend lectures or discussions, at which they could hear and question a guest faculty of students, nurses and lay persons, who have themselves had to meet as best they could, the problem of chronic, 'incurable' diseases?" (Sanes 1979).

However, empathy alone is not enough for the treatment of the patient. Only when we can put it aside from time to time and use our ability to observe and think about the physical history of the patient, his psychological strength and liability, his attitude toward work and leisure time, his relations to his fellows, and his ability to tackle problems on his own, will we be able to estimate how far and in what areas we can help the patient to come to grips with his illness. Hence, the rational relationship between physician and patient must be reinforced as far as possible, in other words, we must achieve a working alliance between patient and doctor (Greenson 1978).

The Association with the Cancer Patient

The association with the cancer patient lasts from the disclosure of the diagnosis until the patient's death and sometimes even longer, as persons close to the patient might also be in need of psychological care. The moment of telling the patient the diagnosis of his condition, the first months of the patient's struggles with the fact that he is suffering from cancer, the time before and after surgical interventions, and chemotherapy and radiation therapy all impose considerable stress upon the patient and his family. Both localized flare-ups and the appearance of metastases are situations requiring special psychological care by the physician (Schmale 1970). It is also important during the time when curative medical treatment is no longer successful and the physician has to try to alleviate symptoms (Schmale 1970; Kubler-Ross 1974).

Telling the Cancer Patient his Diagnosis

The first consultation is important for the future relationship between the patient, his family, and the physician. Again and again the question arises as to whether the diagnosis of "cancer" should be communicated to the patient. There are still proponents of the opinion that the diagnosis of cancer should not be told to the patient under any circumstances (Schmale 1970). Because of the patient's right to information, nowadays the physician is obliged to impart to the patient the diagnosis, its significance, the choice of therapies available, their possible side effects, and the prognosis, using language the patient will understand. However, the patient's right to be informed often misleads the physician into releasing the information in a manner unsympathetic to the feelings of the human being who is the recipient of this information. The physician should be aware that he is not fulfilling his obligations by just imparting the information. During the first interview, somatic, psychological, and social factors should be discussed at length: This is the basis for the working alliance and the patient feels the physician's empathy. By asking the patient about his thoughts, he provides an opportunity for the patient to explain his ideas about the illness. Based on long experience of himself, his body, and his own way of thinking, in most cases the patient will give the physician a definite impression as to whether he rejects the possibility of having a cancer or whether he already suspected it or even was definitely sure of it. This facilitates the physician's approach to the patient. Sometimes the physician presumes the patient is ignorant of the possibility of cancer, but this might reflect his own desire not to discuss this problem with the patient. In fact, such ignorance on the part of the patient is quite rare (Greene 1962; Kastenbaum et al. 1966; Kennedy and Fortung 1974).

On the basis of the success of the first interview, it is much easier for the pyhsician to discuss, for instance, the result of the biopsy. During the initial interview the physician also learns who is most important among the patient's relatives or friends and he may then propose to conduct further discussions in which this person should participate. The patient has the right to insist on absolute discretion toward a third person, but, in most cases, the patient is quite ready to share the knowledge with his or her spouse. This is beneficial to all participants: to the physician because he avoids the risk of imparting different versions of the disease and because it enables him to assess the ability of the spouse to support the patient and the spouse's own needs for support; and to the patient the presence of the spouse offers protection, consolation, and helps to prevent isolation. Such isolation would arise if only the spouse were informed of the diagnosis: The need to keep the diagnosis of cancer secret would result in a break in communication. To inform only one family member would impose a heavy burden on this person who would then have to put up a smoke screen in his or her contact with the cancer patient. But in spite of all pretense, gestures, and words, the patient would see through the attempted dissimulation.

The first interview, if well conducted, brings out clearly that the question is not *whether* the truth should be told, but *how* it should be told (Kübler-Ross 1974; Sanes 1979; Schmale 1970). During the first interview with the patient, without asking suggestive questions the physician should provide the patient with an opportunity to talk about his own ideas of his illness and this, in turn, should alert the physician about important points to consider in 'how' to present the information. Sanes commented that truth is not equal to cruelty provided the truth is also based on emotional support. From his own experiences as a cancer patient, he suggested the following basic rules for the proper attitude of the physician: to establish a personal relationship to the patient and the family; to be available and to arrive on time for an appointment; to have time; to introduce himself, particularly in hospital situations; to organize the discussion in such a manner that interruptions do not occur; to use simple terms instead of medical jargon; to control and observe his own reactions in order not to transfer his own anxieties evoked by the diagnosis to the patient; when the disease is "cancer", to use this word and to explain the nature of the particular kind of cancer, using paper and pencil to illustrate the explanations; to be open to questions put by the patient and his family; to give the patient and the family his telephone number and to explain who will assist in case he is not available; not to get angry about "illogical" questions asked by the patient and relatives or about inquiries into treatment modalities which they have read about in the lay press (Sanes 1979). These principles are often met with the argument that they are too time-consuming, but this argument is inappropriate. The physician who is experienced in carrying out these principles hardly requires more time than the physician who takes down a complete history asking a list of questions with "yes" and "no" answers. Furthermore, if the primary interview is conducted with empathy and a working alliance is achieved, much time is saved later on. The patient and his family will then feel that they are understood by the physician because they can ask questions and receive information not in technical, but in simple, sympathetic language. This will reduce anxiety, there will be much fewer emergency calls, and the amount of time required for the patient will decrease progressively.

Discussion of the Prognosis

The rules for the first interview and the communication of the diagnosis apply equally to the discussion of the prognosis. The physician should be guided in his statements by what is scientificly known and he should discuss the various treatment modalities available, but he should never crush feelings of hope in the patient and he should avoid getting involved in discussions of life expectancy. All patients and all cancers are different and so the prognosis is different in every case. He should also keep in mind that life expectancy data are based on statistics which say little about the individual patient. Experience proves that, in most cases, the patient does not so much desire an exact time prognosis as the assurance that his doctor will be at his side, no matter what the future development may be. According to Sanes, who was both pathologist and patient, many physicians faced with the diagnosis of "cancer" are much too pessimistic because they lack thorough oncological knowledge and equate cancer with rapid destruction and death, instead of taking into account the different development of individual types of cancer and of patients, as well as the progress made in cancer therapy.

Behavior of the Patient During Different Phases of Illness

The care of the cancer patient and his or her family requires knowledge on the part of the physician of the behavior of a human being overwhelmed by news of a condition for which he has been unable to prepare himself. Possible reactions of the cancer patient have been described by Kübler-Ross (1973). They correspond to the reactions observed during mourning (Lindenmann 1944; Milt 1966). A period of shock and disbelief or of absence of feelings and devotion to the automatic routine of daily tasks is followed after hours, days, or even months by a gradual realization of the facts accompanied by anxiety, helplessness, and hopelessness, which alternate with ideas that everything is completely unchanged. Then follows the rebellion against destiny, the anger at being one of those afflicted by cancer. Still later there is a reasonable degree of acceptance of the situation, as well as bargaining for time to be present at some event or other. The final stage is marked by resignation and, with waning physical performance, retreat, isolation from the social environment and the world as a whole, and acquiescence. A total acceptance of fate will certainly remain the exception. It is essential to realize that these phases do not necessarily develop in this order, but that the patient may remain in one phase for a long time or may repeatedly revert from later phases to earlier ones. This may happen after a period of acquiescence, when there is a relapse after the disease seemed to be under control. Sometimes the patient goes through different phases simultaneously.

As far as grief is concerned, the time factor deserves special consideration. The physician cannot influence the various phases, but he must support the patient and his family with much patience, while they adjust in their own personal manner to the various situations arising from the disease. Before medical intervention, the physician often finds himself in the awkward situation that the patient has not yet had sufficient time to accept the information emotionally. It is essential to explain to the patient the consequences of nonintervention, but to let him make his own decision freely. If the patient feels that the physician takes his arguments and indecision seriously, it is easier for him to submit to surgery, which he cannot yet accept emotionally. The patient sees that he is being treated as a partner with definite thoughts and feelings. This reinforces the working alliance. If the physician ignores the patient's grief, the patient might look upon himself as somebody who has "false" emotions, which is equivalent to being mad. This will disturb the patient and can lead to anxiety, anger, and, in short, to behavior that will destroy the cooperative effort.

Once medical therapy has begun, denial, anxiety, and depression mostly diminish and the patient tries to reestablish the routine of his life. But even if the disease does take a satisfactory course, the patient still needs the support of his physician. The patient and his family have to be secure in the knowledge that they always have access to the physician, that they can tell him about any preoccupations, and ask questions. For example, some of the patient's friends and relatives might withdraw from him, even if he feels well, because cancer is generally considered a threat. This experience may result in social isolation. Sanes commented in this regard that for him the possibility of social death was more traumatic than the somatic menace (Sanes 1979).

At the time of a relapse, but, of course, also during the other phases, anger may be the predominant emotion of the patient. It is often misinterpreted by the physician and the family if they do not realize that this is a normal phase in the process of experiencing sadness. In this case, the physician may, in his turn, be angered by the thanklessness and lack of cooperation of the patient or he may withdraw his friendliness and retreat from the patient. Feelings of dissatisfaction and anger may also arise in family members. Because of the long course of the disease and the exacerbation in spite of all the therapy given, the family may become anxious and fearful of losing the patient. This can proceed to such a degree that the patient and/or the family insist on terminating the treatment, on going to another hospital, or on seeking the services of a nature-healer. As soon as the physician becomes aware of this kind of change in emotional relations, he should speak to the patient and his family in something like the following manner: "Mr. X., I don't know whether I am on the right track, but it seems to me that you are now much more tense than usual. Could it be that the lack of progress depresses you or even makes you very angry?" Frequently, doctor and patient then suggest calling in a consultant (Schmale 1970) and, in this way, the patient and family feel that their emotions have been taken into consideration and that the physician does not consider himself the ultimate authority, but is capable of working in cooperation with another physician and does not want to make the patient feel inferior. Then the situation will become less tense and desires for a change of physician will disappear.

When the stage is reached where no further curative procedures can be applied, the physician often withdraws because he thinks he is of no further use. But the patient and his family, who again pass through phases of denial, dispute, anger, and despair, need the

physician just as much as before. In this phase, the patient withdraws more and more and even refuses contact with his next of kin and with friends who want to spend time with him. But even if the physician can now no longer give medical help, he is still in a position to give important support to the patient. It is now no longer a question of saying something clever and educated, but of coping with the situation, sitting next to the patient, perhaps putting his hand on the patient's arm, and remaining silent. Often the patient will then speak of the past or may confess having done something wrong for which he asks pardon.
The physician's duties do not cease with the death of the patient. He must give support to the bereaved who are at risk of losing their psychological and physical balance. He should ask himself the critical question: "Is grief a disease?" (Engel 1951), a question which must be answered in the sense that mourning can add to the appearance and worsening of psychological and physical diseases (Parkes 1976). The treatment of pain in the cancer patient must include the psychological aspects. The comprehension of these psychological factors is based on empathy, the working alliance, as well as on psychological knowledge. The physician to whom "the secret of the care of the patient is in caring for the patient" (Peabody 1927) makes every effort to acquire the necessary knowledge and capacity for this kind of treatment.

References

Adler RH (1981) Die Mißachtung der Gefühle – ein Hindernis für die Entwicklung einer patientorientierten Medizin. Schweiz Med Wochenschr 111: 1245–1249

Engel GL (1961) Is grief a disease? A challenge for medical research. Psychosom Med 23: 18–22

Greene WA (1962) What the cancer patient should be told about his diagnosis and prognosis: "Psychiatrist's recommendation". In: The physician and the total care of the cancer patient. The American Cancer Society, New York, pp 69–73

Greenson RR (1978) Explorations in psychoanalysis. International Universities Press, New York, Chaps 11, 15, 22, 26

Kastenbaum R, Cutler DR, Kalisk RA, Weismann AD (1966) Death and responsibility. Psychiatr Opinion 3: 3–41

Kennedy BJ, Fortung IE (1974) Therapeutic castration in the treatment of advanced breast cancer. Cancer 17: 1197–1202

Kübler-Ross E (1973) On death and dying. Macmillan, New York; Collier-Macmillan, London

Kübler-Ross E (1974) Questions and answers on death and dying. Macmillan, New York; Collier-Macmillan, London

Lindenmann E (1944) Symptomatology and management of acute grief. Am J Psychiatry 101: 141–148

Merskey H, Spear FG (1967) Pain: psychological and psychiatric aspects. Bailliere, Tindall and Cassell, London

Milt H (1966) The roots of suicide: an examination of a major mental health problem. In: Milt H (ed) The experience and the disease GRIEF. Trends in psychiatry, vol 3/1. Merck Sharp & Dohme, West Point

Morgan WL, Engel GL (1969) The clinical approach to the patient. Saunders, Philadelphia

Parkes CM (1976) Bereavement. Studies of grief in adult life. Penguine, Harmondsworth

Peabody FW (1927) The care of the patient. JAMA 88: 877–882

Sanes S (1979) A physician faces cancer in himself. State University of New York Press, Albany

Schmale AH (1970) Coping reactions of the cancer patient and his family. Workshop V: Grief and bereavement. In: Proc. 4th national symposium on catastrophic illness in the seventies. Critical issues and complex decisions, 15–16 Oct 1970, New York, pp 91–105

Sternbach RA (1968) Pain, a psychophysiological analysis. Academic Press, New York

*Hospice Care: The Treatment of Pain in Advanced Cancer**

T. D. Walsh and C. M. Saunders

Department of Clinical Pharmacology, Guy's Hospital,
St. Thomas Street, London SE1 9RT, United Kingdom

Introduction

St Christopher's Hospice, London, was the first of the modern units and is unique amongst them for its commitment to teaching and research in addition to patient care. Stimulated by the philosophy and practice of such units, hospice care in a variety of forms is now a rapidly expanding field in many parts of the world. Essential to such progress and to the provision of humane effective care for the dying has been the emphasis on the patient as a person whose needs must be met by a dedicated, multidisciplinary team, and the realisation that morphine and other opiates (when used correctly) relieve pain safely, effectively and reliably.

Hospice History and Philosophy

The mediaeval hospice was a place of refreshment for pilgrims and travellers which welcomed all who reached its doors, sheltered them until ready to continue their journey, and cared for the sick and wounded. When the Irish Sisters of Charity opened Our Lady's Hospice in Dublin in 1879 and St Joseph's Hospice in London in 1905 they took in many long-stay patients but made the dying so much their special concern that the term 'hospice' came to be equated with this work. The modern hospice has become a skilled community which aims at improving the quality of life remaining for patients with long-term as well as mortal illnesses and sometimes for the frail elderly. It accepts the patient with his family as the focus of its concern, involving them when possible as part of the caring team and supporting them in their bereavement.

The present ideal has grown from the work of those hospices and other similar homes founded at the turn of this century on both sides of the Atlantic for patients with terminal cancer and tuberculosis, some of which acknowledged their debt to the Deaconess hospitals of Europe. As hospitals became more involved with acute care such patients tended to be discharged and could only turn to Poor Law or equivalent institutions if they were unable to remain in their own homes. Hospice therapeutics may be traced back to the classic work *The Care of the Aged, the Dying and the Dead* (Worcester 1935), written by a family doctor for students of Harvard Medical School, to *A Harveian Oration* (Gavey 1952) and to a few articles from the homes. That little of this knowledge was being passed on was made plain by surveys carried out by the Marie Curie Memorial Foundation (1952; Hinton 1963), and

* Supported by DHSS grant number: OCS (A) 3

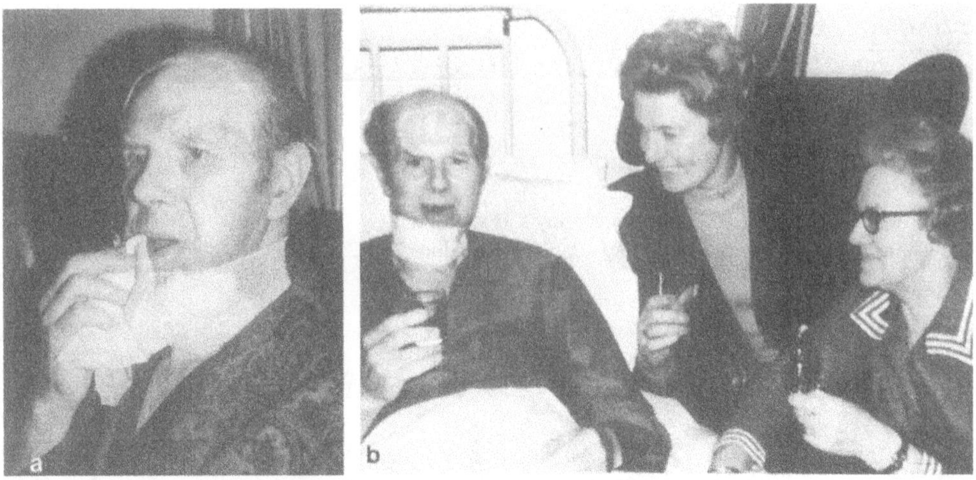

Fig. 1a, b. Mr. B., married, aged 62, had extensive surgery, radiotherapy and chemotherapy for carcinoma of mandible. He was admitted after a week at home with pain, and very anxious and depressed. Foetor from his infected wound was a great humiliation and he was becoming slightly confused (**a** taken shortly after admission). Vigorous treatment of the infection, an increased dose of regular diamorphine given orally, a decrease of the dose of amitriptyline and an increase of chlorpromazine restored his morale as well as relieving his pain and foetor. **b** Was taken at his birthday celebration 5 weeks after admission and 5 days before his death. It was sent to the hospice by his wife, who wrote: "The photograph is to let you see how happy he was just before he died"

others which revealed how much suffering was still endured by dying patients in hospital and in their homes.

Advances in the treatment of malignant disease had offered longer term control, better palliation and sometimes cure to many patients; but for others it had greatly lengthened the time of ill health and dependence and had led to much physical and mental suffering. The trend in Western countries for the patient to die in hospital rather than in his home isolated him from all that was familiar, often without offering him understanding or treatment appropriate to his special needs (Hinton 1963).

Work on the control of terminal pain in advanced cancer carried out in St Luke's Hospital from 1948 onwards was developed in St Joseph's Hospice between 1958 and 1965 (Saunders 1963). It was then possible to begin to exploit the therapeutic advances of the 1950s: new psychotropic drugs, cancer chemotherapy, palliative radiotherapy, the techniques of the new pain clinics and a greater knowledge of family responses to stress and bereavement. The focus of the modern hospice movement thus began with attention to the nature of terminal pain, to its better understanding and therefore more effective treatment. This was accompanied by a revival of the old concept of a "good death" and attention to the achievements that a patient could still make in the face of physical deterioration. A hospice aims by skilled and experienced awareness of a patient's symptoms and feelings to help him live to the limit of his potential in physical strength, mental and emotional capacity and in social relationships (Fig. 1). It offers an alternative form of treatment to the acute care of the general hospital, not in opposition but as a further resource for those for whom that is no longer appropriate. It is the alternative to the negative and socially dangerous suggestion that a patient with an incurable disease likely to cause suffering should have the legal option of hastened death or "euthanasia".

The research and teaching hospices, opened from 1967 onwards, set out to establish recognized standards of care which could be interpreted in the home, was well as in other settings and cultures, and become a part of general medical and nursing teaching. They aimed to identify some of the common problems, to find solutions and to spread this knowledge as widely as possible. As the work spread, a wide variety of interpretations and innovations grew into the "hospice movement". Different titles and ways of working in the palliative or continuing care units, which are an integral part of a general hospital, separate small homes, home care teams, and symptom control or support teams in hospitals all emphasize different approaches and appear under the umbrella term "hospice". Many of these are outside the National Health Service (N.H.S.) in the United Kingdom, but most are closely related in policy and practice and receive considerable financial support. A few are totally within the N.H.S. In none have patients to pay for their care. The present position of terminal care in the N.H.S. in general was recently reviewed (Ford and Pincherle 1978; Hillier and Lunt 1981) and information concerning the movement in the USA is obtainable from the National Hospice Organisation (1311A Dolley Madison Boulevard, McLean, Virginia 22102, USA).

A major aim of any hospice is that its experience and teaching should be so accepted that the profession as a whole will carry out the care needed by dying patients, the majority of whom will always die in their own homes or in general hospitals and not in special centres. In practice, however, it has been found that a few such centres continue to be needed for patients with those intractable problems, physical, emotional or social, that are almost impossible to deal with except by a specially trained staff and, sometimes, in a specially planned milieu. It has been important to define the standard of relief that should be achieved so that those in the general field may assess their own practice and recognize the expertise of the special unit or team and when it should be involved. Only such a standard and such integration will ensure that wherever patients die they will receive the best treatment available (Saunders 1976). A survey comparing places and policies of terminal care records that patients were least depressed and anxious in a hospice, preferring the more frank communication there (Hinton 1979).

Basic Principles of a Hospice

Whether it is a geographically separate unit, part of a hospital campus, a separate ward or a home care or hospital team, a hospice should establish the following principles, some of them common to any branch of medicine or nursing, others specific to hospice care.

1. An integrated clinical team is needed for expert control of symptoms, both common and uncommon. The expertise of oncologists, radiotherapists, anaesthetists and psychiatrists may all be called upon by the hospice doctors, who in turn have special knowledge to offer (Saunders 1976).
2. The hospice team itself will involve the paramedical disciplines. Such a team is not unlike those in any unit which is grappling with complex physical and emotional problems.
3. Skilled and experienced team nursing will call for confident leadership by the ward sister and easy communication among its members. The days are past when doctors could step back and consider that nurses should take over (or even the unsupported family), but nursing is the corner-stone of hospice care.

4. Methodical recording and analysis should be used in monitoring clinical practice and, with relevant research where possible, lead to soundly based practice and teaching concerning the management of terminal distress. Successful practice has been spread widely and various studies completed (Walsh et al. 1982) but more are needed.
5. According to local facilities and customs, home care should be developed and integrated with the community services already established. Although the amount of care the hospice itself should undertake will vary, help must be available 24 h a day and 7 days a week from someone who knows the family. This will normally be in consultation with the patient's own doctor, who remains in charge, using the hospice team as a resource. At least half of the patients of a hospice are likely to be in their own home and, as a patient's condition changes, movement between his general hospital, his home and hospice beds (if available) gives continuity of care. The passage back from terminal to acute care is made more frequently as effective symptom control develops.
6. There must be a bereavement follow-up service. The family has to recover and the hospice team must identify those in special need. Good neighbours, social workers, chaplains and family doctors have been able to fill this role but the need for unhurried listening, especially from a member of a group which helped the family deal with the patient's illness and death, may help to reduce the considerable morbidity recorded in several studies of bereaved people. Many hospices use trained volunteers for this service.
7. Teaching must be given in all aspects of terminal care: the competent control of symptoms first, including the use of analgesics and the many forms of adjuvant therapy. These are passed on in writing (Baines 1978; Twycross 1978) and in lectures and seminars. Hospices are used as a resource in both formal and informal consultation.
8. Imaginative use should be made of architecture. Some hospices work effectively as teams with no beds of their own, others have a few allocated to them in a general hospital; only the minority are likely to be able to build. Buildings old and new must be adapted to combine much-needed privacy for patients, families and staff with the equally important sense of openness and community and to maintain a sense of home alongside efficient and easy operation.
9. A competent and approachable administration, essential to any field of human need, is here required to give security to patients, families and staff. Efficiency is comforting. Hospices have shown that their operation is cost-effective as well as appropriate and humane.
10. Although the current interest in hospice care is especially concerned with the dying cancer patient and his family, a good community is usually a mixed one and hospices may include in their concern those with other long-term progressive illnesses, chronic pain and, in some cases, frailty in old age. There are many disadvantage groups who need the same focus and attention.
11. There must be a readiness for the cost of commitment and a continual search for meaning. Devotion has been an outstanding characteristic of past and present hospices. Willingness to face this demand has a fundamental bearing on the way the work is done and upon the stability and support of the staff. Affirmations of faith may be made but never imposed; each individual has to grow into a fuller (though never complete) realization of the truths he accepts. In such a climate, patients and families are encouraged to reach out towards what they see as true.

To see that such care is available has become an essential part of our commitment to every patient with progressive illness whose care we undertake (Dunphy 1976). Competence in helping the patient and his family to handle the situation that faces them, together with the philosophy outlined above, give to the modern hospice a positive and dynamic atmosphere.

Pain in Advanced Cancer

Pain is a common experience in cancer patients (Annual Statistics of St Christopher's Hospice 1981) and in those with advanced cancer often associated with other symptoms (Table 1). It is now widely recognised that cancer pain is not only a common problem but that it is severe in many patients and often mismanaged by medical and nursing staff (Shimm et al. 1979). There are a number of reasons why this is so, for example misunderstanding of the correct use of opiates in this context and failure to devote attention to symptom control as a worthy end in itself. These problems are compounded by the "cure-orientated" approach of medicine in Western Europe and North America. It is

Table 1. Commonest symptoms in advanced cancer: St Christopher's Hospice 1979 (n = 647)

Symptom	Percentage
Pain	69.5
Anorexia	64.75
Weight loss	59.25
Weakness	49.0
Constipation	45.5
Dyspnoea	42.0
Nausea/vomiting	36.75
Oedema/effusion	30.75
Cough	29.0
Insomnia	27.0

Table 2. Pain management in advanced cancer

1 A team management approach is best
2 All *appropriate* therapies are employed in combination
3 Detailed attention is given to social, psychological and spiritual care
4 All therapeutic interventions employed should have low morbidity and not hasten death
5 A problem-solving analytical approach is used
6 Therapy is individualised
7 Investigations are selective
8 Patients must be carefully selected before any destructive procedure, e.g., cordotomy, are conducted
9 Drugs are the mainstay of therapy, should be given orally whenever possible, are used taking into account their pharmacological characteristics, are preferably given regularly and not „as required“

common to find inappropriate continuation of active, i.e. "curative", therapy long past the point of possible benefit. Given the significant morbidity with much modern cancer therapy, not only does active therapy often fail to prolong life, but it may even contribute to a reduction in the quality of life for that person in the final weeks or months (as well as involving time-consuming and often pointless investigative procedures). There is evidence too that some therapeutic procedures employed in the early treatment of cancer contribute to morbidity in the later stages of disease. Foley (1979) has described the clinical pain syndromes found in cancer patients (see also Hartenstein and Wilmanns, this volume p. 72 ff.). Based on the emerging role of hospice care already described, some principles of management of chronic pain in advanced cancer can be suggested (Table 2).

Oral Opiate Analgesics

Routine parenteral opiate administration is unnecessary, and even inappropriate, in the majority of patients with chronic severe pain from cancer. Oral morphine relieves pain effectively in 85% of patients (Fig. 2). It is essential to administer the morphine regularly in order to keep the brain concentration at a level sufficient for analgesia. A 4-hourly regimen has been found adequate (Table 3). The dose has to be adjusted individually (Fig. 3). In the small group of patients where pain is not sufficiently relieved by oral morphine, combinations of drugs with radiotherapy, nerve blocks etc. will give satisfactory control. A few patients may present difficult therapeutic problems, in particular those with pelvic pain, deafferentation pain and extensive bony metastatic disease. These often occur in the context of "total" pain, usually in younger age groups (Saunders 1978). Favoured drugs for

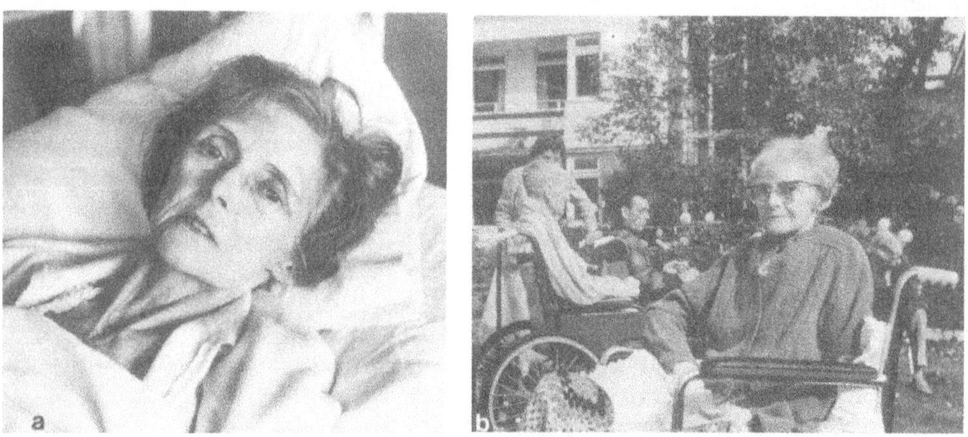

Fig. 2a, b. Mrs. S., a widow aged 63, had a palliative ante colic gastro-jejunostomy for carcinoma of stomach. Three months later, in pain and finding it impossible to cope alone at home, she was admitted to St Christopher's Hospice. She had lost 40 lb in weight and suffered anorexia, occasional nausea and vomiting, periodic diarrhoea and constipation, general weakness and anxiety. **a** Was taken 5 days after admission when her pain had not yet been fully controlled by oral diamorphine and chlorpromazine. Three days later her pain was fully relieved and she had no further increase in dose for the next 8 weeks. She was also prescribed tab. prednisone 5 mg t.d.s. for anorexia and a diuretic. **b** Was taken 4 weeks after admission. In spite of gradually increasing weakness Mrs. S. remained active and alert until she took to her bed a few days before her death. Her drugs were given by injection for the last 48 h with a twofold increase in total dosage

Table 3. Practical use of morphine

1	2.5–180 mg morphine sulphate, five to six 4-h doses/24 h
2	Individualized dose titrated against the pain
3	Aqueous formulation
4	With or without prochlorperazine 5.0 mg 4-hourly
5	With or without adjuvant drugs, e.g., corticosteroids

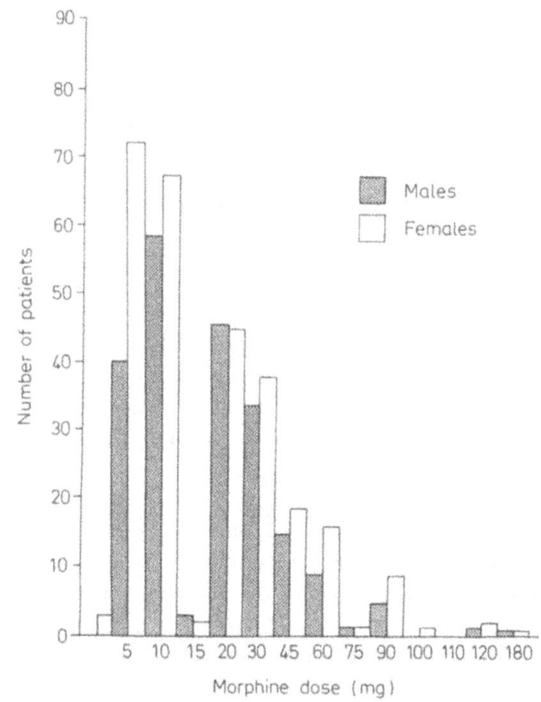

Fig. 3. Histogram of maximum 4-h doses of oral morphine in patients admitted to St Christopher's Hospice in 1979

oral use in severe pain are morphine, diamorphine (heroin), and methadone. Morphine and diamorphine have different milligram potencies but are clinically indistinguishable (Kaiko et al. 1981) in analgesic efficacy and side effects (orally 15 mg morphine = 10 mg diamorphine; parenterally 20 mg morphine = 10 mg diamorphine) for severe chronic cancer pain. Oral morphine is favoured in Britain, methadone in the USA. Methadone is given 8-hourly and may even be effective given once daily (Portnow and Corbett 1982). It has a long half-life and may cumulate when elimination processes are impaired, although it has been successfully employed in patient-controlled analgesic regimes (Sawe et al. 1981). When oral opiates are employed correctly and appropriately, tolerance, dependence and respiratory depression (Walsh and Saunders 1981) are not common problems in this population. Phenazocine is a useful alternative to the above drugs; it may be associated with less gastrointestinal upset and can be given sublingually. Morphine may conveniently be administered orally in an aqueous formulation often in combination with a phenothiazine such as prochlorperazine and it has important advantages over other available drugs (Table 4).

Table 4. Advantages of oral morphine

Flexible dosage – large dose possible in small volume
Easy to swallow
Acceptable taste
Dosage can be changed without patient's knowledge if appropriate
Avoids repeated injections
Can be taken until shortly before death (63% of patients continued to use it within 72 h before death)
Antiemetic/sedative can be given along with it
Rapid dose adjustment
High efficacy
Stable solution
Satisfactory bioavailability

Psychotropic Drugs

Phenothiazines. These are employed as antiemetics, sedatives and coanalgesics. Given intramuscularly, 15 mg methotrimeprazine is equivalent to 10 mg morphine intramuscularly (Bloomfield 1964). Prochlorperazine is the usual phenothiazine employed in conjunction with oral morphine. Chlorpromazine is useful for sedation but methotrimeprazine is favoured for terminal restlessness. The latter drug is associated with a high incidence of side effects. The extent of the coanalgesic effect of these drugs during chronic administration is unclear.

Antidepressant. Clinical depressive syndromes are (surprisingly) relatively uncommon in advanced cancer. Pain complaints may be caused or exacerbated by depression; such complaints will improve with effective antidepressant treatment (Lindsay and Wychoff 1981). The question of whether antidepressants are analgesic in those who are not depressed remains open, despite many anecdotal reports of analgesic benefit and/or opiate-sparing actions in cancer patients.

Non-steroidal Anti-inflammatory Drugs (NSAID)

These seem to give specific and highly effective benefit in pain due to bone metastases used alone or in combination with morphine. Phenylbutazone is perhaps still the most clinically effective drug, although associated with significant side-effects. Presumably, the drugs act via inhibition of prostaglandin synthetase, although some are known to have analgesic actions independent of this mechanism.

Corticosteroids

These are widely used in pain (Table 5) arising from a variety of mechanisms. There is no objective evidence of pain benefit in many of the conditions in which the drugs are employed; the psychological and strength-improving benefits of corticosteroid use are difficult to separate from any analgesic action.

Table 5. Indication for corticosteroid use in advanced cancer

Raised intracranial pressure
Spinal cord compression
Superior vena caval syndrome
Dyspnoea due to lymphangitis carcinomatosis
Lymphoedema
Anorexia
Weakness
Pain due to bone metastases, nerve infiltration, other mechanisms, e.g., lymphoedema
Obstruction of hollow viscus, e.g., colon, ureter
Hypercalcaemia
Vomiting

Table 6. Common nerve block procedures[a]

Total number of patients	74
Total number of procedures	134
Paravertebral	49
Intrathecal nerve root	37
Coeliac plexus	9
Intrathecal saline	7
Hip	6
Interscalene	5
Lumbar plexus	4
Inferior alveolar	2
Obturator	2
Intercostal	2
Caudal extradural	2

[a] St Christopher's Hospice (September 1978–April 1982)

Chemotherapy

Conventional chemotherapy has a limited role in pain control although reduction in pain and improvement in other symptoms may be a welcome benefit of effective chemotherapy. In general hormonal manipulations, e.g., tamoxifen, are most effective and least toxic (particularly for soft tissue disease), as well as having the advantage of oral administration. An important feature is that pain relief from hormonal manipulation may take up to 6 weeks and hormonal therapy is therefore inappropriate for patients with a short prognosis (Bates and Vanier 1978).

Radiotherapy

Single-dose or fractionated radiotherapy is highly effective for isolated, painful bone metastases particularly from carcinoma of the breast or bronchus. Pain benefit may take up to 2 weeks to reach a maximum and, as radiotherapy involves some discomfort for patients, it is unsuitable in those with only a few days to live (Bates 1978).

Nerve Block

Nerve block procedures require careful selection of patients. A common error is that patients are referred for sophisticated procedures before simple measures have been tried. Destructive procedures have significant morbidity and should only be used within the context of a therapeutic program provided by a multidisciplinary team. Effective nerve block procedures often allow reduction of or discontinuation of the use of opiates, although it is usually inappropriate to employ them solely for this purpose (Table 6).

References

Annual Statistics (1981) Department of Clinical Studies, St Christopher's Hospice

Baines MJ (1978) Control of other symptoms. In: Saunders CM (ed) The management of terminal disease. Arnold, London, pp 99–118

Bates TD (1978) Radiotherapy in terminal care. In: Saunders CM (ed) The management of terminal disease. Arnold, London, pp 119–125

Bates TD, Vanier T (1978) Palliation by cytotoxic chemotherapy and hormone therapy. In: Saunders CM (ed) The management of terminal disease. Arnold, London, pp 125–134

Bloomfield S, Wimard-Savoie S, Bernier J, et al. (1964) Comparative analgesic activity of levomepromazine and morphine in patients with chronic pain. Can Med Assoc 90: 1156–1159

Dunphy JE (1976) Annual discourse – on caring for the patient with cancer. N Engl J Med 295: 313–319

Foley KM (1979) Pain syndromes in patients with cancer. In: Bonica JJ, Ventafridda V (eds) Advances in pain pesearch and therapy, vol 2. Raven, New York, pp 59–75

Ford GR, Pincherle G (1978) Arrangements for terminal care in the National Health Service (especially those for cancer patients). Health Trends 10: 73–76

Gavey CJ (1952) The management of the 'hopeless' case. Lewis, London

Hillier R, Lunt B (1981) Terminal care: present services and future priorities. Br Med J 283: 595–597

Hinton J (1963) The physical and mental distress of the dying. Q J Med 32: 1–10

Hinton J (1979) Comparison of places and policies for terminal care. Lancet 1: 29–32

Kaiko RK, Stanley L, Wallenstein MS, Rogers AG, Grabinski PY, Houde RW (1981) Analgesic and mood effects of heroin and morphine in cancer patients with postoperative pain. N Engl J Med 304: 1051

Lindsay PG, Wychoff M (1981) The depression pain syndrome and its response to antidepressants. Psychosomatics 22: 571–577

Marie Curie Memorial Foundation (1952) Report on a national survey concerning patients nursed at home. Marie Curie Memorial Foundation, London

Mount BM (1979) Narcotic analgesics. In: Twycross RG, Ventafridda V (eds) The continuing care of terminal cancer patients. Pergamon, Oxford, pp 97–116

Portnow JM, Corbett RJ (1982) Oral methadone for relief of chronic pain from cancer. N Engl J Med 306: 989–990

Saunders CM (1963) Care of the dying. Practitioner 2: 77–82

Saunders CM (1976) The challenge of terminal care. In: Symington T, Carter RL (eds) Scientific foundations of oncology. Heinemann, London, pp 673

Saunders CM (ed) (1978) The management of terminal disease. Arnold, London

Sawe J, Hansen J, Ginman C, Hartvig P, Jakobsson PA, Nilsson MI, Rane A, Anggard E (1981) Patient-controlled dose regimen of methadone for chronic cancer pain. Br Med J 282: 771–773

Shimm DS, Logue GL, Malbie AA, Dugan S (1979) Medical management of chronic cancer pain. JAMA 241: 2408–2412

Twycross RG (1978) Relief of pain. In: Saunders CM (ed) The management of terminal disease. Arnold, London

Walsh TD, Saunders CM (1981) Oral morphine for relief of chronic pain from cancer. N Engl J Med 305: 1417

Walsh TD, Baxter R, Bowman KB, Grabinski PY, Kaiko RF, Leber B (1982) High-dose oral morphine and respiratory function in advanced cancer. Submitted for publication

Worcester A (1935) The care of the aged, the dying and the dead. Thomas, Springfield, 1935; Arno, New York, 1977

Subject Index

A-beta primary afferent axons 188
A-delta fibers 49, 62, 137
– –, elimination 149
– –, myelinated 47
– nociceptors 111
– primary afferent axons 188
A-fibers 59
A-gamma fibers 137
abdominal cancer 19
– colicky pain 96
– hollow organs, tumor infiltration 39
– pain 179, 180
– wall, somatic pain 127
abuse of euphoric agents 31
accomodation disorders 124
acetylcholine 120
acetylsalicylic acid 5, 6, 7, 60, 157
acid phosphatase, fluoride-resistant 59
acidosis 190
–, local 130
acoustic neurinoma 36
acquiescence 198, 199
activation, antidromic 153
– of second-order neurons 153
acute abdomen 41
– care 204
– dystonic reaction 124
– intestinal toxicity 91
– leukemia 75, 76, 94, 95
– pain 21, 23, 45, 77
– –, physiopathology 20
– – syndromes 89
– radiation enteritis 90
– toxicity 90
– transient pain 86
addiction 10, 22, 23, 101
– to narcotics 140
adipose tissue necrosis 43
adjuvant therapy 204
adrenaline 54, 129
adrenergic transmitters 62
adriamycin 89, 176
advanced cancer 18
– –, chronic pain 206
– –, pain 201, 205
– –, symptoms 205
– –, terminal pain 202
– lesion 16
– malignancies 104
affective impact of pain 13
afferent axons, irritation 45
– fibers 53, 54, 151
– –, myelinated 153
– –, neurophysiological identification 48
– –, nonmyelinated 153
– –, unmyelinated 47
– inhibition in the dorsal horn 55
– inhibitory neurons 60
– nerve fibers 54, 56, 79, 129
– neurons 45, 52, 53, 54
– nociceptive fibers, sensitization 51
– – neurons, chronic irritation 56
– pain pathways, interruption 148
– – system 119
– peripheral nerves 61
akathisia 124
alcohol 9, 128, 132, 137, 138, 144, 145
– block 141
– –, subarachnoid 139, 141, 143
–, chemical neurolysis 149
– injection into the hypophysis 152
–, intrathecal application 137
– neurolysis, intrathecal 129
– treatment 138
algesic substances 6, 49, 51
algesics, narcotic 22
–, non-narcotic 22
algodystrophy 74, 143
algogenesis 75
algogenic psychosyndrome 100
alkaline phosphatase 179, 182
alkylating agents 173

allergic dermatome 69
– reactions 9
allergy 134
– to local anesthetics 134
– to methylparaben 134
alpha- plus betaadrenergic vasoconstrictor 134
amethopterin 173, 176
amide type of local anesthetics 134
aminophenazone 6, 179
amitriptyline 8, 118, 124
ammonium sulfate 137
amputation 81, 89, 162, 169
–, breast 43
– of a limb 90
analgesia 148, 149, 150, 151, 153
–, epidural opiate 107, 109, 110
–, oral administration 10
–, parenteral administration 10, 107
–, regional 112
–, selective 151
–, toxic effects 10
analgesic effect of calcitonin 182
– – of psychotropic drugs 123
– therapy 4, 5, 7, 12
analgesics 31, 32, 66, 67, 127, 204
–, anti-inflammatory 5, 6, 7
–, application intervals 105
–, centrally acting 102, 103, 104, 105
–, enteral administration 111
–, mild 5
–, narcotic 4, 9, 12, 122
–, non-narcotic 6, 7, 8, 110, 122
–, parenteral administration 111
–, peripherally acting 6, 104, 140
–, toxic risks 100
–, underdosage 105
analgetic effect of ionizing radiation 190
– therapy 171
anemia 88
anesthesia 134, 148, 151
–, diagnostic local 2
–, – spinal 140
– dolorosa 149
–, local 150
–, regional 137
–, spinal 9
anesthetics, intravascular injection 133
–, local 110, 127, 129, 130, 134, 140, 144
–, overdose 133
aneurysmal bone cyst 161
anger 19, 95, 195, 198, 199
angina pectoris-like syndrome 92
animal calcitonins 182
anorexia 205, 209
anterior paratracheal technique 132
– roots 138
anterolateral cordotomy 51
anthropological reality of pain and suffering 29
anti-inflammatory agents, nonsteroid 60
– analgesics 5, 6, 7
– drugs 3, 4, 208
– irradiation 190
antidepressant therapy, side effects 124
antidepressants 8, 118, 119, 120, 121, 122, 123, 124, 208
–, anxiolytic effects 122
–, dosage schedules 122
–, tricyclic 8
antidepressive effects 125
antidromic activation of primary afferents 153
– vasodilatation 62
antiemetics 208
antimetabolites 89, 173
antineoplastic chemotherapy 171, 173
– cytostatic therapy 171
– drug therapy 174
– drugs 173
– hormonal therapy 171
antiparkinsonian drug 124
anxiety 3, 7, 18, 77, 95, 100, 119, 124, 133, 195, 198, 199
anxiolytic effects 125
– – of antidepressants 122
– – of neuroleptics 122
– tranquilizers 8
apathy 100
apoplexy 172
ara-C 87, 92, 93
– syndrome 87, 88, 92
arterial embolization 94
– ischemia 76
– occlusion 2, 52
arteritis 40
–, obliterative 41
–, stenotic 41
arthropathy 76
articular pain 179
ascending pathway, degeneration 138
– tract systems, surgical interruption 150
aseptic bone necrosis 69
aspiration tests 133
aspirin 5, 60, 110
atelectase 69
atrophy 80, 90
–, transganglionic degenerative 185, 188

atropine 134
autodigestion 41
autodigestive pancreatitis 41
autogenic training 195
autonomic nervous system 80, 190
axonal degeneration 89
axoplasmic transport, blockade 188, 189

back pain 26, 39
backache 75
Balint group 196
barbiturates 7, 130, 134
behavioral assessment 26
– methods 24
benign bone tumors 157, 160, 161, 162
benperidol 120
benzamide 119
bereavement 202
– follow-up service 204
beta-endorphine 122, 178
beta-lipotropin 178
bioavailability 115
biperidine 124
bipolar stimulation 154
bitterness 19
bladder catheter, permanent 145
– disorders 143
– dysfunction 80, 142, 143
– pain 144
– tenesmus 8
blastomatous processes 79
bleeding 89
block, alcohol 141
–, caudal epidural 132
–, celiac plexus 127, 128, 144
–, diagnostic 127, 128, 142, 143
–, – local anesthetic 140
–, differential 127
–, dorsal root 138
–, epidural 128, 129, 130, 134
–, intercostal 127, 128
–, – nerve 135
–, interscalenus 144
–, intrathecal 142
–, local 129, 130, 135
–, – anesthetic 130, 133, 143
–, lumbar epidural 132
–, – sympathetic 132, 133, 144
–, motor 127, 129
–, neurolytic 137, 144
–, paravertebral 128, 135
–, phenol 141
–, placebo effect 128
–, plexus solaris 144
–, prognostic 127, 128
–, regional 134
–, reversible 129
–, saddle 139
–, sensory 127, 129
–, stellate ganglion 132
–, subarachnoid 137, 138, 140, 145
–, – alcohol 139, 141, 143
–, – neurolytic 141, 142
–, sympathetic 127, 132, 137, 143
–, temporary 129
–, therapeutic 133
–, thoracic epidural 134
blockade of axoplasmic transport 188, 189
–, chemical 149
– of conduction of pain pathways 153
–, neurolytic 113
blocking of dorsal roots 142
– of nociceptive pathways 24
– of regional sympathetic nervous supply 132
– of ventral roots 142
blocks against reflex dystrophies 144
– against vascular disorders 144
blood-brain barrier 101, 111
blood coagulation disorders 77
– flow, disorders 39
– vessels, compression 172
– –, tumor-induced occlusions 41
blunt pain 111
bone cyst, aneurysmal 161
– degradation, osteoclastic 39
– destruction 39, 169
– –, osteoblastic 167
– –, osteolytic 167
–, infiltration 37
– marrow transplantation 91, 94, 95
– metastases 3, 5, 6, 17, 39, 65, 68, 69, 73, 108, 130, 152, 167, 168, 169, 171, 191, 192, 208, 209
– –, osteolytic 180
– pain 3, 87, 148, 152, 174, 179, 180
– protection 4
– regeneration 39
– scan 26, 164
– surgery 11
– tumor clinic 160
– tumors 6, 66, 157, 182
– –, benign 157, 161, 162, 169
– –, malignant 157, 162
– –, primary 37, 157, 162, 167, 169
– –, semimalignant 157, 161, 162, 169
bony metastatic disease 206
borderline insufficiency 142

bowel disorder 143
brachial plexus, interscalenus block 144
– – irritation 167
– – lesions 91
– –, neuropathologic changes 21
– –, paresis 145
– –, radiation damage 148
brachialgia 186
bracing 167
–, orthotic 167
bradycardia 134
bradykinin 5, 33, 49, 50, 51, 52, 60
brain 34, 107, 111, 113, 178
– edema, focal 35
– –, generalized 35
– metastases 74, 75
– nerve damage 192
– stem 55, 60
– tumors 7, 67, 74
– –, primary 81, 191
– –, secondary 81, 191
breast amputation 43
– cancer 15, 65, 73, 75, 91, 167, 171, 190
– carcinoma 167, 174
bromocriptine 153
bronchial carcinoma 35, 41
– –, metastases 38, 39
– –, parvicellular 37
– obstruction 145
bronchitis, chronic 115
bronchogenic cancer 75
– carcinoma 73, 74, 75, 76
bupivacaine 108, 127, 129, 130, 132
buprenorphine 102, 103, 105, 108, 111, 112
–, epidural 111
–, lipophilic 112
–, sublingual administration 103
burning pain 130
busulfan 173
butyrophenones 120

cachectic patient 135
cachexia 100
caffeine 7
calcitonin 178, 179, 180
– analgesia 178
–, analgesic potency 179, 180, 181, 182
–, binding sites 178
–, biologic effects 182
–, central mechanisms 181
–, intracerebro-ventricular administration 182
–, pain relief 181
–, peripheral mechanisms 181
calcium channels 54
calcium-conserving hormone 178
cancellous bone grafting 161, 162
cancer pain centers 25
– –, central mechanisms 46
– –, chemotherapeutic treatment 174
– –, chronic 207
– – control, current status 19
– –, effects 18
– –, generation 45, 46
– –, neurosurgical treatment 148
– –, peripheral mechanisms 46
– –, radiotherapy 193
– –, symptomatology 172
– – therapy, inadequate 20
– –, upper abdominal 132
– statistics 15
cancer-concomitant diseases 76
capsaicin 61, 62, 63
–, local application 62
capsular distension 33
– pain 191
carbamazepine 118
carcinomatous lesions 81, 82
– miningiosis 75
– neuritis 131
carcinosis 41
–, peritoneal 41
–, pleural 41
cardiac arrests 134
cardioactive pressure agents 130
cardiovascular complications 134
– resuscitation 134
– support 134
Carpal-tunnel-like syndrome 92
carrageenan 52
castration 174
catheter, epidural 129
–, permanent bladder 139, 141, 145
–, thoracic 129
cauda equina syndrome 35, 80
caudal epidural block 132
– – catheter 129
causalgia 74, 186
causalgiform pain 149
C-cell carcinoma 182
celiac plexus block 127, 128, 144
cellulitis 88
central gray matter, stimulation 135
– mechanisms of calcitonin 181
– nervous system 5, 45, 51, 60, 61, 62, 91, 94, 118, 119, 121, 122, 178, 189
– – – complications 133
– – –, degenerative alterations 43

central nervous system, lesion 82
– – – stimulators 130
– neurotransmission 63
– pain 81
– threshold 51, 55
centrally acting analgesics 102
centrum medianum 151, 193
cerebral lesions 81
– tumors 81
cervical cancer 14, 20, 66
– percutaneous chordotomy 150
cervicothoracal chain, neurolytic block 144
C-fibers 49, 59
–, elimination 149
–, primary afferent 62
–, unmyelinated 47
chemical blockade of peripheral nerves 149
– – of the sympathetic plexus 149
– injury of nociceptive neurons 59
– interruption of nociceptive pathways 24
– irritants 62
– neurolysis with alcohol 149
– – with phenol 149
– rhizotomy 149
– stimulation of nociceptors 56, 60
– stimuli 47, 49, 62
chemoreceptor trigger zone 101
chemosensibility 51, 54
chemosensitive pain receptors 82
chemosensitivity, abnormal 53
chemotherapeutic drugs 82
– treatment of cancer pain 174
chemotherapy 2, 3, 5, 11, 17, 19, 20, 67, 69, 85, 86, 87, 88, 157, 162, 167, 171, 173, 175, 176, 191, 196, 202, 209
–, aggressive 162
–, antineoplastic 171, 173
–, combined 93
–, intra-arterial 94
–, local 94
–, palliative 176
–, preoperative 162
–, prophylactic 91
chemotherapy-sensitive tumors 176
chest pain 76, 87
chlorambucil 173
chlorocresol 137
chlorpromazine 8, 124, 208
cholangitis 86
cholecystitis 74
cholinergic transmitters 62
cholinesterase inhibitors 120
cholinomimetics 120
chondrosarcoma 160, 161, 162, 163
chordoma of the clivus 37
chordotomy 3, 51, 113, 150, 155
–, anterolateral 51, 150
–, bilateral high cervical 150
–, – open high thoracic 150
–, cervical percutaneous 150
–, percutaneous 4, 149, 150
–, unilateral high cervical percutaneous 150
Christian interpretation of suffering 28
– salvation, practice 30
chronic affection of nociceptive nerve fibers 55
– animal models 55
– bronchitis 115
– cancer pain 207
– inflammation 47, 55
– irritation of afferent nociceptive neurons 56
– lesions of primary afferent fibers 54
–, long-lasting pain 96
– nonhealing ulceration 89
– pain 1, 5, 19, 21, 23, 45, 47, 55, 56, 60, 63, 72, 77, 78, 85, 86, 87, 115, 119, 121, 122, 129, 154, 188, 189, 204
– – in advanced cancer 206
– –, nonmalignant 18
– –, phases 31
– –, physiopathology 20
– persistent pain 18, 100, 153
– – – of benign origin 153
– postsurgical pain syndromes 90
– respiratory disease 116
– severe pain 89, 116
– stimulation of nociceptors 55, 56
– ventilatory failure 116
circulatory depression 102
clinical pain classification 148
clomipramine 118, 122, 124
C nociceptors 111
coagulation of the glossopharyngeal nerve 151
–, high-frequency 152
– of the trigeminal ganglion 151
coanalgesics 208
codeine 7
cognitive methods 24
cold stimulation 188
colicky abdominal pain 90, 91
– cramps 94
– pain 86, 90, 91
colon carcinoma 40
–, distension 50
–, ischemia 50, 52
colorectal cancer 75

colostomy 129, 139, 141, 145
combination antidepressant-neuroleptic therapy 124
– chemotherapy 96
combined chemotherapy and surgery 162
– epidural application of opiates and local anesthetics 130
– osteosynthesis with polymethylmethacrylate 167
complications, cardiovascular 134
– of epidural blocks 134
– of regional blocks 134
– of subarachnoid alcohol blocks 143
compression 33, 35, 79, 81
– fracture 171
– of blood vessels 172
– of lymph vessels 7, 172
– of the nerve plexus 171, 172
– of nerve roots 79, 191
– of nerves 7, 8, 52, 69, 171, 172
– of the spinal cord 69, 171, 172
– of ureter 172
– of veins 7
– of vertebra 172
concomitant treatment of pain 1
congestion 72
congestive organ diseases 75
consolation 197
constant drip infusion of local anesthetics 129
constipation 10, 102, 103, 205
continuous pain 105
contraction 51, 75
convergence phenomena 82
convulsion 133, 134, 144
cord section 153
CO_2-response curve 112
corticosteroid therapy 7
corticosteroids 7, 8, 208, 209
coughing 135
coxalgia 73, 94
cramps 86, 93, 95
–, colicky 94
craniopharyngioma 75
cryogenic nerve blocks 4
cryosurgical measures 152
CSF fistulae 152
CT scan 26
cutaneous hypalgesia 138
– hyperpathia 5
– nociceptive systems 55
– nociceptors 51
– sensibility 142, 144
cyclazocine 122
cystitis 69, 86, 91, 95
cytostatic agents 93, 171, 172, 173, 174, 176
– chemotherapy 172
– drug, local administration 176
– –, oral administration 176
– drugs 81, 87, 95, 171, 176
– therapy 85, 129, 171, 174, 176
cytostatics, misapplication 43
cytotoxic drugs 86, 88, 89, 93, 94

deafferentation pain 79, 148, 154, 206
death rates from cancer 15
decompression of nerve plexus 191
– – roots 191
decrease of sensation 153
decubitis 77
decussating pain pathways 151
deep brain stimulation 4
– lancinating pain 93
– somatic nociceptors 55
– – pain 49, 56
– – structures 45, 47, 49
– tissue 59
– –, chronic inflammation 55
deformation of vertebrae 2
degeneration of the ascending pathway 138
–, axonal 89
–, malignant 163
–, retrograde 62
degenerative processes 52
demyelination 189
denial 199
dependence 10, 101, 102, 105, 118, 202, 207
–, physical 101
–, physiologic 23
–, psychological 101
depersonalisation of pain 119
depositis 81
depression 3, 7, 18, 78, 95, 119, 124, 199, 208
dermal reactions 134
dermatomes 75, 79, 80, 81, 82, 111, 149, 150, 187, 188
–, allergic 69
dermatomyositis 77
descending inhibitory control systems 55, 189
– – neurons 60
despair 19, 77, 199
destruction of the pituitary anterior lobe 193
destructive techniques of neurosurgery 148, 153 , 155
detrusor vesicae, paralysis 139

dextropropoxyphene 105
diabetes insipidus 152, 192, 193
diabetic neuropathy 69
diagnosis communication 198
diagnostic local anesthesia 2
– nerve blocks 9, 127, 128, 140, 142, 143
– – – with local anesthetics 140
– spinal anesthesia 140
diamorphine (heroin) 14, 115, 207
diarrhea 90, 91, 93, 95
diazepam 8, 133, 134
differential block 127
diffuse itching 110
– pain 3, 108
dilatation of the splanchnic vessels 144
dilatations 39
diphosphonates 179
disbelief 198
discharge threshold 51, 55
disorders of micturition 101, 103
dispute 199
dissection, radical neck 90
distension 51, 75
– of the colon 50
– of nociceptive structures 76
–, neck vein 76
–, thoracic vein 76
distress 2
distribution of pain 25
disturbance in the relation of man to himself 28
domperidon 110
dopamine 120
dorsal columns, stimulation 153
– horn 45, 51, 55, 60, 61, 185
– –, afferent inhibition 55
– –, presynaptic inhibition 55
– roots, blocking 138, 142
– –, pain-conducting 138
– –, thermocoagulation 149
dorsal-column stimulation 154
dorsalgia 73, 186
dorsomedian nuclei 151
dosage schedule for neuroleptics 124
– schedules for antidepressants 122
drowsiness 133
drug administration, intra-arterial 176
– –, intravenous 176
– –, oral 176
– –, titrating 23
– rotation 7
– toxicity 173, 176
drugs, anti-inflammatory 3, 4, 5, 6, 7, 208
–, antineoplastic 173
–, antiparkinsonian 124
–, chemotherapeutic 82
–, cytostatic 81, 87, 95, 171, 176
–, cytotoxic 88, 93, 94
–, epidural administration 12
–, hormonal 171
–, inadequate amounts 22
–, narcotic 9, 112
–, – analgesic 9
–, non-narcotic analgesic 5, 8
–, non-steroidal anti-inflammatory 208
–, pain-killing 188
–, psychotropic 4, 8, 22, 103, 118, 119, 122, 123, 125, 191, 202, 208
–, systemic 12, 23
–, titration of doses 116
–, vasoconstrictor 134
dryness of the mouth 103, 124
dying 201
dysesthesia 8, 77, 80, 81, 82, 149, 151
dysfunction, bladder 80
–, monosegmental 80
– of the motor system 82
–, multisegmental 80
–, primary 79
–, rectal 80
–, secondary 79
–, trophic 80
dyskinesia 124
dysregulation of sympathetic nerves 74
dystrophic alterations of skin osteoporosis 131
dysuria 124

economic impact of pain 13
ectopic excitation 130
edema 7, 76, 91, 131, 140
–, cerebral 172
–, facial 76
–, focal pressure-raising 36
–, painful lymph 76
edematous processes 7
educational programs for medical students 24
effects of cancer pain 18
efferent pathways 45
– sympathetic system 9
electric stimulation 5, 62, 150, 153, 154, 178
elephantiasis 43
elimination of the hypophysis 152
– of pain fibers 149
embolectomy 90
embolism 77
emesis 103

emotional impact of pain 13
– morbidity 18
– reactions 18
– support 2
empathy 196, 197, 198, 200
emptiness 195
empyema 41
en bloc tumor resection 162, 163, 167, 168, 169
encapsulated organs 33, 49
encephalopathy 81
endogenous opioid system 119
endoneural infiltration 36
endoprosthetic replacements 163, 165, 166, 167, 168, 169
endorphins 119
endosteum, irritation 39
enkephalin analgesia 122
enkephalinergic interneurons 60
enkephalins 119, 121
enteritis 88, 90, 91
–, acute radiation 90
–, radiotherapy-induced 88
enterochromaffin cells 61
enzymolytic phenomena 75
ephaptic transmission 53, 54
ephedrine 134
epicritic sensitivity 148, 149
epidural administration of drugs 112
– – of local anesthetics 129, 134
– – of opiates 110, 111
– block 128, 129, 130, 134
– –, complication 134
– –, thoracic 134
– buprenorphine 111
– catheter 108, 109, 113, 129
– metastasis 35, 191
– opiates 4, 107, 109, 111, 113, 130
– opiate analgesia 107, 109, 110, 112
epidurals, thoracic 108
epigastric pain 68
epineural infiltration 36
epipharyngeal tumors 192
escape phenomenon 182
esophagitis 91
estrogen receptor 174
– treatment 11
ethanol 138
ether type of local anesthetics 134
ethic perspectives of cancer pain 31
ethyl alcohol 137
etidocaine 129
etiology of pain 2, 26, 87
euphoria 100, 101, 102, 103
euphorica 32
euthanasia 203
Ewing sarcoma 162
excitation, ectopic 130
– of postganglionic sympathetic fibers 54
excitement 102
excochleation 162
– of the metastatic disease 167
excretory ducts, stenoses 41
– –, tumor infiltration 41
excruciating pain 49
exostosis cartilaginea 157
extraosseous tumor 161
– – growth 157
extrapyramidal motor disorders 124
extrasystoles 130
eyelids, flickering 133

facial edema 76
– pain 76, 81, 144, 149
facilitation phenomena 82
faith 30
fall in blood pressure 124
fatigue 102
fear of cancer 13, 66
– of excruciating pain 13
– of life 31
fentanyl 112
fever 87
fibrin-adhesion 162
– system 161
fibrosarcoma 162
fibrosis 42, 43, 90
–, nodular cicatricial 43
–, stenotic intimal 42
fibrous histiocytoma, malignant 162, 164
fila radicularia 138
final phase of suffering 31
first interview 197, 198
fistula formation 90
flare 92
flickering of the eyelids 133
flu-like syndrome 92
fluoride-resistant acid phosphate 59
flushing 182
– of the ears 181
– of the face 181
focal lesions 55
forceful rotation 50
fractionated radiotherapy 209
fractionation, long-term 191
–, short-term 191
fracture, spontaneous 72
fractures of important skeletal parts 191

frequency of cancer pain 64, 65
– of pain 66, 68, 69
frontal cortex 119
frontothalamic system 151
frustration 77
functional lesions 82

gallbladder carcinoma 34
ganglion celiacum 145
–, dorsal root 59
–, stellatum 144
–, trigeminal 59
gastric cancer 14
– distress 60
gastrointestinal hemmorrhage 7
– hormones 178
– toxicity 86
– tract 39, 49
– – tumors 74
gate-control theory 153
genitourinary tract tumors 74
giant-cell tumor 161, 162, 163
glioblastoma 74
glossopharyngeal nerve, coagulation 151
– –, thermocoagulation 149
– neuralgia 76
glucose tolerance 182
glycerine 139
goal-directed medical therapy 195
gonalgia 73
good death 202
graduated spinal block technique 127
graft-versus-host disease 95
granulocyte substitution 96
granulocytopenia 88
grief 199
Group-III fibers 47, 49, 50
Group-IV afferents 50, 52
– fibers 47, 49
gynecologic cancers 171

hallucination threshold 103
hallucinations 100
–, auditory 103
–, visual 103
haloperidol 8, 118, 119, 124
–, chemical structure 120
–, opiate-agonistic effect 120
HCS 11
head cancer 18
– malignoma 76
headache 35, 68, 74, 75, 76, 81, 88, 93, 94, 191, 192
–, tension 75
–, tumor-induced 75
–, vasomotorial 75
Head's zone 82, 83
heat stimulation 188
– stimuli 49
helplessness 77, 198
hematologic neoplasia 171
hematoma 77
–, painfull muscle 88
hematopoiesis 90
hematuria 144
hemiparesis, contralateral 151
hemipelvectomy 160, 161, 164
hemiplegia, homolateral 150
hemoblastosis, acute 171
–, chronic 171
hemopoietic system 188
hemorrhage 39
–, gastrointestinal 7
– in the urinary bladder 40
hepatomegaly 8
heroin 14, 115, 207
–, intravenous application 101
herpes zoster 76, 77, 81, 93
high cervical chordotomy, bilateral 150
– – –, unilateral 150
– thoracic chordotomy, bilateral 150
high-dose medroxyprogesterone acetate 173
high-frequency coagulation 152
– –, stereotactic transnasal 152
– thermocoagulation 151
hip, endoprosthetic replacement 165
– pain 161, 162
histamine 5, 60, 61
–, release 61
Hodgkin's disease 77, 87, 88
– –, side effects of treatment 88
hollow organs, obstruction 67, 69
– viscera, tumor-induced penetration 41
– –, – perforation 41
– viscus, obstruction 209
– –, pain 75
home care 204
– – services (HCS) 11, 12
– – team 203
homolateral hemiplegia 150
hope 195
hopefulness 19
hopelessness 19, 195, 198
hormonal drugs 171
– therapy 2, 4, 11, 171, 174, 176, 191
– treatment of solid tumors 175
hormone-dependent carcinoma 152
hormones 93, 152, 178

hospice, basic principles 203
– care 201, 203
– movement 203
– team 204
hyaluronidase 130, 133
hydroxyproline 179
hypalgesia 80, 139
–, cutaneous 138
hyperalgesia 51, 80, 82
hypercalcemia 69, 180, 182, 209
hypercoagulability 76
hyperemia 62, 89
–, local 187
hyperhydrosis 102
hypernephroma 168, 169, 174
hyperpathia 131
hypersensitivity 86
hyperthermia 94
hypertonic saline solution 137
hyperuricemia 69
hypesthesia 79, 80, 144
hypnosis 23, 195
hypnotics 127
hypobaric alcohol 138, 139
hypochondriasis 18, 19
hypocyclosis 124
hypophyseal tumors 75
hypophysectomy 4, 152, 153
–, transsphenoid microsurgical 152
hypophysis, alcohol injection into 152
–, elimination 152
–, high-frequency coagulation 152
hypotension 134, 144
hypoventilation 23
hypovolemic situations 134
hypoxia 116
hypoxic state 133
hysterectomy 91

IASP 23, 24
iatrogenic impairment 81
ibuprofen 6
ileus 69, 72, 172
imipramine 118, 124
immune modulators 93
– stimulation 94
– system 93
immunomodulation 94
impact of pain 13, 14, 18, 89
implantation of cerebral electrodes 154
– of an endoprosthetic replacement 167
– of radioactive gold seeds 192, 193
– – substances 152
implanted reservoir of opiates 112
implants, metallic 167
impotence 144
inadequate amounts of drugs 22
– cancer pain therapy 20
incidence of pain 16, 17, 67, 69, 89, 93
– of side effects 112
– of therapy-induced pain 87
indomethacin 6
infection 67, 69, 72, 77, 86, 88, 89, 108, 112
–, general 112
–, spinal 112
infectious diseases 93
inflammation 6, 72, 76, 77
– of cancerous tissue 51
–, chronic 55
–, of the joint 52
–, perineural 43
inflammatory diseases 75
– infiltration, perineural 42
– processes 2, 5, 7, 88
– reaction 41, 129
– –, perineural 40
infusion, constant drip 129
inhibitory control systems, descending 55
– mechanisms, descending 51
– –, local 51
– neurons, afferent 60
– –, descending 60
– pathways, descending 122
– –, noradrenergic 124
– –, serotoninergic 124
– system, descending 121
initial interview 197
– paraplegia 169
insomnia 205
insulin secretion 182
intensity of pain 64, 65, 66, 67, 69, 103, 143
– – scales 67, 69
intercostal nerve block 127, 128, 135
– neuralgia 73
intermittent electric stimulation 148, 154
– stimulation with implanted electrodes 154
– – of periaqueductal gray matter 154
– – of the sensory nuclei 154
International Association for the Study of Pain (IASP) 23
– Cancer Research Data Bank (ICRDB) 64
interneurons, enkephalinergic 60
interruption of the descending tract of the trigeminal nerve 151
– of pain pathways 23, 148
– of regional sympathetic nervous supply 131
interscalenus block of the brachial plexus 114

intervertebral foramina 39
intestinal mucosa 61
– toxicity, acute 91
– tumors 18, 39
intra-arterial perfusion technique 176
intracapsular pressure 33
intracerebral neurostimulaton 151, 154
intracranial pressure 7, 8, 35
– tumor 81
intralaminar nucleus 151
intraluminal pressure 52
intramuscular narcotics 112
intraosseous pressure, elevation 37
– tumor growth 157
intrapleural tetracycline 94
intraspinal injections of substance P 61
– tumor 145
intrathecal administration of morphine-like substances 155
– – of neurolytics 144
– alcohol neurolysis 129
– application of alcohol 137
– – of morphine 107, 150
– block of the sacral segments 142
– cytotoxic drugs 94
– injection of neurolytic agents 145
– neurolysis 139
– neurolytics 149, 150
– pain therapy 137
intravasal injection of phenol 144
intravascular injection of anesthetics 133
invasion of nerves 52
invasive penetration of organs 49
ionic channels 54
ionizing radiation 90, 190
– –, analgetic effect 190
iontophoresis, transcutaneous 186, 188
– of vinca alkaloids 185
iontophoretic application of microtubule inhibitors 185
– therapy 187, 188, 189
irradiation, anti-inflammatory 190
– dermatitis 95
– palliative 191
– percutaneous 191
– stereotactic 193
irritation 80
– of afferent axons 45
– of the brachial plexus 167
– of the lumbosacral plexus 160
– of nerve plexus 80
– of nociceptive afferent fibers 74
– – structures 76
– of nociceptors in the periosteum 191
– of organs, mechanical 49
– of pain receptors 74, 75, 82, 148
– of peripheral nerves 80
– of the sciatic nerve 160
– symptoms 80
ischemia 2, 50, 51, 52, 72, 75, 76, 90, 130
–, arterial 76
– of the colon 50, 52
ischemic pain 107
ischialgia 73, 191
iseoplatic-prosthetic replacement 167
isolated tumor 35
isolation 195, 197, 198
isotonic saline 127
itching 111, 134

joint capsule, distension 49
– pain 77, 82

kallikrein 60
kaolin 52
Kibler's zone 83
kidney tumors 18, 34, 167
kinins 178
knee endoprosthetic replacement 165, 166
– exarticulation 163
– joint afferent 49
– – capsule 49

lack of appetite 18
lactic acid 51
lactose malabsorption 93, 96
laminectomy 149, 151
lateral rotation 49
legs, bilateral sympathetic blockade 132
leptomeninges 35
lesions, advanced 16
– of axons in nerves 46
–, benign osteoblastic 157
– of the brachial plexus 91
–, carcinomatous 81, 82
– of the central nervous system 82
–, cerebral 81
–, chronic 54
–, focal 55
–, functional 82
– of the locomotor system 82
–, mechanical 81
– of motor fibers 80
– of the nerve plexus 80, 81
– – root 79
– of nerves 53, 55, 79, 80, 81
–, noxious 127
– in the pain system 151

– of the peripheral nervous system 82
– – neuron 81
–, primary 79
– of the spinal cord 81
–, stereotactic 150, 153
–, structural 79
–, tumor-like 157, 161
– of the vessels supplying the pyramidal tract 150
– of visceral structures 82
leukemia 15, 66, 91, 95, 103
–, acute 75, 76
leukemic infiltration of nerves 74
levallorphan 178
levomepromazine 118, 124
levorphanol 105
life quality 1, 31
lignocaine 129
limb pain 141, 186
– salvage procedures 169
limbic system 60, 119
lipophilic narcotics 112
lips, numbness 133
liquor fistulas 192
lithiasis 75
liver metastases, pain originating 176
– tumor 191
local acidosis 130
– anesthesia 3, 9, 150
– anesthetic block 2, 4, 133, 143
– – –, diagnostic 140
– – –, therapeutic 130
– anesthetics 9, 110, 127, 129, 130, 135, 144
– –. allergy 134
– –, amide type 134
– –, constant drip infusion 129
– –, diagnostic nerve block 140
– –, epidural administration 129, 134
– –, ether type 134
– –, intermittent administration 129
– –, long-acting 130
– –, parenteral injection 135
– –, peridural application 12
– blocks 129, 130, 135
– freezing 9
–'pain 26, 82, 164
– spinal syndrome 82
– tumor recurrence 161
localization of pain 2, 25, 60, 107
localized facial pain 149
– pain symptoms 191
locomotor system, lesions 82
long-acting local anesthetics 130
loss of sensation 149, 153
low-threshold mechanosensitive fibers 54
lower extremities, motor disorders 139
– –, sympathetic block 132
– leg, pain 158
lower-limb disorders 143
lumbago 73, 80, 191
– syndrome 82
lumbar epidural block 132
– pain 159, 160
– sympathetic blocks 132, 133, 144
– – chain 145
– vertebral syndromes 73
lumbosacral plexus, irritation 160
lung cancer 18, 20, 65, 167
– metastases 90
lymph vessels, compression 7, 172
lymphadectomy, retroperitoneal 89, 90
lymphatic edema 81
– flow 61
– tissue 39
lymphatics 37, 41
–, peripheral 43
lymphoedema 209
lymphoma 15, 91, 103
–, malignant 171
lymphoplasmacellular infiltration 40
lymphosarcoma 19

malignancies, advanced 104
malignant degeneration 163
– lymphomas 35, 74, 75, 76
– – in the gastric antrum 39
– – of the gastrointestinal tract 39
– – of the stomach 39
– melanomas 35, 75
– neoplasias 41
– neoplasm 13
– teratoma of the testis 89
– tumors 66, 157
malnutrition 81
mammary carcinoma 35, 36, 152, 153
– tumors 81
maprotiline 118, 124
mastectomy 90
McKenzie's zone 82, 83
mechanical injury of nociceptive neurons 59
– irritation of organs 49
– lesions 81
– occlusion of organs 49
– stimulation 54, 56, 59
– –, afterdischarges 53
– stimuli 47, 52
mechanoreceptive sites 52

mechanosensitive fibers, low-threshold 54
medial rotation 49
medullary tractotomy 151
medulloblastoma 74
melanoma of the extremities, malignant 176
melphalan 173
meningioma 35, 37, 75
meningeal carcinosis 191
meningeosis carcinomatosa 34
meningiosis carcinomatosa 176
– leukemica 176
meningitis 192
meperidine 19, 120
–, chemical structure 120
mesencephalotomy 151
metallic substances 51
metabolic implants 167, 169
metamizol 6
metastases in the bones 67
–, epidural 36, 191
–, macroscopic occult 162
–, osseous 3
–, osteoblastic 192
–, osteolytic 192
– of the spine 81, 167
–, subdural 36
– surgery 11
metastatic advanced cancer 23
– brain compression 172
– cancer 16
– carcinosis 34
– infiltration of the small pelvis 176
– malignancy 100
– skin ulceration 176
methadone 105, 115, 207
methotrimeprazine 208
methylparaben, allergy 134
methylprednisone 134
microfractures 39
microinjections of substance P 61
microtubule inhibitors, iontophoretic application 185
– –, systemically administered 189
micturition, disorders 101, 102
midbrain, stereotactic lesions 153
–, stimulation 153
midline pain 151
mild analgesics 5
misinjections 43
mitomycin C 176
mitosis 188
mobile structures, infiltration 37
monopolar stimulation 154
monosegmental dysfunction 80
mood alteration 9
– elevation 102
morphine 3, 9, 10, 11, 61, 62, 63, 100, 102, 103, 105, 107, 108, 110, 111, 112, 115, 120, 121, 178, 187, 201, 207
–, analgesic effect 120, 122
–, chemical structure 120
– derivatives 102, 105
– dosage 116
–, epidural administration 107, 111
–, hydrophilic 112
–, intrathecal application 107, 150
–, main properties 101
–, oral 3, 103, 115, 116, 206, 207, 208
–, parenteral administration 103, 115
– plasma levels 116
–, psychotropic effects 101
–, respiratory depressant effect 117
–, subcutaneous administration 101
–, systemic application 112
morphine-like substances, intrathecal administration 155
motility disorders 39
motor block 127, 129
– deficits 149
– disorders in the lower extremities 139
– fibers 138
– –, lesions 80
– paresis 142
– pathways 45
– system 49, 79
– –, dysfunction 82
mourning 198, 200
mouth cancer 190
– ulceration 86, 89
mucocutaneous side effects 86
mucosa, ulceration 42
mucosal infiltration 39
mucositis 21, 88, 89
multidisciplinary cancer pain diagnostic and therapy team 25
multimodal therapy 86, 87, 93
multiple bone metastases 108
– myeloma 181
multisegmental dysfunction 80
muscle fibers 37
– hypertone 3
– pain 77, 82
– spasms 82, 90, 130, 135
– twitching 133
– weakness 25
musculoskeletal nociceptors 157
– pain 5
– tumors, pain 157

musculotendinous pain 5
myalgia 87
mycosis 69
myelin loss 89
myelinated fibers 47, 51, 52, 53
myeloma, multiple 180, 181
myelopathy 81
myelotomy 151
myofascial trigger points 9
myogelosis 72, 73
myography, cisternal 26
–, lumbar 26
myopathy, paraneoplastic 81
myotendinosis 82

naloxone 103, 105, 178
narcotic analgesics 4, 9, 12, 19, 22, 122
– therapy 19
narcotics 9, 23, 112
–, addiction 140
–, epidural 111, 113
–, intramuscular 112
–, intravenous 111
–, lipophilic 112
–, oral 111, 113
–, side effects 143
–, systemic 12
National Cancer Institute (NCI) 21
natural stimuli 49
nausea 9, 10, 18, 90, 93, 101, 103, 110, 111, 181, 205
neck cancer 18, 149
– dissection, radical 90
– malignoma 76
– vein distension 76
necrosis 39, 41, 72, 75, 76, 88, 89, 90, 91
–, adipose tissue 43
–, aseptic bone 69
–, painful 43
nefopam 5, 6, 102, 105
neoplasias of the bone 37
–, hematologic 171
–, primary 37
–, secondary 37
neoplastic disease 67
nerve axons, irritation 52
– block procedures 209
– blocks 9, 23, 26, 206, 210
– –, cryogenic 4
– –, diagnostic 9, 128, 140
– – intercostal 135
– – by local freezing 9
– –, neurolytic 4, 5
– –, sympathetic 9, 131
– –, therapeutic 9
– compression 5, 8
– – pain 141
– – syndromes 130
– connections, inadequate 53
– damage 81
– –, partial 8
– – by radiation 153
– destruction 172
– infiltration 209
– innervation, peripheral 132
– –, segmental 132
– lesions 43, 47, 55, 74, 145
– –, partial 53
– plexus 36, 79
– –, compression 171, 172
– –, decompression 191
– –, irritation 80
– –, lesions 80
– –, tumorous infiltration 153
– roots 36, 39, 79, 81
– –, compression 79, 169, 191
– –, decompression 191
– –, irritation 159
– –, lesions 79
– –, stretching 79
– –, tumors 79
– section 153
– stimulation, transcutaneous 4, 5
nerves, compression 69
neural therapeutic procedures 135
neuralgia 5, 69, 74, 186
–, glossopharyngeal 76
–, intercostal 73
–, occipital 75
–, posttherapeutic 5, 8
–, trigeminal 75, 76, 137, 186
neuraxis 24
neurinoma 75
neuritis 69, 76, 144, 186
–, carcinomatous 131
–, secondary 138
neurogenic pain syndromes 74
neuroleptic therapy, side effects 124
neuroleptics 7, 8, 118, 119, 120, 121
–, anxiolytic effects 122
–, dosage schedule 124
neurological pain 93
neurolysis 84, 128
–, bilateral 138
–, chemical 149
–, intrathecal 139
– –, alcohol 129
– of peripheral somatic nerves 144

neurolysis of the sympathetic nervous system 143
neurolytic agents 138, 140, 143, 145
– –, injection 137
– –, intrathecal injection 145
– –, lumbar sympathetic block 144
– –, sympathetic blocks 143
– block 2, 4, 5, 113, 137
– – of the cervicothoracal chain 144
– –, subarachnoid 141, 142
– treatment of peripheral nerves 150
neurolytics 144, 149, 150, 155
–, intrathecal administration 144, 149, 150
–, peripheral application 51
–, sympathetic blocks 144
neuroma 53, 54
– of the sciatic nerve 53
–, stump 53
– of the superficial peroneal nerve 53, 54
–, traumatic 43
neuroma-in-continuity 53
neuro-orthopedic examination 80
neuropathologic changes 21
neuropathy 3, 9, 77, 88, 93
–, diabetic 69
–, paraneoplastic 81
–, peripheral 93
neuropeptides 52, 61
neurostimulation 153
–, intracerebral 151
– of the specific sensory thalamic nuclei 153
–, spinal 151
– techniques 23, 152, 153
– –, nondestructive 155
neurosurgery 2, 129, 148
–, destructive techniques 148
neurosurgical operations 23, 154
– pain treatment 154
– procedures 51, 143
neuroticism 18, 19
neurotomy 149
neurotoxicity 89, 93, 94, 96, 173
– of cancer therapy 93
–, chronic painful 88
neurotransmission, central 63
neurotransmitters 61, 62, 119, 120, 122
nidus, excision 158
–, surgical excision 157
nitrosoureas 176
nociceptive afferent fibers 33, 47, 54, 55, 143
– – –, cutaneous 49
– – –, irritation 74
– – –, polymodal cutaneous 49
– afferents 45, 49, 51, 130
– nerve fibers, chronic affection 55
– –, chemical injury 59
– –, mechanical injury 59
– –, thermal injury 59
– pathways, blocking 24
– –, chemical interruption 24
– reflexes, threshold 178
– stimulation 62
– stimuli 72
– structures, distension 76
– –, irritation 76
– system, cutaneous 55
– threshold 107
– visceral afferent fibers 50, 52
nociceptor excitation 6, 9, 11
nociceptors 6, 49, 59, 61
–, chemical stimulation 60
–, chronic stimulation 55, 56
–, cutaneous 51
–, deep somatic 49, 55
–, irritation 191
–, meningeal 35
–, musculoskeletal 157
–, peripheral 33, 55, 188
–, permanent stimulation 56
–, stimulation 45, 55, 56, 60
–, threshold 76
–, visceral 49, 55
nocturnal apnea 150
nodular cicatricial fibrosis 43
– meningeal metastases 36
–, subdural metastases 35
nonablative methods of neurosurgery 153
nondestructive methods of neurosurgery 153
– neurostimulation techniques 155
nonhealing ulceration 90
noninvasive therapy 185, 188
nonmyelinated afferent fibers 153
non-narcotic analgesics 5, 6, 7, 8, 22, 110, 122
nonnoxious flexion 52
nonparenchymatous pain 140
non-small-cell bronchogenic carcinoma 174
nonsteroid anti-inflammatory agents 60
non-steroidal anti-inflammatory drugs 208
nonvisceral pain 140
noradrenaline 51, 53, 118, 120, 122
nortriptyline 124
noxious lesion 127
– pressure 50
– rotation 50
– stimulation 51, 128, 130

NSAID 208
nucleus limitans 151
numbness of lips and tongue 133
numerical pain scale 127, 128

obliterative arteritis 40
obstipation 111, 124
obstruction of hollow organs 67, 69
– – viscus 209
obstructive jaundice 69
occlusion of blood vessels 76
– of organs, mechanical 49
occlusions, vascular 43
oculomotor disorders 152
oncological therapy 85
oncology, medical 21
–, surgical 21
operation trauma 150
opiate addiction 103
– agonist-antagonist 102, 105
– agonists 102, 103, 119, 120
– analgesics 125
– –, oral 206
– antagonists 178
– applications, epidural 130
– receptors 107, 119, 120
– –, spinal 112
– therapy, oral 11
opiate-agonistic activity 124
opiates 101, 201, 205, 210
–, administration to the spinal cord 148
–, epidural 4, 107, 109, 113
–, – administration 110, 111
–, implanted reservoir 112
–, oral 112, 115, 207
–, overdosage 101
–, parenteral administration 105, 115, 206
–, peridural 2, 12, 55
–, spinal 107
–, synthetic 101
–, systemic 107, 111, 113
–, ventilatory failure 116
opioid therapy 10
opioids 11, 101
–, oral administration 11
–, parenteral administration 11
–, systemic application 105
optic nerve damage 192
oral administration of analgesia 10
– – of narcotic analgesics 4
– – of opioids 11
– medication 105
– – of opiates 112
– morphine 115, 116, 206, 208
– narcotics 113
– opiate analgesics 206
– – therapy 11
– opiates 207
– pentazocine 102
organ cysts 75
– destruction, malignant 176
– infarctions 75
– lesions 172
– tumors 191
organ-specific pain 82
oropharyngeal candidosis 77
orthopedic surgery 157, 167, 169
orthopramide 119
orthoprosthesis 163
orthostatic problems 118
– disorders 124
orthotic bracing 167
osteitis deformans 182
osteoblastic bone destruction 167
– lesion, benign 157
– metastases 192
osteochondroma 157, 158, 159, 160
osteogenic sarcoma 162, 163, 165, 166
osteoid osteoma 157, 158
osteolysis 6, 39
osteolytic bone destruction 167
– metastases 180, 192
osteosarcoma 89
osteosclerosis 39
osteosynthesis 168, 169
osteotropic hypocalcemic hormone 178
ovarectomy 174
ovarian carcinoma 42
overdosage of opiates 101
overdose of anesthetics 133
Oxford cancer registry 66
oxygen 134
oxyphenbutazone 6

Paget's disease 179, 180, 182
pain of the upper abdomen 145
–, abdominal 42, 179, 180
–,– colicky 96
–, acute 21, 23, 45, 77
–,– transient 86
– in advanced cancer 85, 201, 205
– afferent neuron 121
–, anthropological reality 29
–, articular 179
–, assessment 2, 128
– in the back 39
– of benign origin 154
–, bilateral 150, 151

pain, bilateral saddle 141
–, blunt 111
– due to bone metastases 208, 209
– in the bone 2, 3, 148
–, burning 130, 131, 144
–, capsular 191
–, causalgiform 149
– caused by bone metastases 171
– – by stretching of tissue or organs 191
– – by swelling of tissue or organs 191
–, causes 69, 72
–, central 81
– in the upper cervical spine 161
– in the chest 76
– – wall 37
–, chronic 1, 5, 21, 23, 45, 47, 55, 56, 60, 63, 72, 77, 78, 85, 86, 87, 115, 119, 121, 122, 129, 154, 188, 189, 206
–,– long-lasting 96
–,– nonmalignant 18
–,– persistent 18, 100, 153
–,– severe 89, 116
– clinic 202
–, clinical classification 148
– in the coccyx 150
–, colicky 86, 90, 91
–, concomitant treatment 1
– as a consequence of cancer therapy 67, 69, 85
–, continuous 105
–, deafferentation 79, 148
–, deep lancinating 93
–,– somatic 49, 56
–, depersonalisation 119
–, from the descending colon 143
– development, time-course 4
– diagnosis 1, 2, 22, 23
– diary 3, 4
–, diffuse 108
–,– large area 2
– as a direct consequence of tumors 67, 69
–, distribution 25
–, dull 33. 131
–, ethos 28, 29
–, etiology 2, 26, 87
– evaluation 4
– in the extremities 145
– in the upper extremity 143
– in the face 151, 154
–, facial 76, 81, 144
– following chemotherapy 69
– –, radiation 69
– in the fossae infratemporales 76
–, frequency 68, 69
– in the head 143
– in the hip 161, 162
– in a hollow viscus 75
–, impact on the patient 89
–, incidence 16, 17, 67, 69, 89, 93
– as an indirect consequence of tumors 67, 69
–, intensity 67, 69, 103, 143, 173, 179, 180, 181
– –, assessment 3
–, ischemic 107
– in the joint 77, 82
– in the larynx 76
– in the legs 35
–, local 26, 82, 164
–, localization 2, 25, 60, 107
–, localized facial 149
–, low back 26
– in lower abdomen 68
– – extremities 80, 143
– – leg 158
–, lumbar 159, 160
– in the lung 143
–, magnitude 69
– due to malignant diseases 171
– of malignant origin 153, 154
–, measurement 69
–, mechanisms 26
– mediated by trigger points 130
– due to metabolic imbalances 67, 69
–, midline 2, 151
–, muscle 77, 82
–, musculoskeletal 5
– in musculoskeletal tumors 157
–, musculotendinous 5
– in the nasal cavity 76
– in the neck 37
–, nerve compression 141
– due to nerve compression 5
–, neurological 93
–, – diagnosis 79
–, nonparenchymatous 140
–, nonvisceral 140
– in the oral cavity 76
–, organ-specific 82
– originating from liver metastases 176
– – from metastatic infiltration of the small pelvis 176
– of osseous metastases 3
–, palliative therapy 2
– in the paranasal sinus 76
–, parenchymatous 141
–, paraneoplastic 5
– in a parenchymal viscus 75

– of parenchymatous origin 145
–, pathogenesis 2
– after pathologic fracture 168, 169
–, pathological 47
–, pathophysiologic consequences 100
–, pathophysiological 45
–, pathophysiology 100, 105
– pathways, blockade of conduction 153
–, decussating 151
–, interruption 23
–, pelvic 206
– from the pelvic viscera 143
– of the pelvic wall 140, 145
– in the pelvis 68, 151
– in the pelvis-perineum 139
–, perception 60, 120
– in the perineum 139
– due to peripheral-nerve involvement 26
–, persistent 72, 77
– in the pharynx 76, 151
– physiology 148
– in the pleura 143
– due to plexus or cord involvement 26
–, postoperative 87, 89, 90, 107, 112, 160, 162, 163, 166, 168, 182
–, posttraumatic 107
–, prevalence 16, 17
–, projected 73, 127
–, psychodynamics 100, 105
– through psychogenic influences 77
–, psychological dimensions 28
–, psychopathologic consequences 100
–, quantification 127
– questionnaire 3, 4
–, radiating 82
–, radicular 79
–, range of phenomena related 87
–, receptor 82
– receptors 33, 74, 129
– –, chemosensitive 82
– –, endosteal 73
– –, irritation 74, 75, 82, 148
– –, periosteal 73
– –, stimulation 82
– reccurrence 153, 192
–, reccurrent 45, 56
–, referred 26, 49, 82, 83, 127, 128
– in the region of the nasopharynx 151
– without relation to cancer 67, 69
–, relapse 152
– relief, assessment 141
– – scale, verbal 128
– – due to calcitonin 181
– removing effect 119
– research, psychological 4
– resulting from malignant organ destruction 176
– of the retroperitoneum 140, 145
– in the sacrum 150
– scale 127
– –, numerical 127, 128
– –, verbal 127, 128
– –, visual analogue 128
–, self-evaluation 3
–, sequelae 100
–, shooting 81
– in the shoulder girdle 37
– in the shoulders 39
–, shoulder-arm 144
– in the small of the back 68
– – pelvis 139
–, social dimensions 28
–, somatic 62, 127, 130, 141, 148, 154
–, – dimensions 28
–, somatogenic 78
–, spinal projection 113
–, spiritual dimensions 28
–, spondylogenic projected 128
–, stabbing 33
– stimulus 36
–, stretching 75
–, stump 5
–, subscapular 135
– due to sympathetic disturbances 3
–, symptomatic therapy 2
– symptoms, localized 191
– syndromes, acute 89
– –, chronic postsurgical 90
– –, clinical 72
– –, neurogenic 74
– –, specific 89, 92
– –, visceral 82
– system, lesion 151
–, telos 28, 29
–, tension 43
–, thalamic 81
– therapy, intrathecal 137
–, therapy-induced 85, 86, 87, 88, 89, 94, 95
–, thoracic 111
–, of the thoracic wall 145
–, terminal 185, 188, 202
– in the thigh 163
– in the throat 68, 154
– of the trunk wall 140
–, unilateral 2, 150
– when urinating 68
– from the viscera between stomach and colon transversum 143

pain, visceral 49, 51, 56, 62, 127, 128, 130, 141, 144, 145, 149
– from visceral tumors 143
– as a warning signal 31
pain-conducting dorsal roots 138
– pathways 148
pain-inhibiting system, stimulation 148
pain-intensity rating 4
pain-killing drugs 188
pain-mediating structures 73
pain-producing C fibers 137
– meningeal carcinosis 191
pain-sensitive structures 73
painful compartment syndrome 90
– ileus 75
– lymph edema 76
– motility disorder 40
– multiple bone metastases 192
– muscle hematoma 88
– muscle spasms 130, 135
– neuropathy 74
– paraneoplastic syndromes 173
– region, careful examination 26
– side effects of radiotherapy 91
– toxicity 87, 89, 94
Palacos 167
palliative chemotherapy 173, 176
– irradiation 191
– radiotherapy 4, 202
– surgery 4
– therapy of pain 2, 16, 20
– tumor therapy 173
Pancoast carcinoma 39
Pancoast's syndrome 74, 191
– tumor 9, 21, 144, 149
pancreas tumor 144
pancreatic metastases of bronchial carcinoma 41
pancreatitis 74, 89, 92, 180, 182
–, acute 179
–, autodigestive 41
paracetamol 6, 110
parafascicular nucleus 151
paralysis 143, 171, 172
–, bilateral 80
– of the detrusor vesicae 139
–, partial 80
– of the sphincter 139, 150
paraneoplastic conditions 36
– myopathy 81
– neuropathy 81
– pain 5
– syndromes 72, 76, 77, 81, 173, 176
paraplegia 39, 169
pararenal tissue 34
paravasation 89
paravertebral block 128, 135
– tumors 79
parenchyma 34, 41
parenchymal viscus, pain 75
parenchymatous pain 141, 145
parenteral administration of analgesia 10, 107
– – of morphine 115
– – of opiates 105, 115
– – of opioids 11
– local anesthetic injections 135
paresis 143
– of the brachial plexus 145
– of the extremities 142
paresthesia dolorosa 186
–, segmental 138
Parinaud syndrome 151
Parkinson syndrome 124
parotitis 95
partial nerve damage 8
– paralysis 80
parvicellular bronchial carcinoma 34
pathogenesis of pain 2
pathologic fractures 168, 169, 171, 172
pathological pain 47
pathophysiologic consequences of pain 100
pathophysiological pain 45
– processes 52
pathophysiology of pain 100, 105
– of therapy-induced pain 87
pathways, ascending 138
–, pain-conducting 148
patient's right to information 197
peak flow rate 115
pelvic pain 151, 206
– wall, pain 140, 145
pelviperitoneal area, tumors 144
pelvis-perineum, pain 139
pentazocine 102, 103, 105, 122, 180
–, oral 102, 103
–, parenteral 103
peptic ulcer 7
peptidergic transmitters 62
perception of pain 60
percutaneous cannulation 112
– chordotomy 19, 149, 150
– implantation technique 154
– irradiation with ultrahard rays 191
– stereotactic technique 151
– surgery methods 154
perforation 42, 43
periaqueductal gray matter, electric stimulation 154

– – –, intermittent stimulation 154
peridural application of local anesthetics 12
– – of opiates 2, 12, 55
perineum, pain 139
perineural infiltration 37
– inflammation 43
– inflammatory infiltration 42
– Vinblastin cuff 188
periosteum, irritation of nociceptors 191
–, lesion 37
peripheral application of neurolytics 51
– mechanisms of calcitonin 181
– nerve damage 81
– – injury 188
– – lesions 79, 81
– nerves 9, 24, 36, 41, 90, 138
– –, afferent 61
– –, axonal degeneration 89
– –, chemical blockade 149
– –, compression 7, 171
– –, electric stimulation 5, 153
– –, irritation 80
– –, lesions 80
– –, neurolytic treatment 150
– –, transection 149
– nervous system, degenerative alterations 43
– – –, lesion 82
– neuron lesion 81
– neuropathy 69, 74, 93
– nociceptors 55, 188
– somatic nerves, neurolysis 144
peripherally acting analgesics 6
peritoneal carcinosis 41
peritonitis 42
periventricular gray matter, electric stimulation 154
permanent bladder, catheter 139, 141, 145
peroneal nerve, neuroma 53, 54
persistent pain 72, 77
pertrochanteric fracture 168
pethidine 101, 112, 179, 180, 187
phantom limb pain 90
– pain 69, 162, 163, 165
– –, postoperative 164
– sensations 81
– stump pain 81
phenazocine 207
phenol 9, 128, 137, 139, 141, 144, 145, 149
– block 141
–, chemical neurolysis 149
–, intravasal injection 144
– treatment 138
phenol-glycerine 139
phenothiazine 8, 207, 208
phenylbutazon 6
physical deterioration 18
– therapy 3
physiologic dependence 23
– impact of pain 13, 18
physiopathologic noxae 77
physiopathology of pain 20
pimozide 120
pituitary anterior lobe, destruction 193
– gland, radioresection 191, 192
placebo block with saline 128
– effect 173
– – of blocks 128
– iontophoresis 187, 188
plant alkaloids 173
plasma beta-endorphins 178
– extravasation 61
– morphine level 115
plasmocytomas 73, 192
plethora 76
pleurae 41
pleural carcinosis 41
– effusion 41
pleurisy 74
plexus neuropathy 74
– solaris block 144
PMMA 167, 168, 169
pneumonia 86
Polster's device 169
polychemotherapy 87, 89, 93
polymodal neurons 59
polyneuropathia 5
polyneuropathy 81, 173, 176
postganglionic sympathetic fibers, excitation 54
postmastectomy syndrome 69
postneurolytic situation 128
postoperative pain 87, 88, 89, 90, 107, 112, 160, 162, 163, 166, 168
– – in nontumor patients 182
– phantom pain 164
posttherapeutic neuralgia 5, 8
postthoracotomy syndrome 69
posttraumatic pain 107
potassium 60
povidone iodine 108
practice of Christian salvation 30
Pravidel 153
preganglionic axons, stimulation 54
pressure 33, 49, 52, 82, 90
–, intraabdominal 130

pressure, intraluminal 52
–, noxious 50
presynaptic inhibition in the dorsal horn 55
prevalence of pain 14, 16, 17, 21
primary afferent C-fibers 62
– – fibers 45, 55, 60, 61, 62
– – –, chronic lesion 54
– – neurons 45, 51
– afferents, antidromic activation 153
– angiosarcoma 33
–, bone tumors 15, 73
– brain tumors 81
– carcinoma 76
– cerebral tumors 74
– dysfunction 79
– invasion of the carcinoma 108
– lesion 79
– lymphoma 76
– musculoskeletal tumors 157
– nociceptive neurons 59
– sarcoma 76
– sensory neurons 185, 188
– skeletal tumor invasion 74
– thrombotic obstruction 76
– tumor of the peripheral nerves 36
procaine 127, 135
– hydrochloride 179
prochlorperazine 207, 208
proctitis 91
proctocolitis 90
prodromes 133
progestational agents 174
progesterone receptor 174
prognostic block 128
– blocks 127
projected pain 73, 127
proliferative radiation vasculopathy 81
propoxyphene 120
prostaglandin E1 51, 52
– system 178
prostaglandins 3, 5, 6, 33, 39, 51, 52, 60
prostate cancer 20, 167
– carçinoma 36, 73, 152, 153, 174
– pain 144
protein denaturation 138
pseudo-affective reactions 51
pseudoradicular syndrome 82, 83
psychic alteration 7
– dependence 10
psychoactive agents 105
psychodynamics of pain 100, 105
psychogenic influences 77
psychologic assessment of pain 26
– effects of pain 13, 18
– procedures 23
psychological care 196
– factors 77, 78, 89, 95
– pain research 4
– reaction 119
psychometric tests 26
psychopathologic consequences of pain 100
psychosocial evaluation 26
psychosomatic symptoms 18
psychotherapy 195, 196
psychotropic drugs 4, 7, 8, 22, 103, 118, 119, 122, 125, 191, 202, 208
– –, analgesic effect 123
pulmonary metastasis 164

quality of life 2, 157, 169, 173, 201, 206
quantification of pain 127

radiating pain 82
radiation 69, 80, 81, 82
– damage to the brachial plexus 148
– enteritis 42
– fibrosis 69
– injuries 91
–, ionizing 90
– myelopathy 69
–, nerve damage 153
– oncology 21
– therapy 19, 20, 21, 67, 87, 90, 196
radiation-induced complications 91
– fibrosis 81
radical neck dissection 90
radicotomy 149
radicular pain 79
– symptomatology 26
– syndrome 79, 80
radiculitis 113
radioactive gold seeds, implantation 192
– substances, implantation 152
radioenteritis 43
radiofibrosis 42
radiogenic vascular damage 81
radiogold 152
radiologic improvement of tumor lesions 181
– pain therapy, indications 190
– thalamotomy 193
– therapy, indications 191
radionuclide therapy 191, 192
radioresection of the pituitary gland 191, 192
radiotherapy 2, 81, 85, 88, 90, 94, 129, 157, 162, 167, 171, 186, 190, 193, 206, 209
–, fractionated 209
–, painful side effects 91

–, palliative 4, 202
–, prophylactic 91
–, single-dose 209
radiotherapy-induced enteritis 88
radiovasculitis 43
radioyttrium 192
range of pain phenomena 87
Raynaud's disease 74
rebellion 198
receptor pain 82
– populations, deep somatic 51
– –, visceral 51
rectal carcinoma 150, 192
– dysfunction 80
recurrent cancer 16, 23
– pain 56
referred pain 26, 49, 82, 83, 127
reflex dystrophy 135, 145
– –, blocks against 144
– hypertonus 9
– – of skeletal muscle 5
– hypotension 62
regenerative processes 52
regional anesthesia 137
– block, complications 134
– cancer registry 67
– pain relief unit 67
– sympathetic nervous supply, block 132
relapse of pain 152
relation disturbances 30, 32
– of man to God 28
– of man to himself 28
relaxants 134
remineralization 181, 191
renal cancer 75
– carcinoma 73
– injury 144
resection of the metastatic disease 167
resection-plasty 162
resection-rotation-plasty 162
resentment 19
resignation 198
resistance 182
respiratory arrest 101
– depressant effect of morphine 117
– depression 9, 10, 11, 22, 102, 107, 111, 112, 113, 115, 116, 207
– disease, chronic 116
– disorders 150
resting activity 47, 51, 54, 56
restlessness 124, 135
–, terminal 208
resuscitation, cardiovascular 134
retention of urine 124
retreat 198
retroganglionic operations 149
retrograde degeneration 62
retroperitoneal lymphadectomy 89, 90
retroperitoneum, infiltration 37
–, pain 140, 145
reversible block 129
rheumatic disorders 60
rheumatoid arthritis 69, 77, 180
– syndromes 173, 176
rhizotomy 51, 130, 149, 155
–, chemical 149
–, surgical 149, 150
root damage 79
– pain 74
– section 153
root-compression syndromes 73, 74
rotation 52
–, forceful 50
–, noxious 50

sacral segments, intrathecal block 142
sacroiliac joint, osteochondroma 160
saddle block 139
– pain, bilateral 141
sadness 195, 199
saline solution, hypertonic 137
salmon calcitonin 181, 182
– –, intraventricular administration 178
sciatic nerve, irritation 160
– –, neuroma 53
sclerosis of the cortex 158
secondary dysfunction 79
– neuritis 138, 144
– tumors 81, 87, 157
second-order neurons, activation 153
sedation 9, 101, 102, 112
sedatives 110, 208
segmental irritation symptoms 82
– paresthesia 138
selective analgesia 151
self-evaluation of pain 3
semimalignant bone tumors 157, 161
seminoma 191
sensation, decrease 153
–, loss 153
senselessness 195
sensitivity to pain 4
sensitization of afferent fibers 51, 52
– of receptors 56
sensory block 127, 129
– deficits 25
– neuropathy 36
– nuclei, intermittent stimulation 154

sensory stimulation 153
– thalamic nuclei 154
sepsis 86
sequelae of pain 100
serotonin 5, 33, 61, 118, 120, 122
serous mucosa 41
serum calcitonin 182
shock 198
shooting pains 81
shoulder joint, endoprosthetic replacement 165
– pain 167
shoulder-arm pain 144
shoulder-hand pain 74
– syndrome 73
side effects of antidepressant therapy 124
– – of epidural opiate analgesia 110
– – incidence 111, 112
– –, mucocutaneous 86
– – of narcotics 143
– – of neuroleptic therapy 124
– –, toxic 95
– – of treatment of Hodgkin's disease 88
sight disorders 192
single-dose radiotherapy 209
sinusitis 76
skeletal metastases 167, 169, 191
– muscle, hypertonus 3
– –, reflex hypertonus 5
– musculature, infiltration 37
skin, cyanotic 131
– edema 82
– osteoporosis, dystrophic alterations 131
– sensitivity 188
– ulceration, metastatic 176
sleep disturbance 18
sleepiness 102, 103
sleeplessness 19
Sloan-Kettering Cancer Center 66
small pelvis, metastatic infiltration 176
– –, pain 139
small-cell bronchogenic carcinoma 174
smooth muscle spasm 3
social consequences of pain 100
– effects of cancer pain 19
– factors 197
– isolation 2
sociologic effects of pain 13
sodium bicarbonate 134
– ions 119
– –, infiltration 37
soft tissue tumors 17, 157
solid tumors 18, 35, 171, 174, 175
somatic nervous pathway 132
– pain 62, 127, 130, 141, 148, 154
– preoccupation 18
– sensation, loss 149
somatogenic pain 78
somatostatin 59, 63
somnolence 112, 118
spasm of skeletal muscles 9
spasmogenic effects 102
spastic constipation 101
specific drug toxicity 176
– pain syndromes 89
sphincter paralysis 139, 150
spinal anesthesia 9, 140
– block technique, graduated 127
– commissurotomy 151
– cord 35, 38, 39, 51, 54, 55, 56, 60, 75, 82, 107, 111, 122, 140, 143, 149, 185
– –, administration of opiates 148
– – compression 169, 171, 172, 209
– – lesions 81
– –, secondary changes 46
– – stimulation 153, 154
– cord-compression syndromes 74
– ganglion 138, 149
– infections 112
– nerves 9, 39
– neurostimulation 151
– opiate receptors 112
– opiates 107
– projection of pain 113
– syndrome, local 82
spine, metastases 167
spinoreticulothalamic tract, stereotactic destruction 151
spinothalamic tract, stereotactic destruction 151
– –,– interruption 150
splanchnic vessels, dilatation 144
spleen tumor 191
spondylogenic projected pain 128
spontaneous fracture 72, 73
status of cancer pain control 19
stellate ganglion block 132
stenosis 41, 42, 172
stenotic intimal fibrosis 42
stereotactic destruction of the spinoreticulothalamic tract 151
– – of the spinothalamic tract 151
– interruption of the spinothalamic tract 150
– irradiation of the centrum medianum of the thalamus 193
– lesion in the nonspecific nuclei of the thalamus 150

– lesions in the midbrain 153
– operation technique 151
stereotactical thalamotomy 191
– transnasal high-frequency coagulation of the hypophysis 152
stiff neck 75, 80, 93
stiff-neck syndrome 82
stimulation, bipolar 154
– of the central gray matter in the midbrain 153
–, chemical 56, 60
–, chronic 55
–, cold 188
–, deep brain 4
– of the dorsal column 153, 154
–, electric 62, 150, 154, 178
–, heat 188
–, intermittent 153
–, – electric 148
–, intracerebral 154
–, mechanical 53, 54, 56, 59
– of the midbrain 153
–, monopolar 154
–, nociceptive 62
– of nociceptors 45
– –, permanent 56
–, noxious 51, 130
– of pain receptors 46, 49, 82
– of pain-inhibiting systems 148
– of preganglionic axons 54
– of the spinal cord 153, 154
–, transcutaneous nerve 5, 140
stimulator, portable 5
stimuli, chemical 47, 49, 51, 62
–, heat 49
–, mechanical 47, 51, 52
–, natural 49
–, nociceptive 72
–, noxious 128
–, thermal 47
–, tissue damaging 49
stomach cancer 17, 190
stress 150, 202
stretching of nerve roots 79
– pain 75
Strontium-89 192
structural damage 79
– lesion 79
stump neuroma 53
– pain 5, 90, 162, 163, 165
subarachnoid alcohol block 139, 141
– – –, complications 143
– block 137, 138, 140, 145
– injection 142
– neurolytic block 141, 142
subscapular pain 135
substance P 51, 52, 60, 61, 62, 63
–, intraspinal injections 61
–, microinjections 61
–, neurogenic release 62
substantia gelatinosa 107, 189
substrates of cancer pain, anatomic 21
– – –, biochemical 21
– – –, physiologic 21
Sudeck's algodystrophy 180
– atrophy 74
sudomotor disturbances 131
suffering 28, 30, 31, 32, 202
–, anthropological reality 29
–, Christian interpretation 28
–, final phase 31
–, mental 202
–, physical 202
suicide 19
superior vena cava syndrome 76, 209
surgery, palliative 4
–, radical 162
surgical excision 160
– – of the nidus 157
– interruption of the ascending tract systems 150
– intervention 67, 69
– operations 19
– rhizotomy 149, 150
– therapy 20, 43
sweating 124
sympathectomy 149
sympathetic algodystrophy 9, 74
– block 3, 4, 9, 110, 127, 137, 143
– – of one lower extremity 132
– – with neurolytic agents 143, 144
– –, lumbar 132, 133, 144
– blockade, bilateral of the legs 132
– blocking properties 129
– chain 144
– disturbances 3
– dysfunction 5, 143
– efferent system, pathophysiology 3
– ganglia 143, 149
– nerve blocks 131
– nervous system 49, 74, 143, 145
– – –, neurolysis 143
– pathways 45
– plexus, chemical blockade 149
– reflex dystrophy 130, 131, 140, 143
symptom control 204, 205
symptomatic therapy of pain 2
symptomatology, radicular 26

symptoms in advanced cancer 205
–, expert control 203
synaptoneogenetic process 189
systemic antineoplastic therapy 171
– application of opiates 107, 113
– – of opioids 105
– cytostatic therapy 43
– drugs 23
– narcotic drug 12
– opiates 111
– therapy 85, 86, 93
– toxicity 133

tachycardia 124
tachyphylaxis 129
tactile sensitivity 150
tamoxifen 92, 173, 209
temporary block 129
tendinopathy 82
tendon reflexes 80
tension headache 73, 75
– pain 43
terminal cancer 8, 201
– care 112, 203, 204
– distress, management 204
– pain 185, 188
– – in advanced cancer 202
– restlessness 208
– stage of illness 113
test blocks, paravertebral 129
testicles, tumors 191
testicular cancer 74, 75
– tumor 95
testis 49
tetracaine 129
tetracycline, intrapleural 94
thalamic nuclei, specific somatosensory 151
– pain 81
thalamocortical system 55
thalamotomy 151, 155
–, radiologic 193
–, stereotactical 191
thalamus, stereotactic lesion in the nonspecific nuclei 150
therapeutic blocks 9, 133
– deficiencies 20
– local anesthetic block 130
therapy, analgesic 4, 5, 7, 12
–, corticosteroid 7
–, cytostatic 85
–, hormone 2, 4
–, multimodal 86, 87, 93
–, oncological 85
–, opioid 10
–, oral opiate 11
–, palliative pain 2
–, physical 3
–, surgical 43
–, symptomatic pain 2
–, systemic 85, 86, 93
–, – cytostatic 43
therapy-induced neurologic syndromes 93
– pain 85, 86, 88, 89, 94, 95
– –, incidence 87, 88
– –, pathophysiology 87, 88
– –, prevalence 86
therapy-related deaths 91
thermal injury of nociceptive neurons 59
– stimuli 47
thermocoagulation of the dorsal roots 149
– of the glossopharyngeal nerve 149
–, high-frequency 151
– of the trigeminal ganglion 149
thermolesion 150
thioridazine 124
thiotepa 176
thoracic catheters 129
– dermatoma 111
– epidural block 134
– epidurals 108
– pain 111
– sympathetic system 134
– vein distension 76
– wall, pain 145
thoracotomy 89, 90
thorotrastosis 33
threshold, central 55
–, discharge 55
–, mechanical 54
– to mechanical stimulation 54
– of nociceptive reflexes 178
– of nociceptors 75, 76
–, thermal 54
throat, carcinoma 149
thrombectomy 90
thrombopenia 88
thrombosis 77, 90
thrombotic obstruction 76
thymoma 76
thymus 178
thyroid C cells 178
– cancer 167
– carcinoma 73
tiapride 119
tilidine 103, 105
–, abuse 103
tilidine-naloxone 103
time scale 87, 88

time-course of pain development 4
tinnitus 60
tiredness 100, 103
Tissucol 161
tissue damaging stimuli 49
titrating of drug administration 23, 116
TNS 5
tolerance 11, 101, 102, 105, 112, 117, 182, 207
tomography 26
tongue, numbness 133
tooth pulp, electrical stimulation 178
toxic effects of analgesia 10
– – of calcitonin 182
– reactions 133
– risks of analgesics 100
– side effects 95
toxicity, acute 90
–, systemic 133
traction 33, 51, 82
tractotomy 151
tramadol 101, 102
tranquilizers 8, 118
–, anxiolytic 8
transcutaneous iontophoresis 186, 188
– nerve stimulation (TNS) 4, 5, 140
– Vinca iontophoresis 188
transection of a peripheral nerve 149
transganglionic degenerative atrophy 185, 188
transmitter-receiver system 153
transmitters, adrenergic 62
–, cholinergic 62
–, peptidergic 62
transplantation of bone marrow 91, 94, 95
transsphenoid microsurgery 152
– microsurgical hypophysectomy 152
trauma 154
traumatic neuroma 43
tremor 124
tricyclic antidepressants 8
trigeminal ganglion, coagulation 151
– –, thermocoagulation 149
– nerve, interruption of the descending tract 151
– neuralgia 37, 76, 137, 186
trigger points 3, 4, 130, 135
– –, myofascial 9
– –, pain mediated 130
trimipramine 118, 124
trophic dysfunction 80
trunk, somatic pain 141
– wall, pain 140
truth 197
tuberculosis 201
tubulin 188
tumor compression 54, 74
– envelopment 40, 41
– excision 161
– –, marginal 162, 169
– –, wide 162, 169
– growth 81
– –, extraosseous 157
– –, intraosseous 157
– infiltration 33, 74
– – of parenchymal organ 75
– –, perineural 40
– invasion, primary skeletal 74
– lesion, radiologic improvement 181
– pain from the upper extremities 144
– – from the upper thoracic region 144
– recurrence 75, 160, 163, 166, 171, 191
– resection 165, 169
– –, radical 162, 165, 166
– –,– curative 162
– surgery 11, 43
– –, marginal 161
– –, radical 161
– –, wide 161
tumor-induced headache 75
– penetration of hollow viscera 41
– perforation of hollow viscera 41
tumor-like lesions 157, 161, 162, 169
tumor-related distension 74
– reflex dystrophy 135
tumorous bone infiltration 73
– compression 75
– distension 75
– infiltration of nerve plexus 153
– lesions 72
– stretching 75
tumors of the abdominal hollow organs 40
– of blood vessels 76
–, chemotherapy-sensitive 176
– of encapsulated organs 33
– of the head 76
– of the liver 33
– of lymphatics 76
– of the neck 76
– of nerve roots 79
– of the posterior cranial fossa 74, 81
–, primary cerebral 74
– of the testicles 191
– of the urinogenital hollow organs 40

ulcer, peptic 7
ulceration 39, 42, 76, 88, 96, 163
–, chronic nonhealing 89

ulceration of the mucosa 42
–, nonhealing 90
unconsciousness 133
undecapeptide 61
underdosage of analgesics 105
undertreatment of cancer pain 22
unmyelinated fibers 47, 51, 52, 53
upper abdomen, pain 127, 145
upper intra-abdominal visceral cancer pain 144
ureter, compression of 172
urinary bladder carcinoma 40
– retention 111
urogenital cancer 65

vaginal hysterectomy 181
valproate sodium 118
VAS 3
vascular disorders 144
vascular nerves, excitation 41
– occlusions 43
vascular-zone disturbances 131
vasoactive algesic substances 72
vasoconstriction 74, 76, 130
vasoconstrictor 129, 134
–, alpha- plus betaadrenergic 134
– drugs 134
vasodilatation 61, 62, 74, 76
–, antidromic 62
vasomotorial headache 75
vegetative excitability 119
veins, compression 7
vena cava superior syndrome 76
venous engorgement 76
– occlusion 76
ventilatory failure, chronic 116
– obstruction 142
ventral roots, blocking 142
verbal pain relief scale 128
– – scale 127
vertebra, compression fracture 171, 172
–, deformation 2
–, infiltration 39
–, pathologic fracture 171
–, tumor-affected 135
vertebral body metastases, osteolytic 38
– canal 138
– column 39, 130
– compression 73
– metastases 130
– –, osteoblastic 38
Vinblastine 92, 173, 185, 186, 187, 188
– cuff, perineural 188
– iontophoresis 188
Vinca alkaloids 87, 89, 93, 96, 186, 187
– –, iontophoresis 185
– – iontophoretic therapy 189
– –, locally applied 189
– –, transcutaneous iontophoresis 188
Vincristine 89, 92, 173, 186, 187, 188
vindesine 96
visceral cancer 18
– dysfunction 25
– motility, disorders 41
– nociceptors 55
– pain 49, 51, 56, 62, 82, 127, 128, 130, 141, 144, 145, 149
– strucures, lesions 82
visual analogue scale (VAS) 3, 4, 103, 127, 128
vomiting 9, 18, 101, 103, 110, 111, 181, 205, 209

wallerian degeneration 189
weakness 102, 205, 209
weight loss 205
wheezing 134
withdrawal syndromes 102
working alliance 196, 197, 198, 199, 200

X-irradiation 3, 9, 11, 191

yttrium-90 152, 192

Recent Results in Cancer Research

Sponsored by the Swiss League against Cancer. Editor in Chief: P. Rentchnick, Genève

For information about Vols. 1–9, please contact your bookseller of Springer-Verlag

10 NELSON, R. S.: Radioactive Phosphorus in the Diagnosis of Gastrointestinal Cancer.
11 FREEMAN, R. G. and J. M. KNOX: Treatment of Skin Cancer.
12 LYNCH, H. T.: Hereditary Factors in Carcinoma.
13 Tumours in Children, 2nd Edition. Edited by H. B. MARSDEN and J. K. STEWARD.
14 ODARTCHENKO, N.: Production Cellulaire Erythropoïétique.
15 SOKOLOFF, B.: Carcinoid and Serotonin.
16 JACOBS, M. L.: Malignant Lymphomas and Their Management.
17 Normal and Malignant Cell Growth. Edited by R. J. M. FRY, M. L. GRIEM, and W. H. KIRSTEN (Symposium).
18 ANGLESIO, E.: The Treatment of Hodgkin's Disease.
19 BANNASCH, P.: The Cytoplasm of Hepatocytes during Carcinogenesis. Electron- and Lightmicroscopical Investigations of the Nitrosomorpholineintoxicated Rat Liver.
20 Rubidomycin. A new Agent against Cancer. Edited by J. BERNARD, R. PAUL, M. BOIRON, C. JACQUILLAT, and R. MARAL.
21 Scientific Basis of Cancer Chemotherapy. Edited by G. MATHÉ (Symposium).
22 KOLDOVSKÝ, P.: Tumor Specific Transplantation Antigen.
23 FUCHS, W. A., J. W. DAVIDSON, and H. W. FISCHER: Lymphography in Cancer. With contributions by G. JANTET and H. RÖSLER.
24 HAYWARD, J.: Hormones und Human Breast Cancer. An Account of 15 Years Study.
25 ROY-BURMAN, P.: Analogues of Nucleic Acid Components. Mechanisms of Action.
26 Tumors of the Liver. Edited by G. T. PACK and A. H. ISLAMI.
27 SZYMENDERA, J.: Bone Mineral Metabolism in Cancer.
28 MEEK, E. S.: Antitumour and Antiviral Substances of Natural Origin.
29 Aseptic Environments and Cancer Treatment. Edited by G. MATHÉ (Symposium).
30 Advances in the Treatment of Acute (Blastic) Leukemias. Edited by G. MATHÉ (Symposium).
31 DENOIX, P.: Treatment of Malignant Breast Tumors. Indications and Results.
32 NELSON, R. S.: Endoscopy in Gastric Cancer.
33 Experimental and Clinical Effects of L-Asparaginase. Edited by E. GRUNDMANN and H. F. OETTGEN (Symposium).
34 Chemistry and Biological Actions of 4-Nitroquinolin 1-Oxide. Edited by H. ENDO, T. ONO, and T. SUGIMURA.
35 PENN, I.: Malignant Tumors in Organ Transplant Recipients.
36 Current Concepts in the Management of Lymphoma and Leukemia. Edited by J. E. ULTMANN, M. L. GRIEM, W. H. KIRSTEN, and R. W. WISSLER (Symposium).
37 CHIAPPA, S., R. MUSUMECI, and C. USLENGHI: Endolymphatic Radiotherapy in Malignant Lymphomas. With contributions by G. BONADONNA, B. DAMASCELLI, G. FAVA, F. PIZZETTI, U. VERONESI.
38 KOLLER, P. C.: The Role of Chromosomes in Cancer Biology.
39 Current Problems in the Epidemiology of Cancer and Lymphomas. Edited by E. GRUNDMANN and H. TULINIUS (Symposium).
40 LANGLEY, F. A. and A. C. CROMPTON: Epithelial Abnormalities of the Cervix Uteri.
41 Tumours in a Tropical Country. A Survey of Uganda (1964–1968). Edited by A. C. TEMPLETON.
42 Breast Cancer: A Challenging Problem. Edited by M. L. GRIEM, E. V. JENSEN, J. E. ULTMANN, and R. W. WISSLER (Symposium).
43 Nomenclature, Methodology and Results of Clinical Trials in Acute Leukemias. Edited by G. MATHÉ, P. POUILLART, L.SCHWARZENBERG (Symposium).
44 Special Topics in Carcinogenesis. Edited by E. GRUNDMANN (Symposium).
45 KOLDOVSKÝ, P.: Carcinoembryonic Antigens.
46 Diagnosis and Therapy of Malignant Lymphoma. Edited by K. MUSSHOFF (Symposium).
47 Investigation and Stimulation of Immunity in Cancer Patients. Edited by G. MATHÉ and R. WEINER (Symposium).
48 Platinum Coordination Complexes in Cancer Chemotherapy. Edited by T. A. CONNORS and J. J. ROBERTS (Symposium).

49 Complications of Cancer Chemotherapy. Edited by G. MATHÉ and R. K. OLDHAM (Symposium).
50 Cancer Registry, Edited by E. GRUNDMANN and E. PEDERSEN (Symposium).
51 Gliomas. Current Concepts in Biology, Diagnosis and Therapy. Edited by J. HEKMATPANAH (Symposium).
52 The Ambivalence of Cytostatic Therapy. Edited by E. GRUNDMANN and R. GROSS (Symposium).
53 A. CLARYSSE, Y. KENIS, and G. MATHÉ: Cancer Chemotherapy.
54 Malignant Bone Tumors. Edited by E. GRUNDMANN.
55 MATHÉ G.: Cancer Active Immunotherapy, Immunoprophylaxis, and Immunorestoration.
56 Lymphocytes, Macrophages, and Cancer. Edited by G. MATHÉ, I. FLORENTIN, and M.-C. SIMMLER (Symposium).
57 Breast Cancer: A Multidisciplinary Approach. Edited by G. ST. ARNEAULT, P. BAND, and L. ISRAËL (Symposium).
58 B. S. SCHOENBERG: Multiple Primary Malignant Neoplasms.
59 Selective Heat Sensitivity of Cancer Cells. Edited by A. ROSSI-FANELLI, R. CAVALIERE, B. MONDOVI, and G. MORICCA.
60 Tumors of the Male Genital System. Edited by E. GRUNDMANN and W. VAHLENSIECK (Symposium).
61 D. METCALF: Hemopoietic Colonies.
62 Tactics and Strategy in Cancer Treatment. Edited by G. MATHÉ (Symposium).
63 Antitumor Antibiotics. Edited by S. K. CARTER, H. UMEZAWA, J. DOUROS, and Y. SAKURAI (Symposium).
64 Lymphoid Neoplasias I: Classification, Categorization, Natural History.
65 Lymphoid Neoplasias II: Clinical and Therapeutic Aspects.
Lymphoid Neoplasias I & II. Proceedings of the 1977 CNRS-EORTC International Colloquium. Editors: G. MATHÉ, M. SELIGMANN, M. TUBIANA. Devided into two volumes.
66 Carcinogenic Hormones. Edited by C. H. LINGEMAN.
67/68 Adjuvant Therapies and Markers of Post-Surgical Minimal Residual Disease I & II. Proceedings of the 1978 Annual Plenary Meeting of the EORTC. Editors: G. BONADONNA, G. MATHÉ, S. E. SALMON. Divided into two volumes.
67 Markers and General Problems of Cancer Adjuvant Therapies.
68 Adjuvant Therapies of the Various Primary Tumors.
69 Strategies in Clinical Hematology. Edited by R. GROSS and K.-P. HELLRIEGEL.
70 New Anticancer Drugs. Edited by S. K. CARTER
71 Endocrine Treatment of Breast Cancer. Edited by B. HENNINGSEN, F. LINDER, C. STREICHELE.
72 CAWLEY, J. C., BURNS, G. F., HAYHOE, F. G. J.: Hairy-Cell Leukaemia.
73 Thyroid Cancer. Edited by W. DUNCAN.
74 Cancer Chemo- and Immunopharmacology. 1. Chemopharmacology. Edited by G. MATHÉ and F. M. MUGGIA.
75 Cancer Chemo- and Immunopharmacology. 2. Immunopharmacology, Relations and General Problems. Edited by G. MATHÉ and F. M. MUGGIA.
76 New Drugs in Cancer Chemotherapy. Edited by S. K. CARTER, Y. SAKURAI, H. UMEZAWA.
77 K. STANLEY, J. STJERNSWÄRD, M. ISLEY: The Conduct of a Cooperative Clinical Trial.
78 Prostate Cancer. Edited by W. DUNCAN.
79 Chemotherapy and Radiotherapy of Gastrointestinal Tumors. Edited by H. O. KLEIN.
80 Adjuvant Therapies of Cancer. Edited by G. MATHÉ, G. BONADONNA, S. SALMON.
81 H. P. LOHRMANN and W. SCHREML: Cytotoxic Drugs and the Granulopoietic System.
82 Early Detection and Localization of Lung Tumors in High Risk Groups. Edited by P. R. BAND.
83 Colorectal Cancer. Edited by W. DUNCAN.
84 Modified Nucleosides and Cancer. Edited by G. NASS.
85 Urologic Cancer: Chemotherapeutic Principles and Management. Edited by F. M. TORTI.
86 Vascular Perfusion in Cancer Therapy. Edited by K. SCHWEMMLE, K. AIGNER.
87 F. HOLMES: Aging and Cancer.
88 Paediatric Oncology. Edited by W. DUNCAN.
89 Pain in the Cancer Patient. Edited by M. ZIMMERMANN, P. DRINGS, G. WAGNER.